CLINICAL VOICE DISORDERS

Third Edition

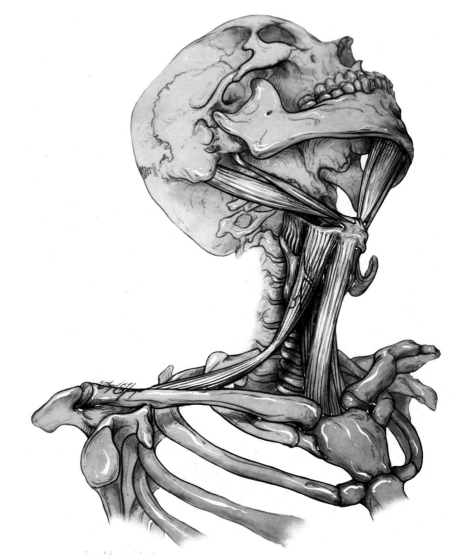

CLINICAL
VOICE
DISORDERS

An Interdisciplinary Approach

Third Edition

ARNOLD E. ARONSON, Ph.D.

Head, Section of Speech Pathology
Department of Neurology, Mayo Clinic
Professor of Speech Pathology
Mayo Medical School
Rochester, Minnesota

1990
Thieme Inc., New York
Georg Thieme Verlag Stuttgart ● New York

Thieme Medical Publishers, Inc.
381 Park Avenue South
New York, New York 10016

CLINICAL VOICE DISORDERS (3rd Edition)
Arnold Aronson

Illustrations by Floyd E. Hosmer

Library of Congress Cataloging in Publication Data

Aronson, Arnold Elvin, 1928–
    Clinical voice disorders.

    Includes bibliographies and index.
    1. Voice disorders. I. Title. [DNLM. 1. Voice
Disorders. WV 500 A769c]
RF510.A76 1985   616.85′5   85–11456
ISBN 0-86577-127-8

Printed in the United States of America.

5   4   3   2   1

TMP ISBN 0-86577-337-8
GTV ISBN 3-13-598802-1

*To my wife and children,
and to the memory of my parents,
with appreciation*

CONTENTS

PREFACE

In the preface to the earlier editions of this book I wrote that voice disorders was speech pathology's stepchild; that, as a profession, we were uncertain about the propriety of delving into disorders of voice; and that this specialty remained an enigma to us because of lack of experience due to insufficient referrals. However, the recent past has been proving these statements to be wrong. Interest in voice disorders is burgeoning. Never before in American speech pathology and otolaryngology circles has more attention been given to patients who have voice disorders than at the time of this revision. The signs come from many different sources. Hardly an otolaryngology conference can be found that does not include clinical and laboratory research papers and seminars on the human voice with speech pathologists as participants. Speech pathology convention programs commonly incorporate the expertise of the otolaryngologist in order to expand its educational offerings. A new journal devoted exclusively to the voice and its disorders has come into existence. Speech pathologists are working increasingly with otolaryngologists in private practice. More than 40 percent of all speech pathologists are now affiliated with hospitals and medical clinics—greater than at any time in our professional history—clinicians who are absorbing increasing referrals of voice patients from otolaryngologists and other physicians for the evaluation and treatment of patients with voice disorders within a medical context.

Meanwhile, the medical specialties of otolaryngology and neurology are drawing closer together. A proliferation of knowledge has taken place in neurologic voice disorders, as evidenced by a relatively new subspecialty, *neurolaryngology,* that has emerged during the life of this textbook and that signifies the common interest between these two specialties when neurologic diseases implicate the phonatory and respiratory systems. Speech pathology is drawn closer to otolaryngology and neurology because of its long involvement with the dysarthrias, of which neurologic dysphonia is a major component.

Our alliance with psychology and psychiatry continues to grow as well because of a mutual recognition of the effects of life stress, interpersonal conflict, and psychoneurosis on voice. It would appear that the question in the preface to the previous editions of this book, "What, in fact, does one need to know and how deeply should one delve?" is closer to finding an answer because of the clarification of our responsibilities to ourselves, to our patients, and to medicine.

The profession of speech pathology has, without doubt, progressed to the point where it is challenged now more than ever before by patients whose voice disorders are caused by common and obscure organic and psychologic illnesses and is responsible to physicians who are coming to depend on us increasingly for diagnostic information, not just therapy. This book, therefore, is intended to draw the student into a serious plumbing of the etiologic depths of voice disorders and their related disciplines. In so doing, it encourages more emphatically than before solid preparation in the basic sciences of gross and neuroanatomy, general physiology and neurophysiology, and in the three medical specialties that can go a long way toward enriching the clinician's understanding of the entire spectrum of voice disorders—namely, *otolaryngology, neurology,* and *psychiatry.*

In the second edition of this book, a chapter on nasal resonatory disorders was added. Professors of speech pathology requested it because they often teach craniofacial defects in the same course as voice disorders. Now, two more chapters have been added: *Anatomy and Physiology of Respiration* and *Normal and Abnormal Respiration for Voice.* Respiration, like resonation, is often taught along with voice disorders because it is impossible to separate phonation from respiration physiologically, and, clinically, they are reciprocally implicated in all voice disorders.

Two chapters were added, but one was withdrawn—*Rehabilitation After Laryngectomy*—a decision made because laryngectomee rehabilitation has evolved to such a considerable extent within the past several years that it has taken on the characteristics of a subspecialty within the subspecialty of voice disorders, requiring the expertise of someone totally invested in laryngecto-mee rehabilitation in order to do justice to this critically important subject.

The author's conviction about the prerequisite knowledge of psychologic interviewing and counseling for anyone preparing to specialize in voice disorders has only been strengthened since this book's inception. The relevance of such knowledge and skill is finally being recognized by our profession, as is evident from continuing education programs and academic courses within our educational institutions. This is one subject that cannot be overemphasized.

As in the previous editions of this book, Chapter 1 introduces the subject of the normal and abnormal voice and classifies voice disorders. Chapter 2 presents the basic anatomy and physiology of the larynx and phonation. A section on the evolution of the larynx in vertebrates reflects my desire to enrich the student's appreciation for the unbroken line of evolutionary development of the larynx as a protective and sound-producing organ. Personally, it has given me a deeper sense of the biologic history of the larynx and a respect for its long, intricate, even tortuous, evolutionary growth in complexity from a primitive sphincter to its present virtuosity.

Chapter 3 is devoted to the normal voice and its development from infancy through old age, with added material on the aging voice. Chapter 4 studies abnormal voice from mass lesions of the vocal folds. Chapter 5 is devoted exclusively to voice disorders that result from diseases of the central and peripheral nervous systems. Because clinical neurologic voice disorders have developed consider-ably between the second and third editions of this book, knowledge of this subject is now imperative for the differential diagnosis of voice disorder unknowns.

Chapter 6, on psychogenic voice disorders, discusses voice as an indicator of personality, of transient emotional states, and as a sign of chronic stress and psychopathology. Nothing could be more important than a knowledge of the relationship between emotions and vocal pathology in view of the fact that there is hardly a patient who develops a voice disorder, regardless of etiology, in whom emotional reaction to the voice and to life stress does not play an extremely important part in diagnosis and therapy. New to this edition, a section titled Supplementary Case Studies in Psychogenic Voice Disorders has been added to this chapter.

Chapter 7 is devoted exclusively to that family of disorders known as the adductor spastic dysphonias. Its message is that adductor laryngospasm during speech, commonly labeled spastic or spasmodic dysphonia, is not a single disorder but can come from either neurologic or psychogenic causes, and that a thorough appreciation and understanding of this fact is indispensable to proper differential diagnosis. The treatment of intractable adductor spastic dysphonia may have to be invasive, and it is important to make sure that the patient has spastic dysphonia of the organic and not the psychogenic type. Appearing for the first time in Chapter 13 is information concerning botulinum toxin injection as therapy for adductor spastic dysphonia, a promising but still experimental treatment, making it all the more important that proper differential diagnosis of spastic dysphonia be secured. Chapter 8 addresses the abductor spastic dysphonias.

Chapter 9 is devoted to the nasal resonatory disorders. Chapter 10 deals with the laryngologic and speech pathology examination of the voice.

Chapter 11 introduces psychologic interviewing and counseling in the diagnosis and treatment of voice disorders, although it is not intended to be a substitute for a much more thorough training that must take place in the student's academic preparation.

Chapter 12 consists of clinical case studies to give the student a conceptualization of how patients with voice disorders present themselves in actual clinical practice. It attempts to provide a realistic representation of the confusion and incompleteness of information with which the clinician has to contend. It is meant to challenge the student's alertness to detail, reasoning, and problem-solving abilities.

Chapter 13, which is devoted to voice therapy, was written with the principle in mind that "cookbook" therapies for voice disorders, in the long run, do not provide clinicians with the versatility they need when confronted by the prodigious individual differences that exist among voice patients; that a knowledge of the *basic principles of therapy,* with the idea that the clinician create his or her own techniques, is more enduring.

As noted earlier, Chapters 14 and 15 are new chapters on respiratory anatomy and physiology and disorders of respiration.

As in previous editions, each chapter contains more detailed, supporting information in smaller type. The usual bibliographic references and suggestions for additional reading with a few lines as to why these references were chosen are included. Readers have commented favorably on these recommendations as a means of expanding their knowledge beyond the contents of this book.

Although no textbook can satisfy everyone, an attempt has been made to include in this one the most comprehensive coverage of phonatory, resonatory, and respiratory disorders possible in order to satisfy the needs of professors and students in courses on voice disorders. One omission, however, pertains to the diagnosis and treatment of singers and actors whose voices have become abnormal and who must be instructed to use their voices with optimum efficiency, an art that still lies within the province of a handful of experts in this field. It would be presumptuous to delve into this realm without the necessary knowledge and experience.

Discussions with practicing otolaryngologists and residents in otolaryngology have made it apparent that this book has attracted a readership that goes beyond the student and clinician in speech pathology. This discovery is gratifying because it demonstrates the needed recognition of the commonality of objectives that exists between speech pathologists and otolaryngologists in the diagnosis and treatment of patients with voice complaints. However, internists, neurologists, and psychiatrists have also shown interest in this book, also a logical development because of their particular stake in patients whose abnormal voices are often early manifestations of general medical, psychiatric, and neurologic diseases. Interestingly and importantly, it is the family practitioner and internist who may be the first to hear a voice change as a sign of general illness. All this interdisciplinary traffic continues to prove that *the highest quality diagnosis and treatment of patients who present with abnormal voices cannot be offered without close communication among speech pathologists, otolaryngologists, neurologists, psychiatrists, and internists.*

If this book advocates the inseparability between abnormal voice and illness, and speech pathology and medicine, it is because it was written based almost entirely on the author's experiences in an interdisciplinary medical institution. It could not have been written without the kindness and willingness of physicians from many different specialties to refer patients for consultation on matters of etiology and therapy concerning patients with voice disorders. I particularly appreciate the years of learning afforded to me by Lawrence W. DeSanto, M.D., Kenneth Devine, M.D., and Bruce Pearson, M.D., otolaryngologists of unusual sensitivity to the importance of voice disorders in medical practice; by the remaining members of the departments of Otolaryngology, Neurology, and Psychiatry at the Mayo Clinic; and particularly by the late Edward M. Litin, M.D., Emeritus Chairman of the Department of Psychiatry at the Mayo Clinic. I thank Judith E. Trost, Ph.D., for her advice on nasal resonatory disorders. I offer my appreciation to Floyd E. Hosmer, M.S., for the aesthetics of his medical art; to Brian C. Decker, B.Sc., for his invaluable advice during the formative stages of the first edition of this work; and to Sylvia Z. Aronson, B.A., for her editorial help in the preparation of the manuscript.

However, I reserve a special place for that individual without whom this book could never have been written—the *patient*. The patient is the real surprise, the inadvertent educator with all the complex physical, cultural, and psychological intricacies that make no two alike, an antidote to complacency, continuously keeping clinical life interesting and rewarding. In the end, it is the patient who makes it all worthwhile and satisfies the objectives that brought us here in the first place.

Arnold E. Aronson

CLINICAL VOICE DISORDERS

Third Edition

SECTION I

Chapter One

INTRODUCTION

It is impossible to know the fundamentals of a phenomenon without having solid knowledge of its origin, development and the chain of causes, conditions and circumstances determining its actual existence.

—Kiml

THE LARYNX IN LIFE

At the crossroads of life is the larynx, a barometer of our physical and mental health, being both an airway through which flows life-sustaining oxygen and a valve that protects the lungs from ingestion of foreign substances. When its powerful musculature shuts off the airway, air can be impounded in the lungs, forming a rigid thorax to support firmly the attached upper extremities during lifting and pushing. Bearing down during laryngeal closure compresses both the abdominal contents for defecation, micturition, and parturition and the thoracic cage for coughing and throat clearing. Yet as vital as these functions are, the larynx manages to shift deftly from protector of life to communicator, generating raw sound for articulation of intellect and as a musical background to language informing the outside world of its owner's personality, emotional state, and cultural heritage.

The mechanics of speech require integration of the respiratory, phonatory, resonatory, and articulatory musculature. This book considers, for the most part, one component of the total speech act, *phonation,* sound generated by rapid vocal fold movement excited by the exhaled airstream. Even though the larynx is but one of four muscular systems that make speech possible, it is not on the same plane with the rest of them. An important and unusual fact about the larynx is that phylogenetically it is eons older than those brain and muscle structures responsible for articulation and language. The latter are synonymous with the intellect, itself a recent vertebrate acquisition, but the larynx and voice owe a disproportionately strong allegiance to the primitive emotions, persuasive proof of which can be found in everyday experience. During emotional arousal, when we are incapable of preventing loss of cortical control over the larynx, it escapes our grasp and drags us back into its primevil depths. Have we not often witnessed such loss of intellectual speech expression as in the following experience? A professor of law, known for his razor-sharp tongue and habit of taunting and ridiculing students (who, incidentally, loved him in spite of it), rose to speak at a farewell banquet.

> He stood motionless for a long time. We observed that his face was different than we had ever seen it before. It had lost its severity. It was flushed and looked pink and kind. The mouth was not a snarl. His voice, too, was different. It was soft without a trace of belligerence or sarcasm. "I cannot bid you all goodbye and leave unsaid that which is the most important thing in my life." He took a deep breath and continued, his voice hoarse with emotion. It grew hoarser as he struggled to eliminate the quiver which was entering it. He then paid tribute to his lovely wife. "I cannot in this leavetaking do other than tell you that I owe all my happiness to her, that she has . . ." He turned. Tears were running down her cheeks. Their gazes met and locked in long silence. Then without another word, he sat down (Nizer, 1978).

We are fascinated by the mystery of how speech and language evolved in the kingdom of the vertebrates and have struggled with a basic question: Are the structure and sound-generating properties of the human larynx mere extensions of its role in lower vertebrates, the ultimate in evolutionary refinement for the expression of ideas? That is to say, is the Darwinian belief correct, that speech is not a product of special creation but only another form of sound-making, more

3

sophisticated because of a quantitative increase in human intelligence? Or, is speech uniquely human, de novo, different in kind, not degree, from lower animals? The answer is unknown.

Another, perhaps less difficult, question is this: Is it the monkey's and chimpanzee's intellect or anatomy that prevents speech in these primates? Some argue that the primitiveness of their laryngeal and articulatory anatomy stands in the way of speech, yet the larynges of the monkey and chimpanzee are remarkably similar in structure and method of sound production to those of humans. The fact is that human speech is not dependent upon a particularly refined larynx, for speech continues despite laryngeal tumor, paralysis, and even total laryngectomy, whereupon the esophagus or even an electronic sound generator can assume the responsibility for sound-making. Most scientists now concur that before primates could talk, a high level of abstract intelligence was required as the governing force.

There is a universal fact about the world of living creatures—almost all make sounds. Insects tap surfaces, snap or rub their wings, or rub leg against wing, as in the case of the grasshopper, producing complex trains of pulses that send messages of courtship and sexual recognition. Admittedly, many lower forms produce sound accidentally, but most do so for a purpose— survival—signalling fear, aggression, mating, territoriality, and pleasure. Situation-specific use of voice in birds, for example, has been firmly categorized into mating, distress, fear, anger, terrorizing, and triumphal calls.

Negus (1929) observed that individual living creatures produce sound as both defense and offense: intimidation, cries for help and food, and decoying of prey. Sound brings and keeps the sexes together for survival of the species, repulsing the opposite sex, and protecting offspring. Sound further enables each species to keep in touch when out of sight, as in grass, in trees, at night, and in lairs or burrows. Sound also aids in the conveyance of special ideas, such as cooperation, calls to food and migration, and entertainment.

Human phonation is linked to much more than the intellectual act of speech. The human voice serves similar sublinguistic purposes of survival. The larynx is an important escape valve for the emotions—anger, grief, and affection—which are essential to the maintenance of psychologic equilibrium.

DEFINITIONS OF TERMS AND CONCEPTS

Terminology

Of the numerous terms that could be defined here, the following have been selected because of their common usage.

Phonation. The physical act of sound production by means of vocal fold interaction with the exhaled airstream. Puffs of air are released within an audible frequency range which resonate in the supraglottic cavities.

Voice. Audible sound produced by phonation.

Vocal Parameters. The elements of voice: pitch, loudness, quality, and flexibility.

   Pitch. The perceptual correlate of frequency.

   Loudness. The perceptual correlate of intensity.

   Quality. The perceptual correlate of complexity.

   Flexibility. The perceptual correlate of frequency, intensity, and complexity variations.

Dysphonia. Abnormal voice, as judged by the listener, involving either pitch, loudness, quality, flexibility, or combinations thereof.

Aphonia. Absence of a definable laryngeal tone. The voice is either severely breathy or whispered.

Mute. Unable to phonate and articulate.

Vocal Folds. Synonymous with vocal cords. Shelves of thyroarytenoid muscle covered with mucous membrane and fibroelastic tissue which project into the laryngeal airway.

Glottis. The space between and bordered by the vocal folds when the latter are partially or fully abducted.

Adduction (of vocal fold). Movement of the vocal folds medially, toward the midline of the laryngeal airway.

Abduction (of vocal fold).   Movement of the vocal folds laterally, away from the midline of the laryngeal airway.

Concepts

NORMAL VOICE

It is more difficult to define normal voice than any other speech or language component because, by nature, voice variety is limitless, and standards for voice adequacy are broad. Moore (1971a) describes the complexity of the task:

> It is obvious that there is no single sound that can be called "normal voice"; instead, there are children's voices, girls' voices, boys' voices, women's voices, men's voices, voices of the aged, and so on. In each of these types of voice both the normal and the abnormal can be recognized. The location of the threshold that separates the one from the other is judged by each listener on the basis of his cultural standards, education, environment, vocal training, and similar factors, but wherever the separation between adequate and inadequate is placed, it is obvious that each individual has acquired concepts of normalcy and defectiveness. This observation should alert the speech clinician to the fact that voice disorders are culturally based and socially determined.

As such, only general standards for normal voice can be stated, exemplified by the following (Johnson et al., 1956):

1. Quality must be pleasant. This criterion implies the presence of a certain musical quality and the absence of noise or atonality.
2. Pitch level must be adequate. The pitch level must be appropriate to the age and sex of the speaker.
3. Loudness must be appropriate. The voice must not be so weak that it cannot be heard under ordinary speaking conditions, nor should it be so loud that it calls undesirable attention to itself.
4. Flexibility must be adequate. Flexibility or variety refers to variations in pitch and loudness that aid in the expression of emphasis, meaning, or subtleties indicating the feelings of the individual.

ABNORMAL VOICE

Abnormal Quality.   Voice quality is the perception of the physical complexity of the laryngeal tone modified by cavity resonation. The printed word cannot convey the multiplicity of pathologic quality variations heard in clinical practice. Hoarseness when used in reference to noisy or atonal voices is a wastebasket term, a concession to the fact that verbal distinctions among the following cannot be validly made: aspirate, breathy, coarse, dead, dull, feeble, flat, gloomy, grating, grave, growling, guttural, harsh, hoarse, hollow, husky, infantile, lifeless, loud, metallic, monotonous, muffled, neurasthenic, passive, pectoral, pinched, rasping, raucous, rough, sepulchral, shrill, somber, strained, strident, subdued, thick, thin, throaty, tired, toneless, tremulous, weak, whining, and whispered (Robbins, 1963).

Fairbanks (1960) tried to distill voice quality defects into three categories—harshness, breathiness, and hoarseness; however, the validity and reliability of these terms were questioned in a study of Jensen (1965). He asked six experienced speech pathologists to rate the voices of cheerleaders who had different degrees and types of dysphonia and found disagreement and inconsistency among their ratings. What certain judges heard as "breathiness" others described as "hoarseness," while still others thought "harshness" best applied. In addition, estimations of voice quality were contaminated by severity. The study unearthed a common problem in clinical practice; individual voices were inconsistent throughout the sample, embodying more than one type of quality. What Jensen concluded experimentally is substantiated clinically: that the traditional labels used to describe voice quality deviations must be viewed with skepticism; one clinician's hoarseness is another's breathiness or harshness. To keep a proper perspective, however, it should be noted that the incongruence between terminology and the actual sound of the voice is not as critical as it was before the advent of sound recording. More important than terminology is the clinician's ability to integrate perceptual, acoustic, physiologic, and psychologic dimensions of abnormal voice, to interpret the abnormal sound in order to determine its cause, and to develop a sensitivity to nuances of voice during therapy.

Abnormal Pitch.   Pitch is the perceptual counterpart of fundamental voice frequency. Disorders of pitch refer to abnormally high or low voices.

Abnormal Loudness.   Loudness is the perception of vocal intensity. The voice may be too weak, or too loud.

Abnormal Flexibility.   The normal voice possesses adequate pitch, loudness, and quality variability during contextual speech to convey more subtle intellectual and emotional meanings. In voice disorders, those fluctuations are either inappropriately flattened or are excessive.

Rarely in clinical practice does abnormal voice vary along a single dimension of quality, loudness, pitch, or flexibility. Most of the time, even though one may predominate, the others are usually present in different combinations and proportions.

VOICE DISORDER

An abnormal-sounding voice provokes most adults to seek the services of a laryngologist or speech pathologist. Even though the voice may not have been a good one previously, it is appropriately alarming that it has changed. Most people are sensitive to voice as an indicator of illness, especially laryngeal malignancy. Although lay persons pay little attention to the specific acoustic parameters of voice that have caught their attention, clinicians and laboratory researchers are more analytic. *A voice disorder exists when quality, pitch, loudness, or flexibility differs from the voices of others of similar age, sex, and cultural group*. However, no fixed, uniform standard of abnormal voice exists, just as no absolute criterion for normal voice can be established.

> It follows that the perceived defectiveness of any one voice will vary among listeners without change in the actual voice. It is apparent that the voice is abnormal for a particular individual when he judges it to be so. Judgment implies a set of standards that are learned through experience and that are related to the judge's own aesthetic and cultural criteria. Judgment also implies that standards are not fixed, that there is opportunity for more than one conclusion. This flexibility in determining the defectiveness of voices does not alter the validity of the basic definition of voice disorders, but it does underscore the observation that vocal standards are culturally based and environmentally determined (Moore, 1971b).

The main implication of this statement is that the definition of a given voice as normal or abnormal depends upon the orientation of the person making the judgment. Child, parent, adult, employer, speech pathologist, and laryngologist all define normal and abnormal according to their own needs and backgrounds, an important point for the speech pathologist to remember, whose judgments about voice must be adjusted according to the purposes of the evaluation.

Perkins (1971) lists five kinds of information that can be extracted from the voice. It is an indicator of the speaker's: (1) physical health, (2) emotional health, (3) personality, (4) identity, and (5) aesthetic orientation. It is also (6) a carrier of connotative and denotative content. This list is important in that it tells us that voice has many meanings for both speaker and clinician and is a rich storehouse of clues to understanding the individual.

ABNORMAL VOICE AS A SIGN OF ILLNESS

Faced with someone whose voice sounds abnormal, the clinician's chief concern should be whether or not the abnormal voice signifies illness. Communicative or aesthetic considerations are, for the moment, secondary. From the laryngology syllabus of a medical school curriculum comes the following statement pertaining to the meaning of abnormal voice in medical practice:

> Hoarseness is not a disease but rather a symptom of disease of the larynx itself or along the course of the laryngeal motor nerves. Thus, hoarseness is the cardinal symptom of laryngeal involvement, often the first

and only signal of dangerous disease, local or systemic, involving this area . . . A thorough examination is necessary in all cases to ascertain the exact cause and prescribe the proper treatment . . . The differential diagnosis may tax the ingenuity of the most exacting physician since many different medical and surgical conditions may result in hoarseness.

The cause or causes of the abnormal voices need to be established, if at all possible. A breathy voice quality that appears gradually and increases in severity may have only minor social, communicative, or aesthetic significance, yet may herald the onset of a brainstem tumor. Once the reason for the voice disorder is known and has been eliminated as a threat to the physical health of the individual, the communicative significance of the voice can then be considered, which falls squarely within the speech pathologist's province. The modern speech clinician must be educated along medical as well as rehabilitative lines, however. Working with physicians, speech pathologists can contribute to the diagnosis of voice disorders as well as to their treatment, a professional philosophy given earlier credence by West et al. (1947).

> The first task of the specialist in speech rehabilitation is to analyze the undesirable elements . . . in the attempt to trace them back to their ultimate causation. It is not enough, for example, to know which sounds are defective; before prescribing . . . speech training, one must inquire why they are defective. Often this inquiry must accompany the early corrective procedures; in many cases necessary diagnostic information can be gained only by testing (the patient's) response to rehabilitory measures; but in every case . . . a thoroughgoing investigation as to the cause of the defect should be completed before a decision is made as to corrective devices to be employed. A search for the cause should not be ended until the basic one has been uncovered; and, if at any time . . . it appears that a reappraisal of its origins would give a clearer picture of its nature, the search for the ultimate cause should be reopened.

ABNORMAL VOICE AS A SYMPTOM OF ILLNESS

Used properly, "symptom" refers to the patient's subjective complaint, real or imagined; whether or not the *clinician* thinks the voice is abnormal is independent of the *patient's* beliefs. Three variations on this theme occur in practice:

1. The voice is judged defective by both clinician and patient, and both advocate a need for its investigation and therapy. Such mutual agreement is ideal for maximum cooperation in clinical diagnosis and therapy. Both parties realize that something needs to be done about the abnormal voice and proceed with optimal effectiveness.
2. The clinician is convinced of a need for voice investigation and therapy, but the patient is not. This situation arises from either (a) the clinician's unrealistic, overdetermined definition of abnormal voice and overemphasis on voice improvement or, (b) the patient's indifference to a genuine problem. In either instance, covert or even overt disagreement between patient and clinician ensues, and efforts at diagnosis or therapy are met with patient disinterest, resistance, or even hostility.
3. The patient's conviction that a voice disorder exists despite the fact that clinicians believe the problem to be trivial or nonexistent. Such conflict is usually a sign of patient overreaction, and frequently, is a sequel to recovery from laryngologic disease or laryngeal surgery. Such reactions are viewed as expressions of hostility, perfectionism, or depression, requiring psychologic assistance.

ABNORMAL VOICE AS A DISORDER OF COMMUNICATION

In addition to abnormal voice as an index of health or illness, it is also valued as an instrument of communication. Within this framework, the following questions are pertinent: (1) Is the voice adequate to carry language intelligibly to the listener? (2) Are its acoustic properties aesthetically acceptable? (3) Does it satisfy its owner's occupational and social requirements? Voice, in other words, has personal, social, and economic significance. The higher one ascends the socioeconomic scale, the greater the emphasis placed on pleasant, effective voices. With few exceptions, the greater the dependence on voice for occupational and social gratification, the more devastating the effects of a voice disorder on the person.

CLASSIFICATIONS OF VOICE DISORDERS

Etiologic

Etiology means the ultimate cause or theory that explains signs and symptoms. Because such a classification encourages the deepest understanding of dysphonia or aphonia, it will be the primary category used in this book. For example, a *neurologic disease,* such as trauma to one recurrent laryngeal nerve, is the etiology of a voice disorder. It causes a pathophysiologic condition, *unilateral vocal fold paralysis,* which in turn causes the *abnormal voice signs* of breathiness, hoarseness, reduced loudness, diplophonia, and reduced variability.

 Etiologic diagnosis of voice disorders is imperative when speech pathology is practiced within the framework of medicine. The teaching that voice symptoms, such as breathiness and hoarseness, are "disorders" in and of themselves is contrary to the purposes of educating the student to *understand the individual behind the abnormal voice.* Attempts to change the voice alone without understanding its underlying cause is the most common reason for failure in diagnosis and therapy, especially within the realm of nonorganic voice signs and symptoms.

Perceptual

Voice disorders can be classified according to their acoustic perceptual attributes: quality, pitch, loudness, and flexibility. Although this system has the advantage of emphasizing the voice characteristics perceived by the listener, if used alone it has the disadvantage of failing to provide sufficient information about the underlying causes and muscular dynamics responsible for the abnormal voice.

Kinesiologic

Exemplified by the terms "vocal hyperfunction" and "vocal hypofunction," this classification categorizes voice disorders according to whether the vocal folds overadduct or underadduct, thus closing the glottis too tightly or incompletely. Although not without merit, this classification, if used exclusively, oversimplifies the complexities of laryngeal diseases, placing excess emphasis on the degree of approximation of the vocal edges rather than on the multiple causes of such approximation defects.

ETIOLOGY OF VOICE DISORDERS

Organic Voice Disorders

A voice disorder is organic if it is caused by structural (anatomic) or physiologic disease, either a disease of the larynx itself or by remote systemic illnesses which alter laryngeal structure or function. Table 1–1 lists various causes of organic voice disorders.

Psychogenic Voice Disorders

A common synonym for "psychogenic" is "functional." Psychogenic voice disorders include disorders of quality, pitch, loudness, and flexibility caused by psychoneuroses, personality disorders, or faulty habits of voice usage (Table 1–2). The voice is abnormal despite normal laryngeal anatomy and physiology.

Voice Disorders of Multiple Etiology

Spastic (spasmodic) dysphonia, including adductor, abductor, and mixed adductor-abductor types, can be neurologic, psychogenic, or of unknown (idiopathic) etiology.

INCIDENCE OF VOICE DISORDERS

Statistics on the incidence of voice disorders in school-age children are fairly abundant in contrast to data on adults. A representative study of the school-age population is that of Senturia and Wilson

Table 1–1 Etiology of Organic Voice Disorders

Congenital Disorders

Cri du chat
Laryngomalacia
Laryngeal web
Cysts
Laryngotracheal cleft
Papilloma
Mongolism

Inflammation

Tumors

Benign
Malignant

Endocrine Disorders

Hypothyroidism
Hyperthyroidism
Hyperpituitarism
Hormonal disorders

Trauma

Neurologic Disease

Lower motor neuron (flaccid) disorder
Bilateral upper motor neuron (spastic) disorder
Mixed lower-upper motor neuron (flaccid-spastic) disorder
Basal ganglia (hypokinetic-parkinsonism) disorder
Cerebellar (ataxic) disorder
Basal ganglia (hyperkinetic-chorea) disorder
Basal ganglia (hyperkinetic-dystonia) disorder
Brainstem (palatopharyngolaryngeal myoclonus) disorder
Brainstem (organic voice tremor) disorder
Gilles de la Tourette's disease
Apraxia of phonation
Akinetic mutism
Pseudoforeign dialect

(1968), who reported that 6 percent of 32,500 children in the St. Louis, Missouri, area had voice disorders. Most other studies place the incidence at a somewhat higher level. Yairi et al. (1974), based on a study of 1500 school-age children, found an incidence of hoarseness in 13 percent. The highest incidence was reported by Silverman and Zimmer (1975), who found voice disorders in 23.4 percent of schoolchildren. Most children with voice disorders have dysphonia related to vocal abuse, either with or without resultant vocal fold nodules or general inflammation. The school-age population is remarkably free of organic voice disorders.

One of the few incidence studies of adults was done by Laguaite (1972), who found that of 428 patients aged 18 to 82, 7.2 percent of the males and 5 percent of the females had voice disorders. In his otolaryngologic practice, Brodnitz (1971), reporting on only "functional" voice disorders, found that in 1851 cases, 25.8 percent had hyperfunctional (musculoskeletal tension) voice disorders, 19.7 percent had polyps, 15.3 percent had vocal nodules, 9.4 percent had polypoid thickening, 5.3 percent had contact ulcers, 4.7 percent had mutational voice disorders, 4.7 percent had spastic dysphonia, 4.4 percent had psychogenic aphonia, and the remaining patients had voice disorders from other causes less common. Cooper (1973), who uses a somewhat different classification system, found in his clinical practice, which includes both adults and children, that 36.6 percent of 1406 patients had voice disorders related to vocal misuse, which includes vocal

Table 1–2   Etiology of Psychogenic Voice Disorders

EMOTIONAL STRESS—MUSCULOSKELETAL TENSION

Voice Disorders Without Secondary Laryngeal Pathology

Voice Disorders With Secondary Laryngeal Pathology

    Vocal nodule
    Contact ulcer

PSYCHONEUROSIS

Conversion reaction

    Mutism
    Aphonia
    Dysphonia

Psychosexual conflict

    Mutational falsetto (puberphonia)
    Dysphonia associated with conflict of sex identification

Iatrogenic

hyperfunction (musculoskeletal tension) disorders; 18.1 percent had vocal nodules; 6.1 percent had contact ulcers; 4.8 percent had polyps; 4.5 percent had polypoid degeneration; 4.2 percent had dysphonia associated with neurologic disease; 3.9 percent had undergone laryngectomy; 3.0 percent had spastic dysphonia; and the remainder had a miscellany of diagnoses.

Representative statistics on the incidence of abnormal voice in otolaryngologic practice were virtually nonexistent until recently. In a study of the prevalence of laryngeal pathologies in medicine according to sex, age, and occupation, Herrington-Hall et al. (1988) investigated 1262 patients drawn from several otolaryngologic practices. They found that the most common disorders were: vocal nodules, 21.6 percent; edema, 14.1 percent; polyps, 11.4 percent; cancer, 9.7 percent; vocal fold paralysis, 8.1 percent; and dysphonia without laryngeal pathology, 7.9 percent. Laryngeal pathologies occurred mostly in the older age groups; 57 percent of patients were over 45 years of age, with 22.4 percent over age 64 years.

Vocal nodules and edema were most common in early adulthood (22 to 44 years); polyps and dysphonia, despite a normal laryngeal examination, were most common during middle adulthood (45 to 64 years); and vocal fold paralysis in late adulthood (over age 64 years). Cancer was evenly distributed between the ages of 45 to 64 and over age 64 years.

In males, vocal nodules were most common between 0 and 14 years, edema between 25 and 44 years, polyps between 45 and 64 years, and vocal fold paralysis primarily after age 64 years.

Of 73 different occupations in the total sample, the most commonly occurring ones were retired persons, homemakers, factory workers, unemployed persons, executives or managers, teachers, students, secretaries, singers, and nurses.

In patients diagnosed as having psychogenic voice disorders, 85 percent were female. With respect to occupational background, 35 percent of psychogenic voice disorders were found in female homemakers. Factory workers were third on the list of the top five occupations with a high incidence of laryngeal pathologies.

SUMMARY

1. The vital functions of the larynx are to protect the lungs from foreign substances, to stabilize the thoracic cage during work done with the upper extremities, and to compress the abdominal contents.

2. Phonation is a secondary laryngeal function and has primitive survival, emotive, and higher linguistic purposes.

3. Normal voice is one in which voice quality, pitch, loudness, and flexibility are reasonably pleasing and audible to the listener.

4. Abnormal voice is defined as deviations in quality, pitch, loudness, or flexibility which may signify illness or interfere with communication.

5. Voice disorders are classified into *organic* types, which consist of dysphonias or aphonia caused by mass lesions or neurologic disease, and *psychogenic* types, which include abnormal voice resulting from psychoneurosis, psychosis, or faulty habit patterns.

6. The incidence of voice disorders in school-age children is 6 to 9 percent and possibly higher. These are mostly dysphonias caused by vocal abuse. The incidence of voice disorders in adults is not well documented, but within this age group is contained the entire spectrum of organic and psychogenic voice disorders.

SUGGESTIONS FOR ADDITIONAL READING

Miller, S.Q., and Madison, C.L.: Public school voice clinics, part I: A working model. Lang. Speech Hear. Serv. Sch., 15: 51–57, 1984.

Miller, S.Q., and Madison, L.L., Public school voice clinics, part II: Diagnosis and recommendations—a 10-year review. Lang. Speech Hear. Serv. Sch., 15: 58–64, 1984.

Both of these articles are interesting for their information on incidence of voice disorders, survey methods and procedures for setting up voice clinics in schools.

Pannbacker, M.: Classification systems of voice disorders: A review of the literature. Lang. Speech, Hear., Serv. Sch., 15: 169–174, 1984.

A worthwhile article on classification of voice disorders.

Senturia, B.H., and Wilson, F.B.: Otorhinolaryngologic findings in children with voice deviations. Preliminary report. Ann. Otol. Rhinol. Laryngol., 77:1027–1042, 1968. One of the few detailed and comprehensive laryngologic studies of school-age children with voice disorders.

Wilson, K.: Voice Problems of Children, 2nd ed. Baltimore, Williams & Wilkins, Co., 1979.

Pages 6 to 11 contain an excellent review of the literature on public school voice disorder surveys.

REFERENCES

Brodnitz, F.S.: Vocal Rehabilitation. Am. Acad. Ophthalmol. Otolaryngol., 75: 1971.

Cooper, M.: Modern Techniques of Vocal Rehabilitation. Springfield, Ill., Charles C Thomas, 1973.

Fairbanks, G.: Voice and Articulation Drillbook. New York, Harper & Brothers, 1960.

Herrington-Hall, B.L., Lee, L., Stemple, J.C., Niemi, K.R., and McHone, M.M.: Description of laryngeal pathologies by age, sex, and occupation in a treatment-seeking sample. J. Speech Hear. Disord., 53:57–64, 1988.

Jensen, P.J.: Adequacy of terminology for clinical judgment of voice quality deviation. Eye Ear Nose Throat Monthly, 44: 77–82, 1965.

Johnson, W., Brown, S.F., Curtis, J.F., Edney, C.W., and Keaster, J.: Speech Handicapped School Children, New York, Harper & Brothers, 1965.

Laguaite, J.K.: Adult voice screening. J. Speech Hear. Disord., 37:147–151, 1972.

Moore, G.P.: Organic Voice Disorders. Englewood Cliffs, N.J., Prentice-Hall, 1971a.

Moore, G.P.: Voice disorders organically based. In Travis, L.E. (Ed.): Handbook of Speech Pathology and Audiology. New York, Appleton-Century-Crofts, 1971b.

Negus, V.E.: The Mechanism of the Larynx. St. Louis, C. V. Mosby Co., 1929.

Nizer, L.: Reflections Without Mirrors. New York, Doubleday and Co., 1978.

Perkins, W.H.: Vocal function: A behavioral analysis. In Travis, L.E. (Ed.): Handbook of Speech Pathology and Audiology. New York, Appleton-Century-Crofts, 1971.

Robbins, S.D.: A Dictionary of Speech Pathology and Therapy. Cambridge, Mass., Sci-Art Publishers, 1963.

Senturia, B.H., and Wilson, F.B.: Otorhinolaryngologic findings in children with voice deviations. Preliminary Report. Ann. Otol. Rhinol. Laryngol., 77:1027–1042, 1968.

Silverman, E.M., and Zimmer, C.H.: Incidence of chronic hoarseness among school-age children. J. Speech Hear. Disord., 40:211–215, 1975.

West, R., Kennedy, L., and Carr, A.: The Rehabilitation of Speech. New York, Harper & Brothers, 1947.

Yairi, E., Currin, L.H., Bulian, N., and Yairi, J.: Incidence of hoarseness in school children over a 1 year period. J. Commun. Disord., 7:321–328, 1974.

Chapter Two

THE ADULT LARYNX

    Cartilages
    Hyoid Bone
    Membranes and Ligaments
    Muscles
    Interior of the Larynx
    Blood and Lymphatic Supply
    Embryology

LARYNGEAL BIOMECHANICS

    Movements of the Larynx and Hyoid Bone
    Movements of the Laryngeal Cartilages

LARYNGEAL PHYSIOLOGY

    Respiratory Functions of the Larynx
    Effort Closure Functions of the Larynx
    Swallowing Functions of the Larynx
    Phonatory Functions of the Larynx
    Vibratory Function of Vocal Fold Mucosa
    Determinants of Loudness and Pitch
    Vocal Registers
    Modes of Vocal Attack

LARYNGEAL EVOLUTION

    African Lungfish
    Salamander
    Frog
    Crocodile
    Lesser Gymnure
    Tree Shrew
    Rhesus Monkey
    Chimpanzee

ANATOMY AND PHYSIOLOGY OF PHONATION

THE ADULT LARYNX

The human larynx is located near the base of the neck. It is attached inferiorly to the trachea and opens superiorly into the pharynx (Fig. 2-1). Not much laryngeal structure can be seen externally except for a prominence in the midline of the neck, the pomum Adami or Adam's apple, formed by the wings of the thyroid cartilage. It is more pronounced in the male because of the wings' larger size and narrower angle. The adult larynx lies anterior to the third to sixth cervical vertebrae (Fig. 2-2). The thyroid cartilage can be felt by placing a forefinger on the thyroid prominence and then moving it a few millimeters superiorly to find the *thyroid notch*. After doing so, the superior border of the thyroid cartilage should be encircled with thumb and middle finger. If, at this point, the fingers are depressed inward, they will sink into the thyrohyoid space and will feel the inferior border of the *hyoid bone*. The hyoid bone can then be encircled with the fingers and followed as far posteriorly as possible. From there the fingers can be moved down to the lower border of the thyroid cartilage, where another space between the thyroid and *cricoid cartilage* will be encountered, the *cricothyroid space*.

In this chapter, the portions of the laryngeal anatomy to be studied include cartilaginous framework, membranes, joints, ligaments, extrinsic muscles, intrinsic muscles, and interior cavity.

Cartilages

The larynx consists of nine cartilages. Three are unpaired—thyroid (1), cricoid (1), and epiglottis (1). Three are paired—arytenoids (2), corniculates (2), and cuneiforms (2) (Fig. 2-3).

THYROID CARTILAGE

The thyroid cartilage is a hyaline type of cartilage derived embryologically from mesenchyme of branchial arch IV. It is the largest in the laryngeal skeleton, consisting of two flat quadrilateral plates, or *laminae,* fused anteriorly to form a 90° angle in the adult male and a 120° angle in the adult female. Along its superior border is a V-shaped notch, the *thyroid notch,* and below it is the *laryngeal prominence*. Posteriorly are the *superior horns* or cornu that serve as attachments to the hyoid bone. The *inferior horns* or cornu articulate with the cricoid cartilage below this bone. An *oblique line* can be found on the lateral surfaces of the laminae marking the position of attachment of the thyrohyoid, sternothyroid, and inferior pharyngeal constrictor muscles. The inner surfaces of the laminae are covered with mucous membrane, and, at the junction of the laminae, this is a place for the attachment of the thyroepiglottic ligament.

CRICOID CARTILAGE

The cricoid cartilage is wider posteriorly than anteriorly and is shaped like a signet ring, from which it derives its name. It is located inferior to the thyroid cartilage and forms a considerable portion of the posterior wall of the larynx. On its lateral aspects are the *articular surfaces* which receive the inferior horns of the thyroid cartilage. These joints are synovial, having capsular ligaments. The

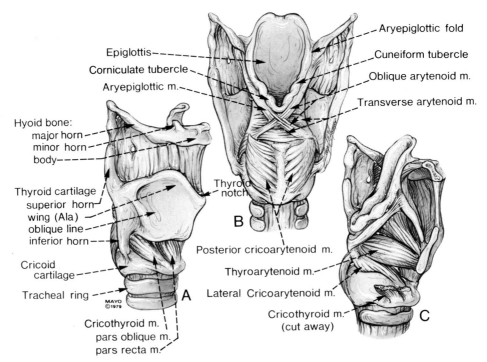

Epiglottis

Corniculate tubercle

Aryepiglottic m.

Aryepiglottic fold

Cuneiform tubercle

Oblique arytenoid m.

Transverse arytenoid m.

Hyoid bone:
   major horn
   minor horn
   body

Thyroid cartilage
   superior horn
   wing (Ala)
   oblique line
   inferior horn

Cricoid
   cartilage

Tracheal ring

MAYO
©1979

Thyroid
notch

B

Posterior cricoarytenoid m.

Thyroarytenoid m.

Lateral Cricoarytenoid m.

Cricothyroid m.
(cut away)

C

A

Cricothyroid m.
pars oblique m.
pars recta m.

Figure 2–1   Lateral and posterior view of the larynx.

movement of the thyroid on the cricoid is primarily rotatory, although sliding motion is also possible. Surfaces for the articulation of the arytenoid cartilages can also be found on the posterior-superior surfaces of the cricoid cartilage. The lower border of the cricoid cartilage attaches to the topmost ring of the trachea by means of the cricotracheal ligament. The superior border of the cricoid cartilage is the site of attachment for the conus elasticus.

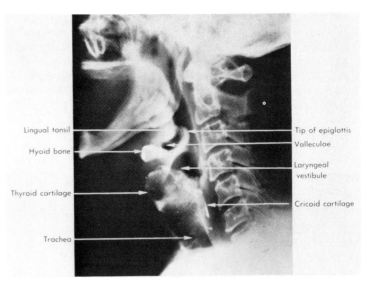

Figure 2–2   Lateral radiograph of the head and neck showing the position of the larynx and hyoid bone in relation to the cervical vertebrae. (*From* Otolaryngologic Clinics of North America, Vol. 3, No. 3, pg. 467 October, 1970, Valvassori, G., and Goldstein, J.C. (Eds.): Radiographic Evaluation of the Larynx. Philadelphia, W.B. Saunders Co.)

Lingual tonsil

Hyoid bone

Thyroid cartilage

Trachea

Tip of epiglottis

Valleculae

Laryngeal
vestibule

Cricoid cartilage

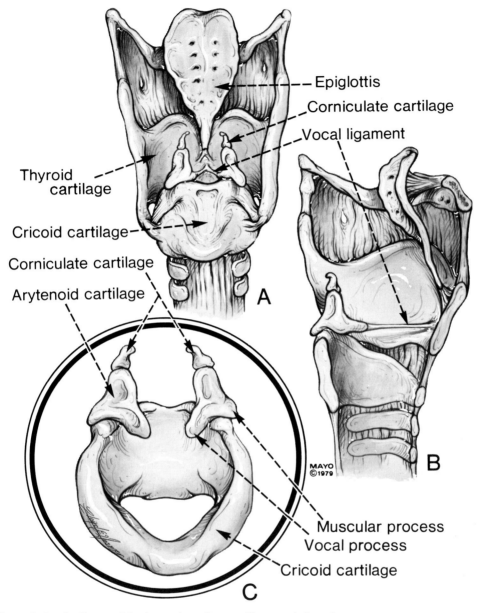

Figure 2–3 Cartilages of the larynx (cuneiform cartilages not shown).

ARYTENOID CARTILAGES

The paired arytenoid cartilages originate from branchial arch VI. Each is shaped like a three-sided pyramid, the bases of which rest upon the articular surfaces of the cricoid cartilage. The apex of each arytenoid cartilage curves posteriorly and medially and is flattened for articulation with the corniculate cartilages. The medial surfaces of the arytenoid cartilages are smooth and covered with mucous membrane. At the base of each arytenoid cartilage is a projection called the *vocal process*, the location of attachment of the vocal ligament that forms the medial aspect of the vocal folds. A second landmark at the base of the arytenoid cartilage is the *muscular process* that points posteriorly. It is given this name because it forms one of the attachments for the anterior (lateral) and posterior cricoarytenoid muscles. The articulation of the arytenoid with the cricoid cartilage is a synovial joint reinforced by capsular ligaments and a cricoarytenoid ligament that restricts forward movement of the cartilage.

CORNICULATE CARTILAGES

Resting atop and articulating with the arytenoid cartilages, either by means of a synovial joint or fused with the cartilages, are the elastic corniculate fibrocartilages, also known as the cartilages of Santorini.

CUNEIFORM CARTILAGES

Within the mucous membrane of the aryepiglottic folds that extend from the apices of the arytenoid cartilages to the epigottis are embedded the small cuneiform cartilages, or cartilages of Wrisberg.

EPIGLOTTIS

The epiglottis is a broad, fibrocartilaginous flat structure whose base is attached to the medial surface of the thyroid cartilage by means of the *thyroepiglottic ligaments,* its free end projecting upward toward the base of the tongue. Its posterior surface is concave, and on its base is found a projection called the epiglottic tubercle. The epiglottis and the base of the tongue are connected with mucous membrane.

Hyoid Bone

Although not technically a part of the larynx, the hyoid bone must be included in any discussion of laryngeal anatomy and, especially, physiology. The hyoid bone is horseshoe-shaped, located immediately superior to the thyroid cartilage and suspended in the neck by means of a sling of muscles and ligaments (Fig. 2-4). It makes no direct physical contact with any other bone or cartilage. The hyoid bone is subdivided into a *body* from which extend posteriorly the larger *major horns* and the smaller *minor horns* (Fig. 2-1A).

Membranes and Ligaments

The *lateral thyrohyoid ligaments* connect the tips of the superior horns of the thyroid cartilage to the posterior ends of the major horns of the hyoid bone. The *thyrohyoid membrane* connects the superior border of the thyroid cartilage to the anterior border of the hyoid bone. It is composed of fibroelastic tissue. The *median thyrohyoid ligament* is a thickening of the central part of the thyrohyoid membrane invested on either side by the internal branch of the superior laryngeal nerve and by the superior laryngeal artery. The *quadrangular membrane* connects the sides of the epiglottis to the arytenoid cartilages. The *conus elasticus* is a tough fibrous elastic material that lines the entire larynx, forming a basement for the musculature.

Muscles

The muscles of the larynx are divided into two types: *extrinsic* and *intrinsic,* The extrinsic muscles are defined as those attached at one end to a cartilage of the larynx and at the other to a bony structure outside the larynx. *The extrinsic muscles are responsible for moving the larynx as a total unit,* thereby changing its position in the neck. The intrinsic muscles attach at both ends to the cartilages of the larynx and *are responsible for moving those cartilages in relation to one another*.

EXTRINSIC LARYNGEAL MUSCLES

Also called the "strap muscles" because of their flat shape, these muscles are subdivided into a suprahyoid and an infrahyoid group (Fig. 2-4). The infrahyoid muscles are those with attachments below the hyoid bone. Their action pulls the larynx and hyoid bone down to a lower position in the

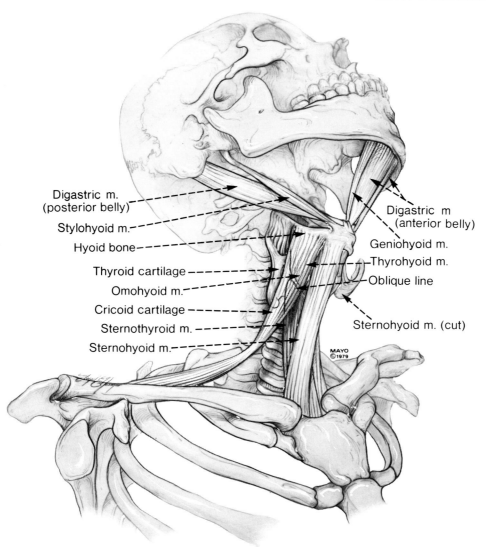

Digastric m.
(posterior belly)

Stylohyoid m.

Hyoid bone

Thyroid cartilage

Omohyoid m.

Cricoid cartilage

Sternothyroid m.

Sternohyoid m.

Digastric m
(anterior belly)

Geniohyoid m.

Thyrohyoid m.

Oblique line

Sternohyoid m. (cut)

MAYO
©1979

Figure 2–4   Extrinsic laryngeal muscles (mylohyoid and stylopharyngeus muscles not shown).

neck. The *sternohyoid* attaches to the manubrium of the sternum and clavicle on one end and to the inferior border of the hyoid bone on the other. The *sternothyroid* attaches to the manubrium of the sternum and first rib on one end and to the oblique line of the thyroid cartilage on the other. The *thyrohyoid* attaches to the oblique line of the thyroid cartilage below and the lower border of the hyoid bone above. The *omohyoid* attaches to the upper border of the scapula and the lower border of the hyoid bone.

The suprahyoid muscles pull the hyoid bone forward, upward, and backward. The *stylohoid* attaches to the styloid process of the temporal bone and to the hyoid. The *mylohyoid* attaches to the inner surface of the mandible and to the hyoid bone. The *digastric* is subdivided into an anterior belly that attaches to the inner surface of the mandible and the hyoid bone, and a posterior belly that attaches to the mastoid process of the temporal bone and the hyoid bone. The *geniohyoid* attaches to the interior surface of the mandible and to the hyoid bone. The *stylopharyngeus* attaches to the styloid process of the temporal bone and to inferior pharyngeal constrictor and posterior border of the thyroid cartilage.

INTRINSIC LARYNGEAL MUSCLES (FIGS. 2-1A AND FIG. 2-11)

The *cricothyroid* muscle is subdivided into two parts: the vertical or pars recta, and the more horizontal, the pars oblique. The vertical fibers attach to the anterolateral surfaces of the cricoid cartilage and to the inferior border of the thyroid cartilage. The oblique fibers attach to the anterolateral surfaces of the cricoid cartilage and to the inferior horns of the thyroid cartilage. The more vertical fibers of the cricothyroid muscle rotate the thyroid cartilage downward. The oblique fibers pull the thyroid cartilage forward.

Two opposing muscles rotate and rock the arytenoid cartilages. The *anterior cricoarytenoid,* also called the lateral cricoarytenoid, attaches at one end to the cricoid cartilage and at the other to the muscular process of the arytenoid cartilage. Upon contraction, these muscles rotate and rock the arytenoid cartilages medially. The *posterior cricoarytenoids* attach to the cricoid cartilage and to the muscular processes of the arytenoid cartilages. They rotate and rock the arytenoid cartilages laterally. The *oblique arytenoids* attach to the posterior surface at the bases of the arytenoid cartilages and to the apices of the opposite arytenoid cartilages; one muscle crosses the other. The *transverse arytenoid* is the only unpaired muscle of the larynx. It attaches to the posterior borders of the arytenoid cartilages similar to the way in which the oblique arytenoids attach, but lies deep to them. Both the oblique and the transverse arytenoids approximate the arytenoid cartilages by sliding and tilting them medially.

The *thyroarytenoid* muscles form the main bodies of the vocal folds. They attach anteriorly to the inner surfaces of the wings of the thyroid cartilage at its angle and posteriorly to the anterolateral surface of each arytenoid cartilage. The muscle passes lateral to the vocal ligaments, forming a broad sheet. Its more medial portion forms the *vocalis* muscle, which is actually a part of the thyroarytenoid and which attaches posteriorly to the vocal process of the arytenoid cartilage and to its lateral surface. The medial edge of the vocalis muscle attaches to the conus elasticus. Contraction of the thyroarytenoid muscle pulls the arytenoid cartilages forward, closing the glottis anteroposteriorly. Finally, the *aryepiglotticus,* which runs from the apices of the arytenoid cartilages to the sides of the epiglottis, contributes to pulling the epiglottis downward over the laryngeal orifice.

Interior of the Larynx

The interior of the larynx can be divided into three levels, or tiers. The *superior vestibule* is that portion that extends from the laryngeal inlet to the level of the ventricular, or false, vocal folds. The middle portion lies between the ventricular and true vocal folds and includes the laryngeal ventricle. The *inferior vestibule* extends from the true vocal folds down to the lower border of the cricoid cartilage and is sometimes referred to as the "infraglottic larynx" (Fig. 2-5). The coronal section of the larynx shows that the laryngeal cavity is hourglass-shaped, wide at the top and bottom and narrower in the middle. The surface of this interior airway is lined with mucosa, under which lies the tough, fibrous *conus elasticus.* The area of the constriction is of special interest. Here there are four shelflike projections into the laryngeal space, two on each side. The superior pair are the *ventricular*, or *false, vocal folds* and the inferior pair the *true vocal folds*. The space between the true and false vocal fold on each side is the *laryngeal ventricle.* Actually, the true and false vocal folds are extrusions of circular thyroarytenoid muscle fibers that, on total contraction, fold or constrict the lumen of the larynx.

A superior view (Fig. 2-6, and see page 396 for color plate) shows that the medial edges of the true vocal folds are yellowish white. These ligamentous medial edges are formed by the vocal ligaments, which are covered by mucous membrane. The epithelium is of the stratified squamous type, having no submucous layer. It therefore has a poor blood supply, imparting to the vocal fold edges their white and shiny appearance.

The horizontal space between the paired vocal folds is called the glottis. Approximately the anterior three fifths of the true vocal fold is called the *intermembranous* or *membranous* portion, and the space between the vocal processes of the arytenoid cartilages is called the *intercartilagenous*

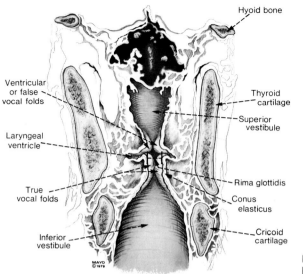

Hyoid bone

Ventricular
or false
vocal folds

Thyroid
cartilage

Superior
vestibule

Laryngeal
ventricle

True
vocal folds

Rima glottidis

Conus
elasticus

Inferior
vestibule

Cricoid
cartilage

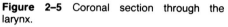

Figure 2–5 Coronal section through the larynx.

portion. Coronal sections through the larynx showing its histologic structure expose the changes in the configuration of cartilage and muscle as the sections progress anteriorly to posteriorly (Figs. 2-7 and 2-8). It is important to note the absence of arytenoid cartilage in the first figure and its appearance in the second.

Blood and Lymphatic Supply

Accompanying the inferior laryngeal nerve into the larynx is the *inferior laryngeal artery,* a small branch of the inferior thyroid artery. The inferior laryngeal artery anastomoses with the *superior laryngeal artery* from the superior thyroid artery to supply the larynx and adjacent regions of the pharynx. The *superior laryngeal vein* empties into the jugular vein. The *inferior laryngeal vein* joins the inferior thyroid vein. The lymphatics of the larynx drain along the vessels both upward and downward into the deep cervical nodes.

Embryology

The larynx develops from branchial (visceral) arches III, IV, and VI. From entoderm arises the epithelial lining of the larynx, and from mesoderm develop connective tissue, voluntary muscles, vascular and lymphatic systems, and skeletal elements of the larynx. The hyoid bone arises from

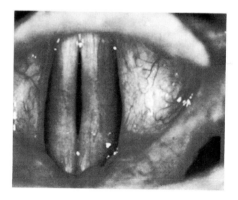

Figure 2–6 Normal larynx during phonation. (See p. 396 for color plate.)

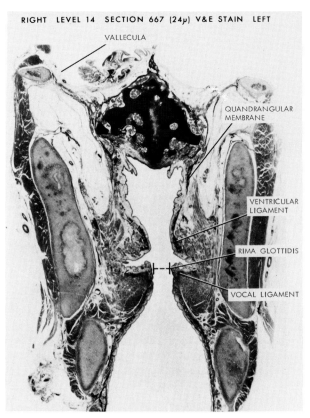

RIGHT   LEVEL 14   SECTION 667 (24μ) V&E STAIN   LEFT

VALLECULA

QUANDRANGULAR MEMBRANE

VENTRICULAR LIGAMENT

RIMA GLOTTIDIS

VOCAL LIGAMENT

Figure 2–7   Coronal histologic section through membranous portion of vocal folds. (*From* Tucker, G.F., Jr.: Human Larynx, Coronal Section Atlas. Washington, D.C. Armed Forces Institute of Pathology, 1971.)

branchial arch III, and the thyroid, cricoid, arytenoid, corniculate, and cuneiform cartilages arise from arches IV and VI. From these arches also come the intrinsic laryngeal and pharyngeal musculature. The superior laryngeal nerve arises from branchial arch IV, and the recurrent laryngeal nerve develops from arch VI.

When the embryo is four weeks old, a primitive laryngeal orifice or slit can be seen lying between branchial arches IV and VI (Fig. 2-9). At five weeks, swellings of mesenchymal tissue can be found lateral to the laryngeal aditus; these are anlage of the arytenoid cartilages. The anterior swelling is the forerunner of the epiglottis. During the fifth and sixth weeks of embryonic life, continued growth of these structures causes the aditus to take on a T-shaped configuration. Between the seventh and tenth weeks, the entrance to the larynx is blind, but in the tenth week its occluding epithelium breaks down and the laryngeal aditus begins to enlarge. The laryngeal ventricles develop, bounded cranially and caudally by anteroposterior folds of mucous membrane, which develop into the false and true vocal folds, respectively. At approximately 10 to 11 weeks of embryonic life, the major topography of the larynx has formed, and the cartilages have hardened.

LARYNGEAL BIOMECHANICS

The larynx and hyoid bone are suspended in the neck by means of ligaments and the extrinsic laryngeal muscles (Fig. 2-10). The laryngeal cartilages are bound together with ligaments and the intrinsic laryngeal muscles. These muscles and ligaments determine the movements and limits of movement of the hyoid bone, the larynx as a whole, and its component cartilages. Suspended as if in a sling, the larynx and hyoid bone can be moved in several different directions, depending upon the components of force exerted on them by the muscles that insert into them. They are suspended

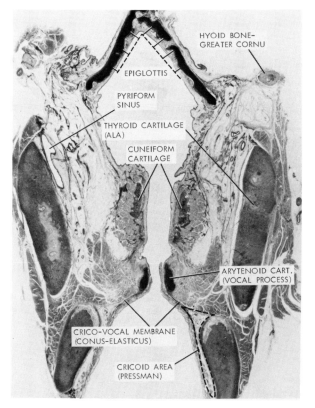

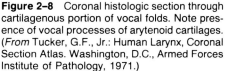

Figure 2-8 Coronal histologic section through cartilagenous portion of vocal folds. Note presence of vocal processes of arytenoid cartilages. (*From* Tucker, G.F., Jr.: Human Larynx, Coronal Section Atlas. Washington, D.C., Armed Forces Institute of Pathology, 1971.)

superiorly by means of the *stylohyoid* ligament, which attaches to the styloid process of the mastoid bone on one end and to the hyoid bone on the other. From the hyoid bone, the thyroid cartilage is suspended by means of the *median* and *lateral thyrohyoid* ligaments. The cricoid cartilage is suspended from the thyroid cartilage by means of the *cricothyroid* ligaments, and the cricoid cartilage is perched on the first tracheal ring. These ligaments are elastic and, therefore, can be stretched as the hyoid bone and larynx are pulled in different directions by the musculature, but elastic recoil causes them to return to their original positions upon muscular relaxation.

Movements of the Larynx and Hyoid Bone

The following effects of extrinsic muscle contraction on the position of the larynx and hyoid bone have been inferred from the direction of the muscle fibers (Fig. 2-10):

1. The hyoid bone is moved superiorly and posteriorly by the action of the stylohyoid, digastric (posterior belly), and medial pharyngeal constrictor muscles.
2. The hyoid bone is moved superiorly and anteriorly by the geniohyoid, genioglossus, mylohyoid, and digastric (anterior belly) muscles.
3. The hyoid bone is moved inferiorly by the thyrohyoid, sternohyoid, and omohyoid muscles.
4. The larynx is moved superiorly by the thyrohyoid muscle.
5. The larynx is moved inferiorly by the sternothyroid muscle.

Movements of the Laryngeal Cartilages

The capsular cricothyroid and cricoarytenoid ligaments that bind the cartilages to one another are capable of being stretched, allowing the intrinsic laryngeal muscles to rotate and slide these cartilages in relationship to one another (Fig. 2-11).

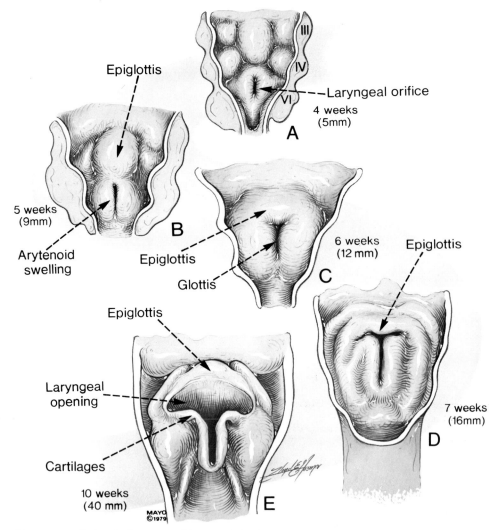

Figure 2–9 Embryologic stages of laryngeal development.

1. Movements between the cricoid and thyroid cartilages.
    a. Rotatory motion. The cricoid and thyroid cartilages rotate around a horizontal axis that
       passes through the cricothyroid joints. The arch of the cricoid cartilage can be rotated
       about 15 degrees superiorly, drawing it closer to the thyroid cartilage. This movement is
       brought about by contraction of the cricothyroid muscle, the pars recta. The effect of such
       action is to move the arytenoid cartilages, perched upon the cricoid cartilage, in a
       posterior direction. Because one end of the thyroarytenoid muscle (vocal folds) is
       attached at the vocal process of the arytenoid cartilage and the other at the angle of the
       thyroid cartilage, such rotary movement passively stretches the vocal folds. In other
       words, *the cricothyroid muscle is the tensor of the vocal ligament and the vocal folds,
       elongating them*.
    b. Sliding motion. The thyroid cartilage can be slid anteriorly, subluxating the joint
       between the inferior horns of the thyroid cartilage and the facets of the cricoid cartilage.
       This sliding action is produced by contraction of the cricothyroid muscle, the pars
       oblique.

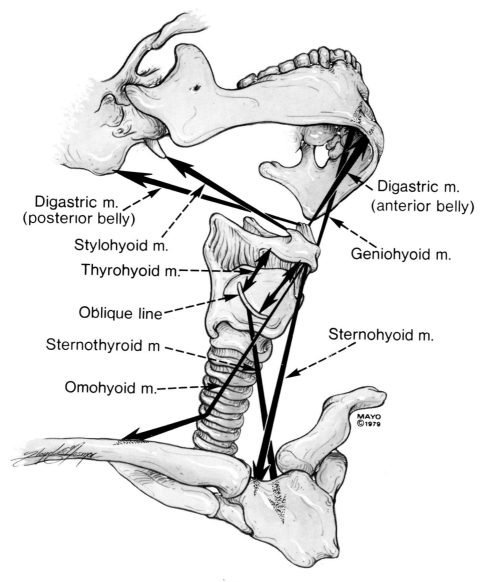

Figure 2-10   Sling suspension of larynx and hyoid bone.

2. Movements between the arytenoid and cricoid cartilages.
   a. Sliding motion. The arytenoid cartilages can be slid anteriorly on the cricoarytenoid joint approximately 2 mm. by means of contraction of the thyroarytenoid muscle. The effect of such action is to shorten the vocal folds.
   b. Rocking motion. The arytenoid cartilages can be rocked anteriorly within a range of about 30 degrees by means of contraction of the thyroarytenoid muscle. The arytenoid cartilages can be rocked medially by the anterior (lateral) cricoarytenoid muscle, aided by contraction of the transverse and oblique arytenoids and producing a vocal fold adduction. The cartilages can be rocked laterally by means of contraction of the posterior cricoarytenoid muscles abducting the vocal folds.
3. Movements between the epiglottis and larynx. The epiglottis can be pulled down over the opening to the interior of the larynx by means of the action of the aryepiglotticus muscle.

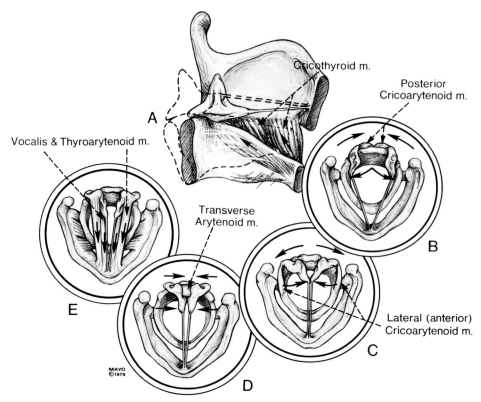

Figure 2–11   Movement relationships of the laryngeal cartilages.

LARYNGEAL PHYSIOLOGY

Respiratory Functions of the Larynx

The larynx devotes more time to respiration than to any other function in order to ensure a free flow of air into and out of the lungs. During quiet inhalation, the vocal folds abduct, moving away from the midline and widening the glottis, and during exhalation they adduct slightly toward the midline, but always maintaining an open glottal airway. Whereas abductor vocal fold movements are small and inconspicuous during quiet inhalation, they are extensive during forced inhalation. The larynx also moves as a body during respiration, downward during inhalation and upward during exhalation. The downward movement increases the airway capacity, admitting a larger volume of inhaled air. According to Fink and Demarest (1978), the larynx lacks muscles to abduct the vocal folds in parallel. Therefore, during inhalation, widening of the glottis to increase the volume flow of air must result from coupling the transverse with the vertical downward excursion of the larynx. The entire bronchial tree, including the larynx, moves downward with every inhalation and upward with every exhalation. Transverse separation of the arytenoids is the net result, due not to active muscular abducting forces, but to passive laryngeal tensions. Not just the glottis widens on inhalation; the entire supracricoid area does.

Effort Closure Functions of the Larynx

A second vital function of the larynx is effort closure, also known as the Valsalva maneuver. In this maneuver, the lumen of the larynx is sealed to prevent air from escaping from the lungs during effortful physical work, such as lifting and pushing, and it compresses the thoracic and abdominal contents during coughing, throat clearing, vomiting, urination, defecation, and parturition. There is a great contrast between the position of the vocal folds during normal phonation and during effort closure. During phonation, only the true vocal folds adduct, but during effort closure, there is massive undifferentiated adduction of the laryngeal walls, including both true and false vocal folds (Fig. 2-12).

The following sequence of events has been observed during effort closure:

1. The arytenoid cartilages are brought to the midline.
2. The false vocal folds are brought together by means of thyroarytenoid muscle contraction.
3. The laryngeal ventricle is obliterated because the false vocal folds are pulled down against the true vocal folds.
4. The thyroid cartilage is elevated, approximating the hyoid bone, as subglottic pressure increases.

Swallowing Functions of the Larynx

The chief purpose of the larynx is to protect the lungs from ingestion of solids or liquids and to admit only air. Consequently, closure of the airway during swallowing is essential if food is to be prevented from entering the lungs. The plug needs to be extremely tight, exerting twice the resistance to pressure from above during swallowing as from below during effort closure. Electromyography shows that intrinsic laryngeal muscle contraction is considerably greater during swallowing than during phonation (Faaborg-Andersen, 1957). The sequence of laryngeal and pharyngeal events during swallowing is shown in Figure 2-13.

1. The larynx rises as the bolus descends onto the back of the tongue; the thyroid cartilage elevates toward the hyoid bone, and the epiglottis is pushed posteriorly against the posterior pharyngeal wall.
2. As the bolus passes through the laryngopharynx, a prominent upward movement of the larynx and trachea is begun by the upward and forward movement of the hyoid bone.
3. As the larynx rises, the epiglottis is forced in the direction of the bolus, its tip tilting backward.
4. The larynx continues to rise as the bolus is squeezed downward.
5. As the bolus passes through the mesopharynx, forward retraction of the larynx stops. The larynx remains closed while the bolus passes through the cricopharyngeal sphincter into the upper esophagus.

The security of the airway against ingestion of foreign substances during swallowing is considerable, nature having provided a strong muscular system with backup capabilities. Clinical experience proves that even though the swallowing musculature may be seriously impaired by neurologic disease, protection of the airway is maintained. Loss of closure protection during swallowing and inhalation of foreign substances happen only during the terminal stages of severe

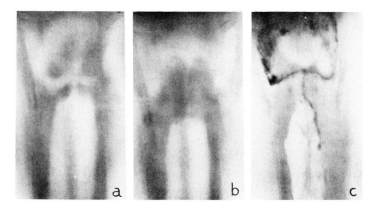

a   b   c

Figure 2-12 Comparison of vocal folds during phonation and effort closure.(a) Prolongation of vowel /i/. (b)Effort closure (bearing down).(c) Effort closure (bearing down), vocal folds outlined with iodized oil. Note the massive, undifferentiated adduction of true and false vocal folds. The lumen of the airway is completely obliterated. (From Ardran, G.M., Kemp, F.H., and Manen, L.: Closure of the larynx. Br. J. Radiol., 26:497–509, 1953.)

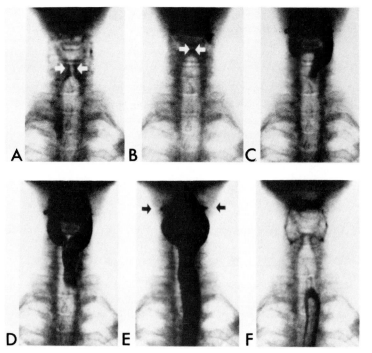

Figure 2–13 Laryngeal action during swallowing. *(a)* Larynx and pharynx at rest. *(b)* Bolus has reached valleculae, spilling over left margin of epiglottis. Larynx has moved upward 1½ vertebral bodies. *(c)* Barium flowing around both sides of epiglottis and aryepiglottic folds. *(d)* Pyriform sinuses and hypopharynx now filled with barium. *(e)* Oral pharynx compressed from side to side. Arrows show outpouching of lateral pharyngeal walls. *(f)* Swallow complete. Larynx and pharynx have returned to resting position. *(From Ramsey, G.H., Watson, J.S., Gramiak, R., and Weinberg, S.A.: Cinefluorographic analysis of the mechanism of swallowing. Radiology, 64:498–518, 955.)*

neurologic diseases, such as bulbar amyotrophic lateral sclerosis, which ultimately require gastric intubation because the weak swallowing mechanism can no longer protect the airway.

Phonatory Functions of the Larynx

Ferrein (1746), from experiments on animal larynges, was the first to prove that vocal fold vibration was responsible for voice. Possibly anticipating the myoelastic-aerodynamic theory by 200 years, he wrote, in the following translation from the French:

> I am not going to offer any new commentary on the opinion of the ancients. On the contrary, I want to show that their theory is not in accord with nature. I want to present a new instrument equally unknown to anatomists and musicians. There are string instruments such as the violin and the harpsicord; there are others—wind instruments—like the flute and the organ. *But we don't know of any which are at the same time both string and wind instruments. This instrument . . . I have found in the human body* [italics mine]. This discovery is based on the experiments that I've done.

Helmholtz (1863) gave us the more accurate explanation, showing that phonation was the product of puffs of air released through the glottis, for we now know that voice is produced by a steady flow of air from the lungs, segmented at the laryngeal level into a series of air puffs at a fundamental frequency that generates higher harmonics in the cavities of the upper airway. Which frequencies will be produced with a minimum attenuation will be determined by the configuration of the supralaryngeal cavities. Such acoustic energy concentrations due to cavity resonation are called "formant frequencies." As Lieberman (1967) states, the relationship between the fundamental frequency of sound produced by vocal fold opening and closing and the configuration of the supraglottic cavities is an independent one; that is, fundamental frequency can be varied, yet the same vowel or vowel formants maintained, or fundamental frequency can be held steady, yet the vowel formants varied by changing the supraglottic cavity configuration.

How the larynx produces sound has been explained according to two contradictory theories, the first of which is rejected and the second accepted.

NEUROCHRONAXIC THEORY (HUSSON, 1953)

The vocal folds, rather than being passively forced open and closed periodically, do so actively by means of rhythmic contractions of the vocalis portion of the thyroarytenoid muscles. These contractions are alleged to occur at the same rate as the fundamental frequency. The theory has been rejected on the following substantive points.

1. There is no evidence that the thyroarytenoid muscle possesses an abductor function.
2. Experiments have proved that the vocal folds of the cadaver are able to produce voice from a subglottic airstream.
3. Unilaterally or bilaterally paralyzed vocal folds are still able to produce voice.
4. Phonation occurs at fundamental frequencies higher than the nerve impulse transmission rates of which the recurrent laryngeal nerve is capable.

MYOELASTIC-AERODYNAMIC THEORY (VAN DEN BERG, 1958)

Periodic opening and closing of the vocal folds is produced by interaction between the mass-tension of the folds and the aerodynamic forces exerted on and around them by the exhaled airstream. The theory's main contention is that the vocal folds, adducted and held passively in the midline, are opened and closed by infraglottic air pressure.

The myoelastic-aerodynamic theory in greater detail follows (Fig. 2-14).

1. The vocal folds are adducted to the midline and firmly held there.
2. As the airstream is forced from the lungs, subglottic pressure rises to a level that overcomes the resistance of the adducted vocal folds, and consequently they open momentarily, releasing a puff of air.
3. At this moment, the airstream is flowing through an hourglass-shaped, cross-sectional area, the wider ends formed by the subglottic trachea and the supraglottic pharynx, with the middle being a narrower channel bounded by the true and false vocal folds.
4. The air pressure within this narrower channel falls during the momentary flow of air through it owing to the *Bernoulli* effect. As the suction produced by the drop in pressure in the region of the folds plus the static tissue forces begins to counterbalance the subglottic pressure from the lungs, the folds begin to move inward, the narrowing channel causing an increase in suction until the folds snap shut. This completes one vocal fold cycle, and the folds are now in position for the cycle to repeat itself.

The physics of the myoelastic-aerodynamic theory of phonation is given by Lieberman (1968) and is summarized below. He reminds us that two forces act on the vocal folds: (1) Aerodynamic-aerostatic forces displacing the vocal folds from their adducted position in preparation for phonation, and (2) tissue forces that act to restore the vocal folds to their adducted position. Figure 2-15 shows that:

1. Positive subglottic air pressure is represented by F_{AS}. When the glottis is closed, this force displaces the true vocal folds outward from their adducted position.
2. The Bernoulli force, represented by F_{AB}, is the negative air pressure in the region of the glottis created by the high-velocity airflow there.
3. Tension of the vocal ligaments that restore the vocal folds to their neutral position is represented by F_{TO} and F_{TC}.

Interaction among the forces is as follows.

4. The aerostatic force F_{AS} resulting from the subglottic air pressure against the adducted vocal folds is maximum at the beginning of the cycle.

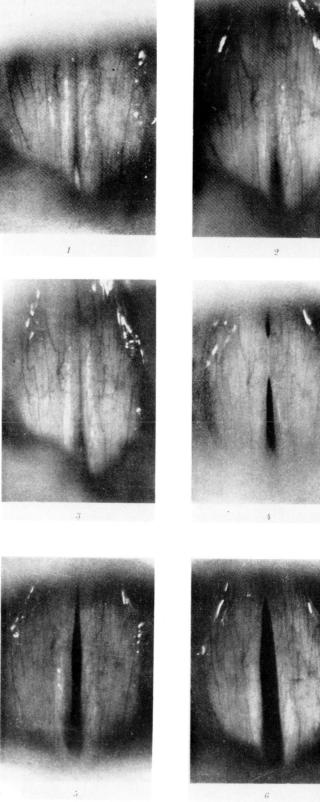

Figure 2–14 Photographic sequence of one complete vocal fold cycle. (*From* Smith, S.: Remarks on the physiology of the vibrations of the vocal cords. Folia Phoniatr. 6:166–178, 1954.)

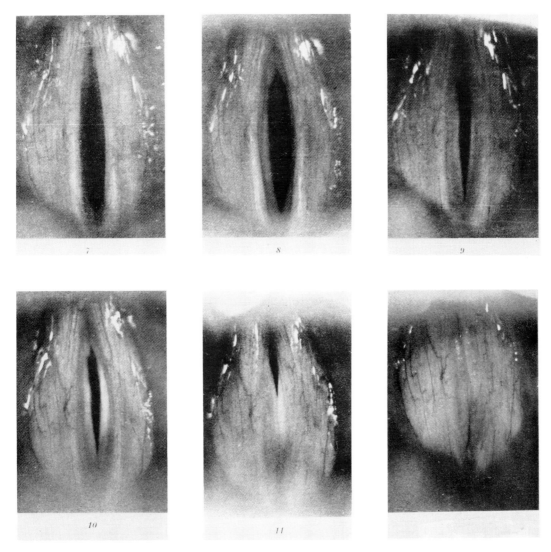

Figure 2–14   (continued)

5. The Bernoulli effect, which is responsible for force F_{AB}, is an example of the conservation of energy; as the velocity of a gas or liquid increases as it flows from a point of lesser constriction to one of greater constriction, its pressure decreases. Assuming that the glottal constriction contains a uniform frictionless flow of an incompressible fluid (Fig. 2-16):
   a. The rate of fluid flow across A_1 is equal to $A_1 V_1 p$, where p is the density of the fluid, A_1 is the cross-sectional area of the trachea, and V_1 is the velocity of the fluid.
   b. If the stream is steady, the same mass must travel per unit of time through the constricted portion of the pathway, so that

$$A_1 V_1 p = A_2 V_2 p$$

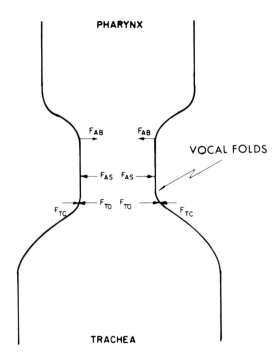

Figure 2–15 Schematic diagram of forces acting on the vocal folds, in open position.

F_{AS}, Force exerted by subglottal air pressure, displacing vocal folds outward.

F_{TO}, and F_{TC}, Forces acting to restore vocal folds to neutral position, owing to action of vocal ligaments.

F_{AB}, Bernoulli force generated by airflow through glottal constriction, acting to pull vocal folds inward. *From* Lieberman, P.: Vocal cord motion in man. Ann. N.Y. Acad. Sci., 155:28–38, 1968.)

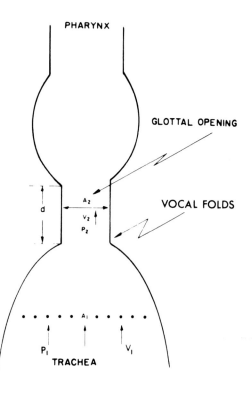

Figure 2–16 Schematic diagram of forces acting on the vocal folds.

$d :$ = Length of glottal constriction.

A_2 = Cross-sectional area of glottal constriction.

V_2 and P_2 = Particle velocity and air pressure at the glottal constriction.

A_1 = Cross-sectional area of the trachea.

V_1 and P_1 = Particle velocity and air pressure in the trachea. (*From* Lieberman, P.: Vocal cord motion in man. N.Y. Acad. Sci., 155:28–38, 1968.)

where A_2V_2 is the cross-sectional area times the particle velocity at the glottal constriction. Since the density p is constant, $A_1V_1 = A_2V_2$. The particle velocity in the glottal constriction will thus be larger than the particle velocity in the pharynx V_1 because

$$V_2 = \frac{A_1V_1}{A_2}$$

where A_2 is the cross-sectional area of the constriction. The kinetic energy of the fluid in the constriction

$$1/2p \left(\frac{A_1V_1}{A_2} \right)^2$$

will, therefore, be higher in the constricted portion of the air passage. The potential energy must decrease as the kinetic energy increases, since the sum of the kinetic and potential energies must remain constant. Physically, this means that the pressure of the fluid in the constriction, P_2, decreases.

   c. The pressure in the constriction falls below atmospheric pressure as the cross-section of the constriction decreases as the vocal folds begin to come together again and are sucked together by the pressure differential between P_2 and atmospheric.

Timcke et al. (1958, 1959) pioneered the frame-by-frame analysis of ultraspeed photographs of the vocal folds during phonation showing the opening and closing of the glottis during each vibratory cycle. In Figure 2-17 of a normal vibratory cycle, glottal width is displayed on the vertical axis, and duration of the cycle is shown on the horizontal axis. Each cycle is divided into an opening, a closing, and an approximation phase. In a normal voice, the vocal folds abduct at a higher rate of speed than they adduct. An equation expressing the ratio of abductor to adductor duration is called the Speed Quotient:

$$S.Q. = \frac{\text{Duration of Abduction}}{\text{Duration of Adduction}}$$

In normal voices the S.Q. is always less than 1.0 but as vocal intensity increases the S.Q. increases; i.e., duration of the opening phase is increased.

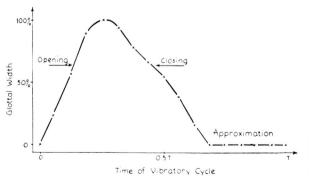

Figure 2–17 Opening, open, and closed phases of one vocal fold cycle. (*From* Timcke, R., von Leden, H., and Moore, P.: Laryngeal vibrations: Measurements of the glottic wave. A.M.A. Arch. Otolaryngol., 69:438–444, 1959.)

A second measure of vocal fold behavior during the glottic cycle is the ratio of the duration of the open period of the vocal folds to the total period of the cycle called the open quotient.

$$O.Q. = \frac{\text{Duration of Glottal Opening}}{\text{Duration of Entire Cycle}}$$

In normal voice, the O.Q. ranges from 0.6 to 0.8 and increases with vocal intensity. What is important about these measures and the profile of the curve is that they change radically when the voice becomes dysphonic.

Vibratory Function of Vocal Fold Mucosa

Mobility of the margins of the vocal folds is now considered to be essential for clear phonation. Hirano (1974) developed the concept of the mucosa as a "cover" of the vocal folds, which produces a wavelike movement during phonation. The importance of the undulatory function of the mucosal covering of the vocal folds for normal phonation has been demonstrated in patients who have scarred or dry vocal folds in which the mucosa has lost its mobility, resulting in breathiness and elevated pitch, which may be also due to an increase in stiffness of the folds.

Determinants of Loudness and Pitch

Vocal intensity (loudness) increases as subglottic air pressure increases. For constant loudness during speech, subglottic pressure must be held constant.

Frequency (pitch) increases as (1) subglottic pressure increases; (2) the larynx rises in the neck, shortening the pharyngeal dimensions; and (3) vocal fold length and tension increase. In a study of excised human larynges, Kitajima et al. (1979) found that vocal pitch increased almost linearly with approximation of the cricoid and thyroid cartilages. Photographic and x-ray studies have proved that fundamental frequency of phonation increases systematically with increased vocal fold length (Hollien, 1960; Hollien and Moore, 1960; Hollien et al., 1969; Soninen, 1954). Vocal fold length increases and thickness decreases with rising frequency in the modal register (Hollien, 1962; Hollien and Coleman, 1970; Hollien and Colton, 1969; Hollien and Curtis, 1960).

Vocal Registers

Although conceding that there are possibly more than three vocal registers, Hollien (1974) recognizes the following:

1. Pulse register. The lowest range of phonation along the frequency continuum.
2. Modal register. The range of fundamental frequencies normally used in speaking and singing.
3. Loft register. The higher range of fundamental frequencies, including the falsetto.

In the untrained singer, transitions between registers are heard as changes in quality and even as a "break" in the voice.

Modes of Vocal Attack

Vowels especially, but consonants also, can be produced in isolation or in contextual speech by three different kinds of vocal fold initiation or attack.

1. The hard, glottal, or stopped attack. Voice is produced by first adducting the vocal folds to the midline, building up infraglottal pressure, and then initiating the vowel. The explosive sound that results is called the *glottal stop* or *glottal coup*.
2. The even or static attack. The vocal folds are nearly approximated as exhalation beings. Voice onset is smooth and instantaneous.

3. The breathy attack. The vocal folds are abducted as exhalation begins and adduct after exhalation has begun. The effect is a moment of breathiness heard just before voicing.

LARYNGEAL EVOLUTION

The first vertebrate larynx appeared in the lungfish of the Devonian era some 300 million years ago, well before *Homo sapiens* entered the vertebrate kingdom no more than four to five million years ago. The frog is at least 200 million years old, and the monkey and chimpanzee go back at least 20 million years. Larynges homologous to the human larynx can be followed back to these early vertebrates.

A continuity has been traced through the phylogenetic series from the larynx of the lungfish to that of man. The number of hyaline cartilages in the framework of the larynx increases progressively from the fish to the primitive mammal, while the laryngeal aperture preserves a relatively constant position near the base of the skull until the early primates. In the primate series, a tendency to displacement in a caudal direction is noticeable. The low station of the larynx in man is determined by the recession of the jaws; the tongue retains its length for the purpose of mastication and pushes the larynx caudally (Fink, 1975).

African Lungfish

The African lungfish is a primitive bony fish that originated during the Devonian period, apparently a direct ancestor to amphibia. It has lungs as well as gills, enabling it to adapt to terrestrial habitats by embedding itself in mud and thus surviving during drought. Its larynx serves to protect the airway to its lungs during aerial oxygenation. It consists of a small median slit in the floor of the pharynx held closed by a simple sphincter and capable of being pulled apart by transverse muscle fibers inserted into its margins. The organism produces a squeaking or catlike mewing during expiration, but it is doubtful that these sounds have communicative importance.

Salamander

The salamander is a primitive amphibian and is mainly aquatic. Its larynx is similar to the lungfish but is more highly developed. The laryngeal entrance is located on top of a small eminence, has sharp edges, and acts as a valvular system. It has two pieces of cartilage; a paired *pars arytaenoidea* and a specialized paired dilator muscle that inserts into cricotracheal cartilages alongside the trachea. A weak, croaking sound is produced during the mating season as the salamander emerges from the water.

Frog

The frogs belong to the subclass of anurans (tail-less amphibians) and are more terrestrial than the salamander. For example, frogs have drowned when prevented from surfacing. The entrance to the frog larynx is located just behind its tongue. In *Ranidae esculenta,* the long axis of the larynx is tilted 45 degrees. It consists of two arytenoid cartilages which support mucous membrane tissue and which serve as vocal folds. The cartilaginous laryngeal skeleton consists of two arytenoids, one cricoid, and four accessory cartilages, the paired apicals and basals. In *Ranidae catesbiana,* the larynx possesses a strong, paired dilator, originating from the cricoid and the hyoid and inserting into the arytenoid, and three U-shaped sphincter muscles. Voice communications have been classified into warning calls made by both sexes, three kinds of territorial calls, and release calls made by both sexes when successful in being clasped.

Crocodile

The crocodile is better adapted to land than the amphibians but is able to pass a great part of its life in the water. It has no capability for skin respiration, and oxygenation is entirely dependent upon pulmonary respiration. The crocodile's laryngeal entrance is a triangular opening caudal to the tongue. It has an epiglottis-like structure formed by the anterior edge of a large hyoid cartilage which reaches the palate, allowing air to pass through the nostrils and choanae directly into the larynx. Its laryngeal skeleton consists of two U-shaped arytenoids and a circular cricoid. Its laryngeal musculature consists of sphincter and dilator fibers. The paired dilator muscles originate on the cricoid cartilage and are attached to the arytenoid cartilages. In contrast to amphibians, which swallow air, inhalation in crocodiles occurs according to the same principle as in higher vertebrates, including man; by increasing the thoracic diameters and by the action of the diaphragm. The crocodile produces a hissing sound as a means of intimidation and a roaring noise during the mating season. Cries have been recorded in newborn alligators.

Lesser Gymnure

The lesser gymnure is an insectivore, considered to be the most primitive placental creature that is entirely terrestrial. Its larynx, located close to its nasopharynx, is typically mammalian. It has arytenoid cartilages, well-developed corniculate, cricoid, and thyroid cartilages; and an epiglottis. Its sound consists of a shrill squeak or series of squeaks.

Tree Shrew

The tree shrew is considered the ancestor to the primates, is partly arboreal, and has effective digits for grasping. Its larynx consists of an epiglottis and arytenoid, corniculate, thyroid, and cricoid cartilages. The tree shrew has a repertory of sounds specific to different situations.

Rhesus Monkey

The rhesus monkey is the ancestral primate to Hominoidea, is arboreal, and is a brachiator with hands and feet effective for grasping. The larynx of the rhesus monkey is typically mammalian in appearance, built of the same components as the tree shrew but with the addition of cuneiform and corniculate cartilages. There is an important evolutionary difference however. Whereas the inner surface of the tree shrew larynx shows only a slight, paired prominence caused by the presence of the thyroarytenoid muscles, monkeys are provided with two pairs of clearly inbending folds, parallel to the thyroarytenoid muscles and enclosing a small space, the ventricle. The cranial or upper folds are presumably analogous to the false or ventricular folds in humans but, unlike in humans, *project caudally*. This configuration ensures fixation of the air within the lungs, thereby producing a stable thorax for attachment of the upper extremities during brachiation; i.e., because of the downward angle of the ventricular folds, the larynx can act as more of a valve than it already is because air pressure on the undersurface of the folds will cause them to close even more tightly. The sound-producing capabilities of the rhesus monkey are prodigious, depending upon the social situation.

Chimpanzee

The chimpanzee belongs to Hominoidea, resembles humans most closely and is both terrestrial and arboreal. To a considerable extent, its larynx is similar to that of humans and differs from that of the monkey in that it does not intrude as far into the pharynx. Because the epiglottis does not reach the soft palate, a gap exists between the two structures, strongly resembling the human vocal tract. The laryngeal cartilages are highly similar to the human larynx.

The chimpanzee has a rich variety of vocalizations, used differently depending upon social situations. Researchers have documented as many as 32 different sounds, each having special meaning, and some of which are accompanied by articulations similar to those of humans.

Differentiated vocalizations as a means of communication in primates have been well documented at the signal or alarm level of symbolic abstraction. As to whether primates use vocalization to communicate, the answer can be affirmative if we accept Scheflan's (1964) definition that communication includes all behaviors that form, sustain, mediate, correct, or integrate relationships; communication occurs when any form of behavior on the part of one participant serves to notify another participant of its status in a relationship. Nevertheless, primate vocalizations are different from human language in that they seem to be limited to the expression of mood, motive states, and interactions more as a part of a total reaction pattern in response to the situation than as a separate, volitional act.

Neurophysiologically, cortical stimulation studies of vocalization in primates establish different neural mechanisms subserving primate cries than those resulting in human speech. In monkeys, no sound can be elicited when bilateral cortical areas homologous to humans are electrically stimulated. Only when the limbic system of the forebrain is stimulated are cries produced in monkeys. In this regard, it is interesting that aphasic patients, when emotionally aroused or upset, undergo temporary language facilitation, evidence perhaps of a surge of power from their evolutionarily primitive limbic systems, and not from the damaged neocortical language areas of the brain.

Research on primates has established that their vocalizations are differentiable and have specific meaning, however crude. Carpenter (1964) studied the vocalizations of howler monkeys in different situations. When disturbed by an enemy or another threatening stimulus, animate or inanimate, the males produce a voluminous low-pitched and ferocious roar, and females produce a terrible bark. On the other hand, mildly disturbing apprehensive situations evoke a series of gurgling grunts and cracking sounds or inhalation. When a young has fallen, a wail ending with a grunt and groan is made. Contact with a mother yields a purr of several seconds' duration. A situation characterized by strange or novel elements produces rapid grunting similar to "Who! Who!"

Vocalizations coordinate the social behavior of primates; Carpenter's (1964) observations on this subject are worth noting.

> In howlers and gibbons marked evolutionary specialization has occurred in the organs for sound production. In these arboreal types, through the medium of calls, inter-group social behavior may be coordinated over distances of more than a mile through dense tropical forests. The most conspicuous verbalizations of howlers and gibbons are related to the inter-group exhanges and particularly to the possession and maintenance of territorial ranges. Coincident with the approach to, or entry of, the territory of one howler group by another, the barking roars of this species are normally exchanged between the two groups. A truly vocal battle between the males of the groups, supported by whines of females and young, ensues and continues usually without actual fighting until one group retreats. Most often the retreat is made by the encroaching group, i.e., the home team usually wins. The territory is defended and inter-group dominance is asserted through the medium of strong and persistent production. These relatively loud inter-group calls of monkeys and apes in natural groups serve as a sound buffer which substitutes for, or actually prevents, fighting which would often result in the wounding and killing of group members. The functions of a League of Nations is at least as old as the nonhuman primate family, and even on this level of evolution local expressions of aggression may substitute for actual battle!

SUMMARY

1. The larynx is phylogenetically much older than the neuromuscular systems of articulation and language. The larynx's role in speech production is an evolutionarily recent one.

2. The vital functions of the larynx are to protect the lungs from foreign substances; to enable the organism to clear the airway by coughing and throat clearing; to impound air in the thoracic cage, providing a rigid platform for the upper extremities; and to enable compression of the abdominal contents for defecation, micturition, and parturition.

3. Embryologically, the larynx arises from branchial arches III, IV, and VI. Its first signs of development can be seen at four weeks of embryonic life, and by the end of the tenth or eleventh week, the major structures of the larynx have formed.

4. The completely formed larynx consists of nine cartilages, excluding the hyoid bone. The muscles of the larynx are subdivided into extrinsic and intrinsic types. The membranes and ligaments that connect the laryngeal cartilages enable them to slide and rotate on one another, returning them to their original positions after release of muscular forces.

5. Phonation is the process of sound production by means of the release of air puffs through glottal opening and closing as a result of the interaction between muscular and aerodynamic forces.

6. Vocal intensity (loudness) is proportional to infraglottal air pressure, and frequency (pitch) is related to both infraglottal air pressure and vocal fold length.

SUGGESTIONS FOR ADDITIONAL READING

Bouhuys, A. (Ed.): Sound production in man. Ann. N.Y. Acad. Sci., 155; 1, 1968.
  Packed with articles by some of the world's experts on physiology and acoustics of phonation and respiration during speech and singing. Especially recommended is the article "Vocal Cord Motion in Man" by Lieberman (pp. 28–38).
Fink, B.R.: The Human Larynx: A Functional Study, New York, Raven Press, 1975.
  An excellent book on laryngeal physiology, including phonation. Some revolutionary ideas on how the larynx opens and closes, from the vantage point of an anesthesiologist. A rich bibliography for the research student.
Hollien, H.: Vocal fold thickness and fundamental frequency of phonation. J. Speech Hear. Res., 5:237–243, 1962.
  A research study illustrating the anatomic-physiologic basis of laryngeal frequency/pitch change.
Kahane, J.C.: Postnatal development and aging of the human larynx. Semin. Speech Lang., 4:189–204, 1983.
  Should be read by those interested in morphologic changes in the larynx from infancy through adulthood.
Lieberman, P.: On the Origins of Language, New York, Macmillan, 1975.
  For the student interested in anthropology and evolution of speech and language. Also contains basic information on speech physiology and acoustics.
Moore, K.L.: The Developing Human. Philadelphia, W.B. Saunders Co., 1977.
  Of the few references available on laryngeal embryology, this is one of the better ones. See pages 160–162, and 188–190, especially. (Incidentally, there are excellent sections on the embryology of the remaining speech muscles and skeletal structures.)
Negus, V.E.: The Mechanism of the Larynx, St. Louis, C.V. Mosby Co., 1929.
  This shortened form of the original out-of-print version of Negus' epic studies of the comparative anatomy of the larynx from lungfish to humans has great historical as well as zoologic importance.
Van den Berg, J.W.: Myoelastic-aerodynamic theory of voice production. J. Speech Hear. Res., 1:227–244, 1958.
  The key article on the accepted theory of voice production. Should be read by all students of voice disorders.
Wind, J.: On the Phylogeny and the Ontogeny of the Human Larynx. Gröningen, Wolters-Noordhoff Co., 1970.
  Out of print, but if one can obtain a copy it will open one's eyes to the mystery of laryngeal evolution—from lungfish to humans—with ample drawings and photographs, not to mention a superb bibliography on the comparative anatomy of the larynx.

REFERENCES

Carpenter, C.R.: Naturalistic Behavior of Nonhuman Primates. University Park, Pa. Pennsylvania State University Press, 1964.
Faaborg-Andersen, K.: Electromyographic investigation of intrinsic laryngeal muscles in humans. Acta Physiol. Scand., 41 (Suppl. 40) 1, 1957.
Ferrein, A.: Memoires de Mathematique et de Physique, de L'Academie Royale des Sciences de L'Année MDCCXLI, A Amsterdam, Chez Pierri Mortier, M. DCCXLVI.
Fink, B.R.: The Human Larynx: A Functional Study. New York, Raven Press, 1975.
Fink, B.R., and Demarest, R.J.: Laryngeal Biomechanics, Cambridge, Mass. Harvard University Press, 1978.
Helmholtz, H.M.: Die Lehre der Tonempfindungen als Physiologische Grundlage für die Theorie der musik, Braunschweig, F. Vieweg u. Sohn, 1863.
Hirano, M.: Morphological structure of the vocal cord as a vibrator and its variations. Folia Phoniatr., 26:89–94, 1974.
Hollien, H.: Vocal pitch variations related to changes in vocal fold length. J. Speech Hear. Res., 3:150–156, 1960.
Hollien, H.: Vocal fold thickness and fundamental frequency of phonation. J. Speech Hear. Res., 5:237–243, 1962.
Hollien, H.: On vocal registers. J. Phonet., 2:125–143, 1974.
Hollien, H., and Coleman, R.F.: Laryngeal correlates of frequency change: A STROL study. J. Speech Hear. Res., 13:272–278, 1970.
Hollien, H., and Colton, R.H.: Four laminagraphic studies of vocal fold thickness. Folia Phoniatr., 21:179–198, 1969.
Hollien, H., and Curtis, J.F.: A laminagraphic study of vocal pitch. J. Speech Hear. Res., 3:362–371, 1960.
Hollien, H., and Moore, P.: Measurements of the vocal folds during changes in pitch. J. Speech Hear. Res., 3:157–165, 1960.
Hollien, H., Damsté, H., and Murry, T.: Vocal fold length during vocal fry phonation. Folia Phoniatr., 21:257–265, 1969.

Husson, R.: Sur la physiologie vocale. Ann. Otolaryngol., 69:124–137, 1953.

Kitajima, K., Tanabe, M., and Isshiki, N.: Cricothyroid distance and vocal pitch. Ann. Otol. Rhinol. Laryngol., 88:52–55, 1979.

Lieberman, P.: Intonation, Perception and Language. Cambridge, Mass., MIT Press, 1967.

Lieberman, P.: Vocal cord motion in man. Ann. N.Y. Acad. Sci., 155:28–38, 1968.

Scheflan, A.E.: The significance of posture in communication systems. J. Psychiatry, 27:316–331, 1964.

Soninen, A.: Is the length of the vocal cords the same at all different levels of singing. Acta Otolaryng. (Stockh) 118, 219–231, 1954.

Timcke, R., von Leden, H., and Moore, P.: Laryngeal vibrations: Measurements of the glottic wave. Part 1. The normal vibratory cycle. A.M.A. Arch. Otolaryngol. 68:1–19, 1958.

Timcke, R., von Leden, H., and Moore, P.: Laryngeal vibrations: Measurements of the glottic wave, Part II, Physiologic variations. A.M.A. Arch. Otolaryngol., 69:438–444, 1959.

Van den Berg, J.W.: Myoelastic-aerodynamic theory of voice production. J. Speech Hear. Res., 1:227–244, 1958.

Chapter Three

NORMAL VOICE DEVELOPMENT

But what am I? An infant crying in the night: An infant crying for the light: And with no language but a cry.

—Alfred, Lord Tennyson

INFANCY

The Postnatal Larynx

By the third month of fetal life the larynx has the same features recognizable at birth. However, only gross vertical movements of the larynx are possible during the neonatal cry. Liberman et al. (1971) has observed that these limited movements and the uniform cross-sectional configuration of the supralaryngeal tract bear a striking resemblance to those of primates. At birth, the neonate's larynx occupies a position higher in the neck, relative to the skull, than at any other time in life. Almost immediately after birth, it begins its descent in the neck. Figure 3–1 shows that at birth the lower border of the cricoid cartilage is level between cervical vertebrae three and four (C_3 and C_4). By age five, the larynx has descended almost to the level of C_7. Between ages 15 and 20, it remains at C_7. After that, it continues to descend throughout life. There is a direct relationship between the descent of the larynx and the decrease in average voice pitch: The pharyngeal tube elongates in order to resonate lower fundamental frequencies.

At birth the thyroid cartilage is contiguous with the hyoid bone. The laryngeal skeleton then separates in a craniocaudal direction. The infant's epiglottis is bulky at this stage when seen superiorly. Together with the aryepiglottic folds, it is omega-shaped and lies over the dorsum of the tongue. The configuration of the alae of the thyroid cartilage changes from a rounded shield during fetal life to an angle of about 110 degrees in the male and 120 degrees in the female at birth. During puberty, the angle in the male thyroid alae narrows to 90 degrees, whereas in the female it remains the same. During the first years of life, the opening into the larynx widens, changing from its T-shape to one more rounded or oval.

The soft cartilages of the neonatal larynx and lax supporting ligaments predispose the infant's larynx to collapse if negative air pressures become excessive within the internal vocal tract. Because the subepithelial tissues are less dense and more abundant and vascular, they have a tendency to accumulate tissue fluids, accounting for the high incidence in infants of infraglottic and supraglottic obstruction due to inflammatory edema. Ossification of the hyoid bone begins by age two years; the thyroid followed by the cricoid cartilage ossifies between ages 20 and 23 years; and the arytenoid cartilages ossify in the late 30s. By age 65 years, all the laryngeal cartilages except the cuneiforms and corniculates have ossified.

Vocal fold length, glottal width, and infraglottal sagittal and transverse dimensions at infancy, puberty, and adulthood are given in Table 3–1. The membranous and cartilaginous portions of the vocal folds are equal in length in infancy, but by adulthood, the membranous portion has elongated to approximately two-thirds of the total glottal length. Glottal width and infraglottal dimensions also increase with age.

Infant Cries

The birth cry after the neonate has emerged from the womb signals the first conventional appearance of voice in humans. Nevertheless, human cries from the fetus *in utero* are known to have occurred.

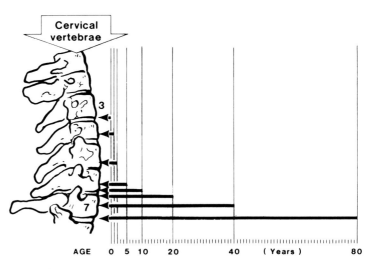

Figure 3–1 Vertical descent of the larynx during life. Shows relationship of lower border of cricoid cartilage to cervical vertebrae at various ages. (*Adapted from* Wind, J.: On the Phylogeny and the Ontogeny of the Human Larynx. Gröningen, Wolters-Noordhoff Publishing, 1970, p. 105.)

Thiery et al. (1973) documented such a case in a 31-year-old woman in her fifth pregnancy. When the fetal head was 3 cm. above the ischial spines the membranes ruptured, releasing 2000 ml. of clear fluid. According to Thiery, "While the fetal head was being displaced to allow the drainage of as much amniotic fluid as possible, the fetus started crying. This sound was clearly heard by the mother, three physicians, and two midwives. The crying recurred six to seven times at intervals of up to 20 seconds."

Do normal infants have distinctively different cries, and, if so, are they indicative of definitive physiologic and emotional states? Is it possible to differentiate types of infant cries from acoustic spectrographic data and by listening to recordings? Are the cries of infants who are ill distinguishable from normal infant cries, based on spectrographic data and listener judgment? In perhaps the most complete study done of normal infant cries, Wasz-Höckert et al. (1968) obtained spectrographic and listener judgment data based on 419 cries of 351 healthy infants. Listeners were able to identify four distinctive types of cries from birth through seven months.

1. Birth signal: ± 1 sec. in duration; flat or falling melody; usually voiceless; always strained or strident; contains glottal plosives.
2. Pain signal: long duration; usually falling melody; high-pitched; strident.
3. Hunger signal: pitch rising-falling; frequent glottal plosives.
4. Pleasure signal: flat pitch; hypernasal; greater pitch variability than the other types of cries; rare glottal plosives; never voiceless; never strident.

As early as infancy, cries illustrate a universal fact about the larynx: The true and false vocal folds respond differentially, depending upon psychophysiologic state. The pain cry is strained, tense, harsh, and forced owing to massive, tight, effortful closure of the entire laryngeal tract, i.e., it is an undifferentiated adduction of both the true and false vocal folds. The pleasure cry, more sonorous, lax, and devoid of strain or tension, is produced by the true vocal folds alone. Throughout life, the voice is smooth, clear, sonorous, devoid of strain or effort, and filled with rich inflectional patterns during pleasure and freedom from anxiety, fear, hostility, or depression. However, it is harsh, strained, and lacking in inflectional patterns during times of situational stress both in normal persons and in persons with some psychiatric illnesses.

FUNDAMENTAL FREQUENCY

Life begins with a voice fundamental frequency 300 to 400 Hz above that which is ultimately achieved by adulthood. In a study by Wasz-Höckert et al. (1968), 77 birth cries averaged 500 Hz.

Between birth and one month, 60 pain cries averaged 530 Hz, and 74 hunger cries averaged 470 Hz. Between one and seven months, 60 pain cries averaged 530 Hz, 74 hunger cries averaged 500 Hz, and 72 pleasure cries averaged 440 Hz. Ringel and Kluppel (1964) found that the fundamental frequency of pain cries from ten normal infants was 413 Hz. Ostwald (1968), in a study of the pain cries of five infants, obtained initial, highest, and final mean fundamental frequencies of 418 Hz, 506 Hz, and 393 Hz, respectively, for each cry.

Greene (1972) studied recordings of infant vocalizations during the first nine months and noted a progressive increase in the range of inflectional glides during cooing and babbling. The earliest appearance of the upward glide, C_3-C#, was in a two-week-old girl, whose range increased from C_3 to E_3 by seven weeks of age. The voice of an infant male at five weeks ranged from C# to F# in one breath, and at 16 weeks his musical inflection varied, rising and falling between C_2# and E. Upward glides appeared first, then rising and falling glides increased in quantity and range up to an octave at six to seven months of age.

DURATION

Wasz-Höckert et al. (1968) found that between birth and one month of age, 77 birth cries averaged 1.1 sec. in duration, 60 pain cries averaged 2.6 sec., and 74 hunger cries averaged 1.3 sec. Between one and seven months of age, 60 pain cries averaged 2.7 sec., 74 hunger cries lasted 1.2 sec., and 72 pleasure cries lasted 1.1 sec. Ringel and Kluppel (1964) and Ostwald (1968) both found that pain cries averaged 1.5 sec. in length.

Listener Identification of Infant Cries

Apparently, listeners are able to identify birth, pain, hunger, and pleasure cries beyond chance odds, and training improves this skill. Wasz-Höckert et al. (1968) had 349 women identify and categorize 24 infant birth, pain, hunger, and pleasure cries. The results showed that pleasure cries were identified most accurately, followed by hunger, pain, and birth cries. However, the accuracy of judgments depended upon the rater's background. Ranked according to decreasing order of accuracy were: (1) midwives; (2) children's nurses; (3) mothers; (4) registered nurses; (5) other women experienced in child care; (6) women with no experience in child care. Overall, there was a high degree of accuracy with all raters, even though rater groups differed significantly from one another.

Hollien and Müller (1973) took issue with the conclusions of Wasz-Höckert et al. that certain cries are associated with specific stimulus situations and that recognizable perceptual differences exist between cries. They argued that: (1) Birth cries and "pleasure" vocalizations ought not have been juxtaposed in the design of the study. (2) Preselection of "typical" samples of cries for listener judgments may have biased the listeners. (3) Cry duration and infant age ought to have been controlled experimentally and statistically. In their own study, Hollien and Müller recorded cries in response to pain, auditory, and hunger stimuli from four male and four female infants, aged three to five months. Two groups of mothers listened: One, the real mothers of the eight infants, and the other, mothers of infants of comparable age. Although statistical analysis proved that some of the hunger cries were correctly identified a significant number of times, the listeners over-identified cries of all types as hunger cries, possibly revealing a bias toward judgments of this kind. From the study, the authors concluded that the acoustic characteristics of normal infant cries carry little perceptual information to the mother about the situation that evoked the cry response. However, the experimenters were less than completely confident in their conclusions, calling them "tentative" and advocating the need for "additional investigations." An interesting finding of this study was that the mothers of the infants in the study had little difficulty recognizing which samples were produced by their own infants.

Facial Expression Associated with Infant Cries

Infant cries and other vocalizations are inseparable from associated facial expressions and bodily movements. Young and Décarie (1977) coded the facial/vocal behavior and body movements of 75 male and female infants, aged 9 to 14 months, who were exposed to six different types of emotionally arousing situations. From their study, they were able to identify two main classes of vocalizations:

1. Positive vocalizations. Those associated with smiling facial expressions, e.g., babbling, cooing, laughing, and squealing.
2. Negative vocalizations. Those associated with grimacing, trembling of the lips and frowning, e.g., harsh wailing, wailing without harsh voice quality, and soft wailing.

They then categorized these vocalizations into the following:

1. Babbling. Vocalization of low intensity, moderate pitch, and a soft-sounding sequence of consonant-vowel combinations, generally pleasurable to the listener, produced during prolonged exhalation and in quick sequence.
2. Coo. Sustained, moderately high-pitched voice of moderate intensity, having a smooth onset, pleasant to the listener, and produced during prolonged exhalation.
3. Laugh. Rapid repetitions of short exhalations of moderate pitch and harsh quality; pleasant to hear.
4. Squeal. Extremely high-pitched, of moderate intensity, variable in duration, positive, and produced during extended exhalation.
5. Harsh wail. Begins with breath-holding of sudden onset and has a rhythmic piercing sound, a definitely negative quality, and is harsh, irritating, and painful to hear.
6. Soft wail. Begins with breath-holding, has a soft but negative quality.
7. Wail. Hard, high-pitched, discordant.

Physiologic Bases of the Infant Cry and Intonation

Little is known of the aerodynamic, respiratory, and electromyographic bases of the infant cry. Fluctuations from periodic to aperiodic acoustic spectra in such cries have been noted by Lieberman et al. (1971), who attributed these variations to the infant's inability to adjust the vocal folds to rising subglottic air pressures, the soft laryngeal tissues being unable to withstand such pressures.

In normal children and adults, the fundamental frequency of the voice drops toward the end of a sustained utterance or breath group owing to the decline of infraglottal air pressure as exhalation progresses. Lieberman (1967) traces the origins of this universal human tendency to early infancy. Citing Bosma et al. (1964), he notes that the shape of the fundamental frequency contour of the cry is similar to that of the typical esophageal pressure contour. The amount of expiratory muscle activity is directly related to the infant's excitability; as greater thoracic contraction produces greater subglottal air pressure, infant cries show higher fundamental frequency and intensity. The fundamental frequency falls as the breath group ends, the lungs being depleted of air at the end of the exhalation. There thus appears to be an innate physiologic basis for intonation. According to Lieberman (1967), "The infant's hypothetical innate referential breath-group furnishes the basis for the universal acoustic properties of the normal breath-group that is used to segment speech into sentences in so many languages."

Infants respond to intonation of voice before they are able to comprehend language. This has been demonstrated by Lewis (1936), who showed that a ten-month-old male and a 13-month-old female changed the fundamental frequencies of their voices depending upon whether they were playing with their mother (higher pitched voice) or their father (lower pitched voice). Thus, early in language development, before the actual appearance of distinctive linguistic features, intonation apparently takes on symbolic meaning. Lewis identified three intonational stages in the development of language.

1. At an early stage, the child shows broad discrimination between different patterns of expression in intonation.
2. When the total pattern (phonetic form plus intonational form) emerges because of language learning, intonation, not the phonetic pattern, dominates the child's response at first.
3. Finally, the phonetic pattern becomes the dominant feature. Although the intonational pattern is subordinated, it never completely disappears.

CHILDHOOD

Fundamental Frequency

The fundamental frequency of the human voice descends with age. The most notable changes occur between birth and adolescence, paralleling the descent of the larynx in the neck. Studies of fundamental frequency during childhood are incomplete; we do not yet have an unbroken continuity of data. Because each study varies in methodology—some employing oral reading and others contextual speech—interpretation of results must be guarded. Mean fundamental frequency of seven-year-old children was found to be 286.5 Hz (Fairbanks et al., 1949), and for those eight years old, it was 275.8 Hz (McGlone and McGlone, 1972).

Frequency Range

Phonational frequency range is the difference in frequency between the lowest sustainable tone in the modal register and the highest falsetto. Studies of children's frequency (pitch) ranges are also incomplete and are complicated by mixed purposes and methodologies, some being designed for gathering musical information and others for physiologic data. VanOordt and Drost (1963) studied 126 children, dividing them into two groups: birth through five years of age (45 children) and six through 16 years of age (81 children). The children aged six through 16 were asked to sing from an arbitrary tone up to the highest they could reach, and then down to the lowest one. From this method the researchers derived: (1) highest musical tone—the highest tone having musical quality; and (2) highest physiologic tone—the highest tone attainable, regardless of musical quality or clarity. The lowest musical tone and the lowest physiologic tone were based on similar judgments. Figure 3–2 shows the comparison between the physiologic voice (frequency) range and the musical voice (frequency) range. This figure illustrates that the physiologic voice range remains constant from ages six to 16—about 2½ octaves—whereas the musical voice range expands.

PUBERTY AND ADOLESCENCE

Anatomy and Physiology of Adolescent Voice Change

Until puberty, the larynx is of equal size in the male and the female. Although both begin to enlarge at puberty, the male larynx outdistances the female, especially in the growth of its anteroposterior dimensions. As shown in Table 3–1:

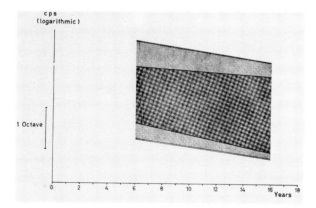

Figure 3–2 Comparison between physiologic and musical voice frequency range. Physiologic frequency range (PVR) is represented by total area, musical frequency range (MVR) by darker area. Both are bordered by regression lines of highest and lowest registered physiologic and musical tones plotted logarithmically. (*From* van Oordt, H.W.A., and Drost, H.A.: Development of the frequency range of the voice in children. Folia Phoniat., 15:289–298, 1963.

Table 3–1   Dimensions of the Larynx*

	INFANCY (mm)	PUBERTY (mm)	ADULT MALE (mm)	ADULT FEMALE (mm)
Vocal Cord—Length	6–8	12–15	17–23	12.5–17
Membranous portion	3–4	7–8	11.5–16	8–11.5
Cartilaginous portion	3–4	5–7	5.5–7	4.5–5.5
Glottis—Width at Rest	3	5	8	6
Maximum	6	12	19	13
Infraglottis—Sagittal	5–7	15	25	18
Transverse	5–7	15	24	17

*From Ballenger, J.J.: Diseases of the Nose, Throat and Ear. Philadelphia, Lea & Febiger, 1969, p. 275.

1. By adulthood, the membranous portions of the male vocal folds range from 11.5 to 16 mm. in length, a 4- to 8-mm. increase from puberty. However, the female membranous vocal folds increase in length to only 8 to 11.5 mm., a 1- to 3.5-mm. increase.
2. The dimensions of the infraglottal sagittal and transverse planes grow in the male to 25 mm. and 24 mm., respectively, and in the female, to 18 mm. and 17 mm., respectively.
3. The angle of the male thyroid lamina decreases until it becomes 90 degrees, whereas in the female larynx, the angle remains approximately 120 degrees.
4. The laryngeal mucosa loses transparency and becomes stronger; the epiglottis flattens, increases in size, and elevates; and the tonsils and adenoids partially atrophy.
5. The larynx descends in the neck. The neck itself elongates. Because of the greater enlargement of the thorax in the male, there is a more prominent increase in vital capacity.

Age of Onset and Duration of Adolescent Voice Change

Evidence indicates that onset of puberty occurs earlier in warmer climates. In temperate climates, onset of puberty in females ranges from ages 12 to 14, and in males, from ages 13 to 15. Near the equator, onset is accelerated one to two years, and near the poles it is delayed one year.

The average time from onset to completion of adolescent voice change is three to six months, one year at most. In females, the voice change is complete by age 15, and in males by age 14 or 15. Although the onset of voice change occurs earlier in females, males and females complete the change at approximately the same age.

Adolescent Fundamental Frequency Change

No differences have been found between male and female voices from birth until puberty according to the measures of average frequency/pitch and frequency/pitch range. Frequency/pitch distinction between male and female begins during puberty and continues throughout adolescence. These voice changes, the result of growth of the phonatory, resonatory, and respiratory anatomy, roughly parallel the appearance and development of the secondary sex characteristics. The pitch and quality changes that occur at puberty are much more apparent in males than in females because of the greater magnitude of the pitch drop. The voice at puberty begins with a husky quality and an unsteady pitch, oscillating perhaps one to two tones. Although the pitch fluctuates from day to day, the general trend is downward. With time, the high tones become less steady, the low tones more stable.

A study of pitch change by McGlone and Hollien (1963) found that female voices dropped 2.4 semitones between ages 7 or 8 to 11 to 15 years. In a study of 15-, 16-, and 17-year-old females, Michel et al. (1966) found average fundamental frequencies of 207.5, 207.3, and 207.8 Hz respectively, their similarities indicating that by age 15 mutational change of voice is essentially completed in females.

Comparison of the frequency/pitch in the male at puberty and at the termination of adolescence indicates that the male voice drops approximately one octave. Voice breaks are uncommon, and they almost always occur in males, rarely in females. Pitch breaks can span an entire octave, transcending vocal registers from high-pitched falsetto to bass. Hoarseness from chronic laryngitis is common if vocal abuse occurs during the period of voice change. Apparently, there is a high prevalence of transient dysphonia during adolescent voice change, if Curry's (1949) figures are indicative, for he found that the voices of 80 percent of 14-year-old boys were of hoarse-husky quality. Curry (1940) found the median fundamental frequency in 10- and 14-year-old boys to be 269.7 Hz and 241.5 Hz, respectively, whereas in 18-year-old males the frequency had dropped to 137.1 Hz. Hollien and Malcek (1967) found the median fundamental frequency in 18-year-old males to be 126.3 Hz.

Stormy Voice Mutation

Stormy voice mutation refers to pervasive sudden voice breaks from high to low pitch, or the reverse, or excessively husky or hoarse voice associated with adolescent voice change. It should be emphasized that the majority of male adolescents have uneventful voice change.

ADULTHOOD

Fundamental Frequency

Research on the fundamental frequency of the speaking voice for the age continuum in adults is also far from complete, and the instrumentation and procedures used to obtain fundamental frequency vary among studies. Despite these limitations, the fundamental frequency values obtained by independent researchers are similar within both adult male and adult female groups. We have arbitrarily taken the age of 69 years as a cut-off point in our discussion of adult fundamental frequency because we wish to discuss a succeeding category that might be designated "older age." A summary of several major studies of the fundamental frequency of the speaking voice in adult males is found in Table 3–2. From this table, it can be seen that most studies have been of males

Table 3–2 Male Mean Fundamental Frequency (Hz) as a Function of Age: Comparative Studies

AGE RANGE (YEARS)	NO.	MEAN FUNDAMENTAL FREQUENCIES (Hz)	INVESTIGATORS
20–29	175	120	Hollien and Shipp (1972)
	27	119	Hanley (1951)
	157	128	Hollien and Jackson (1973)
	24	132	Philhour (1948)
	6	132	Pronovost (1942)
	103	138	Majewski et al. (1972)
30–39	175	112	Hollien and Shipp (1972)
40–49	175	107	Hollien and Shipp (1972)
	39	113	Mysak (1959)
50–59	175	118	Hollien and Shipp (1972)
60–69	175	112	Hollien and Shipp (1972)
70–79	175	132	Hollien and Shipp (1972)
	39	124	Mysak (1959)
80–89	175	146	Hollien and Shipp (1972)
	39	141	Mysak (1959)

within the 20- to 29-year age group. The group mean fundamental frequency for all studies within this age group is 128 Hz, and the range is 119 to 138 Hz. A study by Hollien and Shipp (1972) shows a downward trend in fundamental frequency in males through age 69. It is explained later in this chapter, however, that thereafter the fundamental frequency begins to rise.

Data on the fundamental frequency of the speaking voice in adult females indicate that as a group, their voices average 1.6 times higher than those of males. Kelley (1977) studied 70 females, aged 20 to 90 years, whose mean fundamental frequencies and ranges are given in Table 3–3.

> An important finding of this study was a systematic decrease in mean fundamental frequency in females throughout the age range 20 to 70 years, yielding a Pearson correlation coefficient r = −0.62 (significance at the P = 0.0001 level of confidence) between age and mean fundamental frequency. These data are at variance with the results of studies by McGlone and Hollien (1963), who found no significant change in mean fundamental frequency in females from early adulthood through advanced age. In addition, Saxman and Burk (1967) found that in females, mean fundamental frequency decreases during the middle years and then increases in old age.

OLDER AGE

Having documented the decline in the fundamental frequency of the human voice from infancy through adulthood, we now ask, "What happens to the voice of the aged?" Does it attest to signs of an aging organism? Can we hear differences between younger and older voices? Are there physical changes in the structure of the larynx or its innervation that might account for such voice changes? Information accumulated to date indicates an affirmative answer to all of these questions.

Physical Changes

Several studies show structural changes of the vocal folds with age. Atrophy of the intrinsic laryngeal muscles, thinning and dehydration of the laryngeal mucosa, loss of elasticity of ligaments, calcification of cartilages, flaccidity and bowing of the vocal folds, and edema have been documented by Ferreri (1959), Jackson and Jackson (1959), and Keleman and Pressman (1955).

> In a study of men and women aged 69 to 85 years, Honjo and Isshiki (1980) saw a yellowish or dark grayish discoloration of the vocal folds in 39 percent of the men and 47 percent of the women. Edema of the vocal folds was noted in 74 percent of the women and 56 percent of the men. Vocal fold atrophy was found in 67 percent of the men and 26 percent of the women, inferred from either bowing of the edges of the vocal folds, visibility of the ventricle, or prominence of the contour of the vocal processes of the arytenoid cartilages. Glottal gap was observed in 67 percent of the men as either semicircular (22 percent), linear (28 percent), or partial (17 percent). However, this finding was less common in women, 58 percent, among

Table 3–3   Female Mean Fundamental Frequency (Hz) as a Function of Age*

AGE RANGE (YEARS)	NO.	MEAN FUNDAMENTAL FREQUENCY (Hz)
20–29	10	227
30–39	10	214
40–49	10	214
50–59	10	214
60–69	10	209
70–79	10	206
80–90	10	197

*From Kelley, A.: Fundamental frequency measurement of female voices from twenty to ninety years of age. (Unpublished manuscript.) Greensboro, University of North Carolina, 1977.

whom the semicircular gap was particularly rare. Vocal sulcus was noted in about 10 percent of both men and women.

These authors concluded that the discoloration of the vocal folds found in approximately one half of the subjects was due to either fat degeneration or keratosis of the mucous membrane lining the larynx. Vocal fold atrophy and glottal gap in men were attributed to senescent changes of the entire thyroarytenoid muscle and mucous membrane. Edema of the vocal folds in women was attributed to general endocrine changes after menopause. This increase in the mass of the vocal folds may be the cause of noticeable lowering of average fundamental frequency and roughness and hoarseness of voice in aged women.

Morrison and Gore-Hickman (1986) found that it is the older men with atrophy and the older women with polypoidal degeneration who usually complain about their abnormal voices. These authors found that older patients have a tendency to misuse their voices, their phonation commonly associated with hyperactivity of the ventricular folds. They speculate that this vocal misuse or abuse may have psychogenic bases or may be due to an attempt to compensate for atrophy or polypoidal changes.

They raise the strong possibility that psychologic distress may make an important contribution to dysphonia in older persons, owing to tension, hypochondriasis, and depression. This neglected population, although they may not complain of depression or anger, are nevertheless reacting to loneliness, isolation, family separation, and conflicts with spouses who are also aging.

In a study of the stroboscopic movements of the vocal folds in 20 young adult women aged 22 to 28 years and 20 older women aged 60 to 77 years, Biever and Bless (1989) found aperiodic vibration in 85 percent of the older women but in only 30 percent of the younger ones.

Perceptual Studies

Listeners can accurately detect differences in chronologic age by the sound of the voice, based on ratings of contextual speech and vowel prolongation (Ptacek and Santer, 1966; Shipp and Hollien, 1969; Ryan and Burk, 1974; Ryan and Capadano, 1978). Studies have also shown that the acoustic physical properties of voice change with advancing age (Kent and Burkhard, 1981). Sustained phonation in older age groups has been described as hoarse, breathy, and tremorous by Ptacek and Santer (1966), Hartman and Danhauer (1976), and Ryan and Capadano (1978).

However, the common assumption that voice deterioration as we age is inevitable was challenged by Ramig and Ringel (1983), who found that whether or not the voice of an aging person was judged abnormal depended on that person's general physical health. Older subjects in poor physiologic condition had statistically significantly more jitter, shimmer, and spectral noise in their voices than those in good physical condition.

In a subsequent study, Ramig (1986) compared speakers' physiologic condition with listeners' ratings of age according to resting heart rate, systolic blood pressure, diastolic blood pressure, forced vital capacity, and adjusted forced vital capacity. She found no statistically significant relationship between ratings of age and actual chronologic age in patients 25 to 75 years who were in good physiologic condition. However, she did find a statistically significant relationship between age and judgment of voices as poor in patients who were in poor condition. Listeners were more accurate in their ratings of age when judging connected speech in comparison with vowel prolongations. However, they were more accurate in identifying aged speakers on the basis of vowel prolongation who were in poor physiologic condition in comparison to older speakers who were in good condition. These data seem to support the importance of good general health in the preservation of youthful voice in older age groups.

It would appear, then, that an older sounding voice is not inevitable as we age, and how we sound may be closely tied to the general health and physiologic reserve of the person. What also needs to be studied in greater depth, however, is the effect of psychologic changes on voice in the elderly. Physical and social isolation restricting the amount of daily voice use often produces depression, which is known to have deleterious effects on voice.

Fundamental Frequency

It was already noted that Hollien and Shipp (1972) demonstrated a progressive lowering of fundamental frequency in males from early adulthood to the 40- to 50-year age range, but above this range there was a reversal of this downward trend. The saucer-shaped scatterplot of 175 male subjects can be seen in Figure 3–3. The same trend has been demonstrated in a study by Mysak (1959) of 12 males, aged 65 to 79 years, and 12 males, aged 80 to 92 years. He obtained mean impromptu speaking voice fundamental frequencies of 120.1 Hz for the 65- to 79-year age group and 137.1 Hz for the 80- to 92-year age group. The males aged 80 to 92 years had statistically significantly higher fundamental frequencies than those in the 65- to 79-year age group. Similarly, in a study by Honjo and Isshiki (1979), the average fundamental frequency of 20 males aged 69 to 85 years was 162 Hz, considerably higher than that for young males (120 to 130 Hz).

Fundamental frequency of the speaking voice as a function of age in females does not follow the same trend as in males. In a group of females aged 65 to 79 years studied by McGlone and Hollien (1963), the average frequency was 196.6 Hz, and in another group aged 80 to 94 years, 199.8 Hz was the average. This does not represent a rise in fundamental frequency over younger females, as is true for males. In the study by Kelley (1977), not only did fundamental frequency fail to rise in older aged females, but it declined. In the study by Honjo and Isshiki (1979) of 20 females aged 69 to 85 years, fundamental frequency also showed a failure to increase; it actually decreased from about 260 Hz in young females to an average of 170 Hz in the older age group. The increase in fundamental frequency in males and its failure to increase in females remains unexplained.

Frequency Range

A study by Hollien et al. (1971) of 534 subjects—332 males and 202 females—is probably the most extensive available on phonational frequency range in adults. The males ranged in age from 16 to 59 years, and the females from 18 to 75 years. Subjects had to match voice pitches to a series of pure tones downward and upward from a predetermined frequency. Figure 3–4 shows the frequency ranges for each subject. Individual ranges extended from approximately one octave (13 semitones) to more than 4.5 octaves (55 semitones). Females produced a greater range than males, extending from nearly two octaves (23 semitones) to more than four octaves (50 semitones). Mean phonational frequency ranges for males and females were 38 semitones and 37 semitones, respectively, and each group produced a large standard deviation. There appeared to be no age-related trend. These ranges are slightly greater when compared with the studies of fewer subjects done by Ptacek et al. (1966), Hollien and Michel (1968), and Colton (1959).

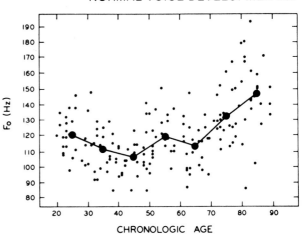

NORMAL VOICE DEVELOPMENT/**53**

Figure 3–3 Male fundamental frequency as a function of age. Scatterplot of the mean fundamental frequencies of 175 subjects' speaking voices. Solid line connects mean values for each age decade. (*From* Hollien, H., and Shipp, T.: Speaking fundamental frequency and chronologic age in males. J. Speech Hear. Res., 15:155–159, 1972.)

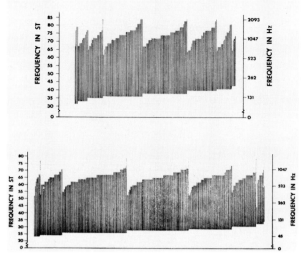

Figure 3–4 (A) Phonational frequency ranges of 202 adult females. (B) Phonational frequency ranges of 332 adult males. (From Hollien, H., Dew, D., and Philips, P.: Phonational frequency ranges of adults. J. Speech Hear. Res., 14:755–760, 1971.)

SUMMARY

1. Birth, pain, hunger, and pleasure cries can be differentiated from one another.

2. From birth, the larynx enlarges and descends in the neck, and with it the fundamental frequency (pitch) of the voice decreases.

3. Male-female fundamental frequency differences are insignificant until puberty, at which time the male voice descends a full octave, whereas the female voice drops three to five semitones.

4. In male and female adults, the fundamental frequency of the voice descends throughout life. However, in older age the fundamental frequency of the male voice begins to ascend, whereas in the female voice it does not.

5. The vocal folds undergo structural changes during older age, consisting of atrophy, thinning, edema, and dehydration of the mucosa covering the vocal folds.

6. Perceptual studies prove that listeners can identify older subjects by the sound of the voice. However, studies have also shown that the voices of older persons who are in good health are difficult to distinguish from the voices of younger speakers.

SUGGESTIONS FOR ADDITIONAL READING

Lind, J. (Ed.): Newborn infant cry. Acta Paediatr. Scand. (Suppl.), 163:1–128, 1965. A collection of four excellent articles on cry sounds and cry motions in normal infants and in those who have cranio-facial anomalies.

Wasz-Höckert, O., Lind, J., Vuorenkoski, V., Partenen, T., and Valanne, E.: The Infant Cry. London, William Heineman Medical Books, 1968.
The most comprehensive study of normal and abnormal infant cries available. Contains tables of frequency and durational cry characteristics and their sonograms, and comes with a narrated disc recording illustrating the cries discussed in the book.

Wilson, K.: Voice Problems of Children. Baltimore, Williams & Wilkins Co., 1979.
See pp. 71–74 for an excellent review of the literature on fundamental frequency characteristics of school-age children.

Young, G., and Décarie, T.G.: An ethology-based catalogue of facial/vocal behavior in infancy. Anim. Behav. 25:95–107, 1977.
This unusual article will broaden the student's horizons, showing how voice is linked with emotional response and facial expression as early as infancy, suggesting that intonation later in life has reflex, inborn roots.

REFERENCES

Biever, D.M., and Bless, D.M.: Vibratory characteristics of the vocal folds in young adult and geriatric women. J. Voice, 3:120–131, 1989.

Bosma, J.F., Lind, J., and Truby, H.M.: Respiratory motion patterns of the newborn infant in cry. *In* Kay, J.L. (Ed.): Physical Diagnosis of the Newly Born. Report of the Forty-Sixth Ross Conference on Pediatric Research. Columbus, Ohio, Ross Laboratories, 1964, pp. 103–116.

Colton, R.H.: Some acoustic and perceptual correlates of the modal and falsetto registers. Doctoral dissertation. Gainesville, University of Florida, 1959.

Curry, E.T.: The pitch characteristics of the adolescent male voice. Speech Monographs (Research Annual), 7:48–62, 1940.

Curry, E.T.: Hoarseness and voice change in male adolescents. J. Speech Dis., 14:23, 1949.

Fairbanks, G., Herbert, E., and Hammond, E.: An acoustical study of vocal pitch in seven and eight-year-old girls. Child Dev., 20:71–74, 1949.

Ferreri, G.: Senescence of the larynx. Ital. Gen. Rev. Otorhinolaryng, 1:640–709, 1959.

Greene, M.C.L.: The Voice and its Disorders. Philadelphia, J.B. Lippincott Co., 1972.

Hanley, J.D.: An analysis of vocal frequency and duration characteristics of selected samples of speech from general American, Eastern American and Southern American dialect regions. Speech Monographs, 18:78–93, 1951.

Hartman, D., and Danhauer, J.: Perceptual features of speech for males in four perceived age decades. J. Acoust. Soc. Am., 59:713–715, 1976.

Hollien, H., and Jackson, B.: Normative data on the speaking fundamental frequency characteristics of young adult males. J. Phonet., 1:117–120, 1973.

Hollien, H., and Malcek, E.: Evaluation of cross-sectional studies of adolescent voice change in males. Speech Monographs, 34:80–84, 1967.

Hollien, H., and Müller, E.: Perceptual responses to infant crying: Identification of cry types. J. Child Lang., 1:89–95, 1973.

Hollien, H., and Shipp, T.: Speaking fundamental frequency and chronologic age in males. J. Speech Hear. Res., 15:155–159, 1972.

Hollien, H., Dew, D., and Philips, P.: Phonational frequency ranges of adults. J. Speech Hear. Res., 14:755–760, 1971.

Hollien, H., and Michel, J.: Vocal fry as a phonational register. J. Speech Hear. Res., 11:600–604, 1968.

Honjo, I., and Isshiki, N.: Laryngoscopic and voice characteristics of aged persons. Arch. Otolaryngol., 106:149–150, 1980.

Jackson, C., and Jackson, C.L. (Eds.): Diseases of the Nose, Throat and Ear. Philadelphia, W.B. Saunders Co., 1959.

Keleman, G., and Pressman, J.: Physiology of the larynx. Physiol. Rev., 35:506–554, 1955.

Kelley, A.: Fundamental frequency measurements of female voices from twenty to ninety years of age (Unpublished manuscript). Greensboro, University of North Carolina, 1977.

Kent, R., and Burkard, R.: Changes in the acoustic correlates of speech production. *In* Beasley, D.S., and Davis, G.A. (Eds.): Aging Communication Processes and Disorders. New York, Grune & Stratton, 1981.

Lewis, M.: Infant Speech, a Study of the Beginnings of Language. New York, Harcourt Brace, 1936.

Lieberman, P.: Intonation, Perception, and Language. Cambridge, Mass., M.I.T. Press, 1967.

Lieberman, P., Harris, K.S., Wolff, P., and Russell, L.H.: Newborn infant cry and nonhuman primate vocalization. J. Speech Hear. Res., 14:718–727, 1971.

Majewski, W., Hollien, H., and Zalewski, W.: Speaking fundamental frequency of Polish adult males. Phonetica, 25:119–125, 1972.

McGlone, R., and Hollien, H.: Vocal pitch characteristics of aged women. J. Speech Hear. Res., 6:164–170, 1963.

McGlone, R.E., and McGlone, J.: Speaking fundamental frequency of eight-year-old girls. Folia Phoniatr., 24:313–317, 1972.

Michel, J., Hollien, H., and Moore, P.: Speaking fundamental frequency characteristics of 15-, 16-, and 17-year-old girls. Lang. Speech, 9:40, 1966.

Morrison, M.D., and Gore-Hickman, T.: Voice disorders in the elderly. J. Otolaryngol., 15:231–234, 1986.

Mysak, E.: Pitch and duration characteristics of older males. J. Speech Hear. Res., 2:46–54, 1959.

Ostwald, P.F.: Diagnostic use of infant cry. Biol. Neonator., 13:68–82, 1968.

Ptacek, P., and Sander, E.: Age recognition from voice. J. Speech Hear. Res., 9:273–277, 1966.

Philhour, C.W.: An experimental study of the relationships between perception of vocal pitch in connected speech and certain measures of vocal frequency. Doctoral dissertation, Iowa City, University of Iowa, 1948.

Pronovost, W.: An experimental study of methods for determining natural and habitual pitch. Speech Monographs, 9:111–123, 1942.

Ptacek, P., Sander, E.K., Malone, W.H., and Jackson, C.C.R.: Phonatory and related changes with advanced age. J. Speech Hear. Res., 9:353–360, 1966.

Ramig, L.A.: Aging speech: Physiological and sociological aspects. Lang. Commun., 6:25–34, 1986.

Ramig, L., and Ringel, R.: Effect of physiological aging on select acoustic characteristics of voice. J. Speech Hear. Res., 26:22–50, 1983.

Ringel, R., and Kluppel, D.: Neonatal crying: A normative study. Folia Phoniat., 16:1–9, 1964.

Ryan, E., and Capadano, H.: Age perceptions and evaluative reactions toward adult speakers. J. Gerontol., 33:98–102, 1978.

Ryan, W., and Burk, K.: Perceptual and acoustic correlates of aging in the speech of males. J. Commun. Disord., 7:181–192, 1974.

Saxman, J.H., and Burk, K.W.: Speaking fundamental frequency characteristics of middle-aged females. Folia Phoniatr., 19:167–172, 1967.

Shipp, T., and Hollien, H.: Perception of the aging male voice. J. Speech Hear. Res., 13:703–710, 1969.

Thiery, M., Yo Le Sian, A., Vrijens, M., and Janssens, D.: Vagitus uterinus. J. Obstet. Gynecol. Br. Commonwealth, 80:183–185, 1973.

vanOordt, H.W.A., and Drost, H.A.: Development of the frequency range of the voice in children. Folia Phoniatr., 15:289–298, 1963.

Wasz-Höckert, O., Lind, J., Vuorenkoski, V., Partenen, T., and Valanne, E.: The Infant Cry. London, William Heinemann Medical Books, 1968.

Young, G., and Décarie, T.G.: An ethology-based catalogue of facial/vocal behavior in infancy. Anim. Behav., 25:95–107, 1977.

Chapter Four

VOICE DISORDERS DUE TO MASS LARYNGEAL
LESIONS IN CHILDHOOD

Cri du Chat
Laryngomalacia (Congenital Laryngeal Stridor)
Congenital Laryngeal Web
Congenital Subglottic Stenosis
Congenital Cysts
Laryngotracheal Cleft
Papilloma
Inflammation
Malnutrition
Mongolism (Down's Syndrome)
Trauma

VOICE DISORDERS DUE TO MASS LARYNGEAL
LESIONS IN ADULTHOOD

Chronic Nonspecific Laryngitis
Chronic Hypertrophic Laryngitis
Cricoarytenoid Arthritis
Malignant Tumors
Endocrine Disorders
Trauma
Esophageal Reflux
Bowing

OBJECTIVE MEASUREMENT OF VOICE DISORDERS
DUE TO LARYNGEAL MASS LESIONS

High-Speed Motion Picture Analysis
Pitch Perturbation
Phonation Quotient
Mean Flow Rate and Maximum Phonation Time
Acoustic Spectrography

ORGANIC VOICE DISORDERS: MASS LESIONS OF THE VOCAL FOLDS

VOICE DISORDERS DUE TO MASS LARYNGEAL LESIONS IN CHILDHOOD

Mass lesions of the vocal folds at any age produce one or more of the following pathologic changes:

1. Increase the mass or bulk of the vocal folds or immediately surrounding tissues.
2. Alter their shape
3. Restrict their mobility
4. Change their tension
5. Modify the size or shape, or both, of the glottic, supraglottic, or infraglottic airway
6. Prevent the vocal folds from approximating completely along their anteroposterior margins
7. Result in excessive tightness of approximation

Cri du Chat

Infants who are ill cry differently from normal infants, and although certain types of cries are associated with specific illness in the newborn, *nonspecific distress cries are produced at higher than normal fundamental frequency* (Mallard and Daniloff, 1973).

> The attendants in the newborn nursery had nicknamed the child "kitten" because of her weak, high-pitched mewing cry (Ward et al., 1968).
> A telephone repairman, not seeing the crying child . . . remarked to the foster mother than she had "an awfully angry cat" (Dumars, 1964).

The syndrome of cri du chat in neonates and children was so named because the voice has a distinctive, high-pitched plaintive wail resembling the cry of a cat. The voice signature of this syndrome is a prime example of the diagnostic usefulness of voice. Three cases of cri du chat were first reported by Lejeune (1963), a professor of genetics at the University of Paris. The unusual voice is only one of many genetic defects. In addition to abnormal laryngeal development, the syndrome presents with micrognathia, a bird- or beak-like profile, microcephaly, hypotonia, hypertelorism, downward slanting palpebral fissures, mental retardation, low-set ears, strabismus, midline oral clefts, and failure to thrive. These defects have been traced to partial absence of the short arm of a B-group chromosome (Fig. 4-1).

1. Overall fundamental frequency invariably higher ($\overline{X}$ = 860 Hz) than for pain ($\overline{X}$ = 530 Hz) and hunger ($\overline{X}$ = 500 Hz) cries of normal infants.
2. Cry durations characteristically longer than normal ($\overline{X}$ = 2.6 sec.) and similar to normal pain cries ($\overline{X}$ = 2.7 sec.).
3. Flat or rising melody patterns.
4. Strained quality rarely containing glottal plosives.

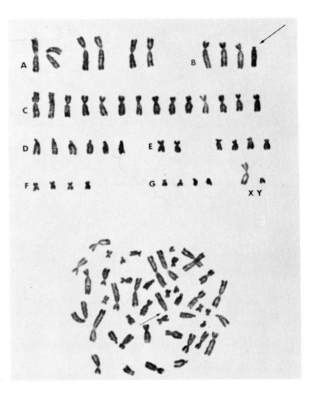

Figure 4-1. Defective B-group chromosome in patient with cri du chat. Arrows show the partial short-arm deletion of a B-group chromosome. (*From* Ward, P.H., Engel, E., and Nance, W.E.: The larynx in the cri du chat (cat cry) syndrome. Amer. Acad. Ophthalmol. Otolaryngol., 72:90–102, 1968.)

5. Crying on inhalation with inhalatory stridor (rare in normal infants).

Listeners had difficulty in determining whether the cry at a particular moment was occurring on inhalation or on exhalation, with the inhalatory-exhalatory cry signals failing to demonstrate the normal 'on-off' phenomenon.

Laryngomalacia (Congenital Laryngeal Stridor)

Stridor means involuntary sound made during inhalation or exhalation. Stridor can occur from any laryngeal disease—not just laryngomalacia—which produces partial obstruction of the airway either subglottally, glottally, or supraglottally. Although obstruction can occur at any age, detection of stridor is especially critical in the newborn because it signals impending asphyxiation. Laryngeal masses, inflammation, and paralysis are its most common causes. Different-sounding types of stridor offer clues to their anatomic sources along the airway, according to Pearson (1979).

In laryngomalacia, the voice on exhalation, during crying, and during other types of phonation may sound normal, but on inhalation there is a *low-pitched vibratory fluttering* or a *high-pitched crowing,* more often intermittent than constant. The stridor is more common when the infant is supine than prone. It usually goes unnoticed at birth but becomes apparent a few weeks after discharge from the hospital. Following is the physical appearance of the larynx in laryngomalacia on examination:

1. The epiglottis is low and narrow and has curled edges (omega-shaped).
2. The aryepiglottic folds are approximated, obscuring the glottis; sucked into the glottis on inhalation; and blown out on exhalation.
3. The mucosa over the arytenoid cartilages is redundant.

All these features, it should be pointed out, can be found in the normal infant larynx, the difference between the normal larynx and laryngomalacia being one of degree Prognosis for the disappearance of laryngomalacia within a few months to one year is good.

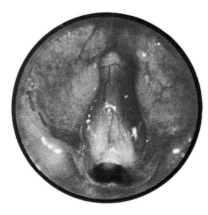

Figure 4–2   Membranous laryngeal web. (See p. 396 for color plate.)

Congenital Laryngeal Web

A web of tissue covering part or all of the glottis may be present at birth because of its failure to separate during the tenth week of embryonic laryngeal development. If the web is complete, asphyxiation and death are imminent unless the web is recognized and surgically divided. Figure 4-2 shows an extensive laryngeal web, but the configuration varies: Some are concave posteriorly (illustrated), others are thick, and still others are so thin and transparent that vocal fold movement can be seen underneath. A small web near the anterior commissure may go unrecognized for years. Approximately 75 percent of laryngeal webs occur at the level of the vocal folds, the remainder being equally distributed in the supraglottic and infraglottic larynx. The voices of infants and children who have laryngeal webs vary depending upon the location and extent of the latter. Both the cry and the speaking voice are abnormal, ranging from *hoarseness to aphonia. Inhalatory stridor* will be heard in cases of near-glottal occlusion.

Congenital Subglottic Stenosis

Arrested embryonic development of the conus or maldevelopment of the cricoid cartilage will produce an obstructive narrowing of the airway from the level of the vocal folds down to the cricoid area, the point of maximum obstruction being 2 to 3 mm. below the glottis. The voice will be *stridorous* from birth, but sometimes this will be noted only during respiratory infections. The voice during crying is usually normal (Ferguson, 1970).

Congenital Cysts

Sessile, nonpedunculated, fluid-filled cysts can arise from any of the laryngeal soft tissues; however, they almost always arise from the laryngeal ventricle, displacing the true and false vocal folds and causing glottic and supraglottic obstruction. The voice or cry will be *feeble or aphonic* but not differentially diagnostic from other obstructions. These lesions are potentially remediable.

Laryngotracheal Cleft

Embryonic failure of fusion of the dorsal cricoid lamina leaves an interarytenoid cleft and an open larynx posteriorly. Few cases have been described, and correct identification of the defect is reportedly difficult. The cry is *weak, feeble, or aphonic,* but feeding difficulties may overshadow the voice disorder.

Papilloma

Laryngeal papillomas are common, benign neoplasms in children, have a tendency to recur despite repeated surgical removal, and inevitably produce an abnormal voice. They usually regress with age, disappearing during puberty. The etiology is viral. Morphologically, papillomas are tumorlike

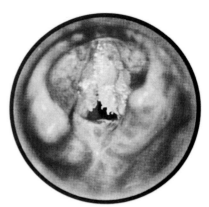

Figure 4–3 Papilloma of the larynx. (See p. 396 for color plate.)

frond-shaped proliferations of squamous cell epithelia, are exophytic, and have a cauliflower or raspberry appearance (Fig. 4–3). These growths frequently extend to include the laryngeal ventricles as well as the true vocal folds, which remain mobile. Lesions may spread to the supraglottic and subglottic regions and even into the trachea and bronchi. If untreated, they can produce asphyxiation and death.

Voice signs and symptoms are *hoarseness, abnormal cry, aphonia,* and *wheezy respiratory stridor.*

The lesions occur between the first and eighth years of life, although they are most common between ages 4 and 6 years.

Laser surgery is the technique of choice for removing the lesions; however, one complication can be laryngeal webbing after repeated surgeries. Tracheostomy may be required as a temporary measure to preserve the airway and, because of this respiratory restriction occurring in the young child, *delayed speech and language development* can be one of its sequelae.

Inflammation

An extensive group of inflammatory reactions of the vocal folds and surrounding tissues can cause aphonia or dysphonia.

ACUTE LARYNGITIS

Hoarseness, cough, and sore throats are common signs of acute laryngitis caused by viruses, bacteria, or chemical irritants. Pharyngeal and laryngeal erythema are found on examination.

CROUP

Several inflammatory laryngeal conditions produce a triad of *hoarseness, barking cough,* and *inhalatory stridor* called "croup." Acute laryngotracheo-bronchitis, also known as viral croup, is the most common form. Acute epiglottitis, which has a similar triad of signs, occurs abruptly and is most often caused by *Haemophilus influenzae.* Diphtheritic croup, although now rare, is still another type. Each of these can progress to respiratory obstruction and death unless an adequate airway is maintained.

In contrast to those with acute laryngitis, croup patients have systemic malaise in addition to dysphonia and stridor. Acute laryngotracheobronchitis, epiglottitis, and diphtheria all cause fever and dysphagia. In diphtheria, the initial respiratory and phonatory difficulties are caused by the appearance of a thick, adherent necrotic membrane. Patients who survive this stage often develop a toxic neurologic syndrome of vocal fold and soft palate paralysis due to vagus nerve involvement. Even if the glottic obstruction is overcome, the paralysis can extend to the respiratory musculature, requiring ventilatory support to avoid a fatal outcome.

Malnutrition

The cries of malnourished infants strongly resemble those of infants with central nervous system disease (see Chapter 5) according to Lester (1976), who described the cries of 12 malnourished infants to be of *high pitch, low intensity* and *excessively long duration,* with an *abnormally long latency between the first and second cry.*

Mongolism (Down's Syndrome)

The cry of Down's syndrome has a *flat melody, lower than normal pitch,* and a *tense or strident, harsh, rough, pressed, howling,* and *guttural* quality. The tenseness or stridency has been attributed to hyperadduction of the ventricular as well as true vocal folds during phonation (Wasz-Höckert et al., 1968; Novák, 1972).

Trauma

The larynges of neonates and infants are susceptible to external and internal trauma of the blunt and penetrating variety, as well as that caused by caustic substances. (See section below on adult voice disorders.)

VOICE DISORDERS DUE TO MASS LARYNGEAL LESIONS IN ADULTHOOD

Chronic Nonspecific Laryngitis

Dysphonia, vocal fatigue, and cough are produced by chronic laryngitis consisting of vasodilation and edema of the vocal folds. Persistent epithelial tissue changes occur in which the mucosal glands atrophy. The resulting dryness of the mucosa is called *laryngitis sicca.* Laryngologists believe that cigarette smoking, air pollution, alcohol, and vocal abuse are contributory factors.

Chronic Hypertrophic Laryngitis

Hypertrophy of the laryngeal mucosa is a common result of excess smoking and alcohol. *Leukoplakia,* a thickening of the epithelial and subepithelial layer, is characterized by the appearance of white patches on the vocal folds, which can be premalignant. *Simple chronic laryngitis* is manifested by *hoarseness,* an urge to clear the throat, diffusely red or pink mucosa, rounded rather than sharp vocal fold margins, and strands of mucus bridging the glottis from one vocal fold to the other. Submucosal edema eventually loosens the mucosa from the underlying vocal

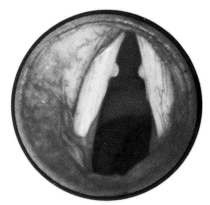

Figure 4–4a Bilateral polypoid vocal nodules. (See p. 396 for color plate.)

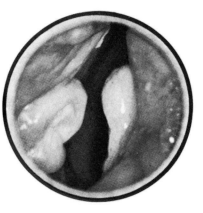

Figure 4–4b Contact ulcer. (See p. 396 for color plate.)

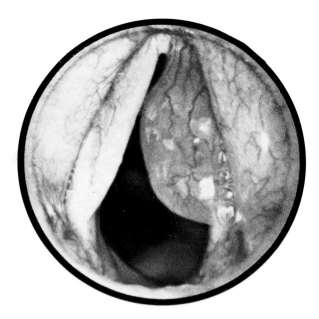

Figure 4-5 Sessile polyp of the vocal fold.

ligament. In the diffuse form, this change is called *polypoid degeneration*. If its occurrence is limited to the midpoint of the membranous vocal fold, it is called a vocal nodule (Fig. 4–4). If the localized form becomes so voluminous that the mass is larger than its base, it is called a vocal fold *polyp* (Fig. 4–5).

Cricoarytenoid Arthritis

Hoarseness and *stridor,* as well as throat pain during phonation, during swallowing and from medial compression of the thyroid cartilage radiating to the ears, can be signs of rheumatoid arthritis. Laryngoscopy shows edema or redness, or both, of the mucosa surrounding the cricoarytenoid joints, and reduced or absent cricoarytenoid joint and vocal fold motion unilaterally or bilaterally. Patients with rheumatoid arthritis or ankylosing spondylitis and cricoarytenoid arthritis can become dyspneic because of vocal fold fixation and can require tracheostomy and arytenoidectomy. At least one such patient experienced a relief of symptoms following corticosteroid therapy (Bienenstock and Lanyi, 1977).

Malignant Tumors

According to English (1976), approximately 80 percent of all laryngeal tumors are malignant (although this estimate may be low), occur most often between ages 50 and 70, are more common in men than women, and are causally linked to cigarette smoking, alcohol, and other sources of chronic laryngeal tissue irritation. The most common malignant lesion is by far *squamous cell carcinoma* (Fig. 4–6). *Adenocarcinoma,* the next most common malignancy, is rare. The relative frequency of squamous cell carcinoma according to site of lesion is shown in Figure 4–7. Approximately 50 percent originate on the true vocal folds and spread to structures beyond. Within the vocal folds themselves, 75 percent originate from the anterior half of the true vocal fold, or near the anterior commissure. *Hoarseness* is initially the only sign of laryngeal cancer when it involves the vocal folds. A lump in the neck or throat pain indicates spread. *Inhalatory stridor* from obstruction of the airway is a very late sign. Throat pain, shortness of breath, difficulty in swallowing, a mass in the neck, weight loss, ear pain, cough, and fetid breath also occur, depending upon the growth pattern of the tumor.

Early detection of laryngeal carcinoma cannot be overemphasized. Because *hoarseness* is its only early sign, its presence for more than six weeks should arouse suspicions of cancer until proved

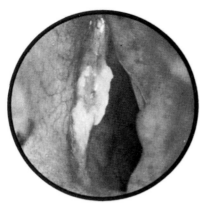

Figure 4–6   Carcinoma of the larynx. (See p. 396 for color plate.)

otherwise. If discovered early, the cancer may be kept from invading surrounding tissues supplied by the lymphatic system and thereby metastasizing to other organs.

Endocrine Disorders

HYPOTHYROIDISM

Hypothyroidism is caused by insufficient secretion of thyroxin by the thyroid glands. The term "hypothyroidism" is used in reference to the hormonal deficit when the disease is mild, and "myxedema" to the physical changes that appear when the disease is severe. Its onset in adults is insidious, taking months or years to develop; because of this, missed diagnosis is common.

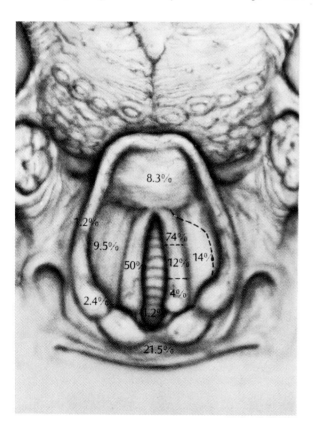

Figure 4–7   Relative frequency of site of origin of squamous cell carcinoma of the larynx. (*From* English, G.M.: Malignant neoplasms of the larynx. *In* English, G.M. (Ed.): Otolaryngology. Hagerstown, Md., Harper & Row, 1976.)

Lethargy, intolerance to cold, puffiness around the eyes, dryness of skin, and loss of frontal hair are classic physical signs. In more severe hypothyroidism the central nervous system may be affected, particularly the cerebellum, resulting in ataxia and *ataxic dysarthria*. As hypothyroidism becomes severe, the clinician may find intellectual, language, and personality changes. As a consequence, such patients are occasionally mistaken to be demented from primary central nervous system disease.

The dysphonia of hypothyroidism is characteristically *hoarse,* sometimes described as *coarse* or *gravelly,* and of *excessively low pitch*. These voice signs are typical effects of mass loading of the vocal folds by their infiltration with myxomatous material. The importance of the dysphonia in the detection and diagnosis of hypothyroidism is illustrated by the following histories.

*   *   *

A 67-year-old widow from Chicago asked her orthopedic surgeon if she could see someone about her voice. She had last been examined six months previously after hip joint surgery. One of her complaints was that she felt tired and fatigued and that her *voice had become hoarse or husky*. Her vocal folds and remaining laryngologic examination were normal, and a diagnosis of "functional" voice disorder was made.

Interview with the patient about her voice revealed that it was hoarse most of the time and worse when tired. On voice evaluation she was *mildly hoarse and the pitch of her voice low,* even after her age was taken into consideration. She volunteered that she found herself sleeping more than usual—three or four hours a day—in addition to eight hours at night, was *chilly* much of the time in her apartment, and was keeping her thermostat high. She complained that her *skin was dry*. A neurologist tested her Achilles reflexes and found that her muscles were slow in returning to their relaxed state. He ordered an evaluation of her total serum thyroxine level and found that it was abnormally low. He made a diagnosis of hypothyroidism and instituted thyroid hormone therapy.

*   *   *

Following surgery for rectal carcinoma, a 57-year-old male elementary school teacher complained of cold intolerance in his feet and hands, loss of sensation in his feet—as if there were "pads" under his soles—and weakness of the lower extremities. These symptoms progressed over a 13-year period from the time of his surgery. He complained of difficulty in climbing stairs and arising from a squatting position, and inability to lift modest weights. Although the weakness varied from day to day, there was no daily fluctuation, and the weakness was not related to amount of physical exertion. He had an unsteadiness of gait—a tendency to stagger more to the left than to the right—and noted loss of hair over his lower extremities, loss of sweating, and impotency.

Neurologic examination showed minimal distal sensory loss with moderate proximal weakness. Deep tendon reflexes were mildly decreased and were slow. There was a slowing and an irregularity of rapid alternating movements and a mild unsteadiness of gait. Nerve conduction studies confirmed mild sensorimotor neuropathy and mild proximal myopathy.

General physical examination revealed dry coarse skin, sparse hair, and puffy facies. He had periorbital edema, dry skin, scaling, and decreased deep tendon reflexes with a slow return phase.

*   *   *

Although the patient and family were not aware of any change in the patient's speech, *the pitch of his voice was hoarse and deep, particularly when he was asked to sing down to the bottom of his pitch range. Articulation was performed with irregular articulatory imprecision brought out by alternate motion rate testing of /p ʌ /, /t ʌ /, and /k ʌ /. The tip and blade of his tongue protruded between the teeth for the production of /s/ and /z/ sounds*. The patient was facetious throughout the examination, making jokes about questions put to him concerning his illness, particularly his speech, which he said was a source of humor in the classroom.

On laryngologic examination, his vocal folds were myxedematous.

A diagnosis of myxedema with myxedematous dysphonia, associated ataxic dysarthria, and lingual articulatory imprecision due to edema of the tongue was made.

*   *   *

In addition to the more typical myxedematous dysphonia, the clinician needs to be alert to distortions of articulation, particularly anterior lingual sounds due to increased tongue size caused by accumulation of myxomatous material in the tongue, and to ataxia dysarthria.

Hyperthyroidism

The dysphonia associated with *hyperthyroidism* has not been carefully described. *Breathy voice quality* and *reduced loudness* have been noted, presumably due to weakness of the respiratory and phonatory musculature. Associated with the dysphonia are anxiety, irritability, and fatigability.

Hyperpituitarism

A tumor in the region of the pituitary gland can cause oversecretion of the pituitary growth hormone somatotropin, producing an untimely enlargement of bone, cartilage, and soft tissue. The result is a condition known as *acromegaly*. When the condition begins in childhood, before epiphyseal fusion, *gigantism* results, in which the patient grows to an abnormally great height.

The dysphonia of acromegaly is an *excessively low pitch* and *hoarseness,* the consequences of enlargement of the vocal folds and laryngeal cartilages. The reduced fundamental frequency of the voice is augmented by enlarged pharyngeal and oral cavities. Because the tongue becomes enlarged and the mandible prognathic, articulation defects are common.

Amyloidosis

Systemic amyloidosis is an uncommon disease in which an abnormal fibrous protein, amyloid, infiltrates the extracellular compartments of connective tissue. The larynx is an occasional site for the localized expression of the disease. Laryngeal amyloidosis occurs as an atypical laryngeal nodule or subglottic stenosis. It is usually misdiagnosed as a vocal nodule or ideiopathic subglottic stenosis. Patients with laryngeal amyloidosis have *breathy*, *strained breathy, or hoarse voices.*

Virilization

Virilization refers to the development of male sex characteristics in females. For example, in a condition known as *perverse mutation,* the larynx grows to a larger-than-normal size during sexual maturation in the female because of excess secretion of the androgenic hormones. The voice is of *abnormally low pitch.* Females treated for menopausal symptoms with drug preparations containing androgen often develop virilization and *low voice pitch* and *hoarseness* in addition to facial hair. Damsté (1967) also noticed *falsetto pitch breaks.* Like myxedema, the dysphonia of virilization can develop insidiously and remain unnoticed. Estrogen or testosterone can produce laryngeal edema, causing *reduced pitch* (Gould, 1972).

Several studies indicate that voice may be affected by the menstrual cycle; *hoarseness* and *reduced pitch* may be caused by vocal fold edema (Smith, 1962). Singers and actresses claim to be severely affected by these periodic episodes of dysphonia, which interfere with their performances.

Trauma

Diffuse laryngeal trauma causes dysphonia or aphonia when the vocal folds and surrounding area are damaged by (1) blunt or penetrating injuries from automobile accidents in which the victim is thrown forward, striking the larynx against the dashboard of the car and causing compression fracture; (2) penetrating wounds of the larynx from gunshot wounds or stabbings; and (3) striking of the neck against wires and cables during skiing, motorcycling, and water-skiing accidents. Edema, hematoma, fractures, dislocations, lacerations, and paralysis are simultaneous tissue reactions to such injuries. The laryngeal surgeon attempts to restore damaged tissue to its normal configuration in order to allow phonation, but the initial consideration is maintaining a patent airway. Once out of danger, the patient's deglutition and voice become of concern. The voice, swallowing, and airway compete for whatever degree of functional-structural restoration is possible.

Laryngeal lesions due to trauma can be classified into supraglottic, glottic, and subglottic types.

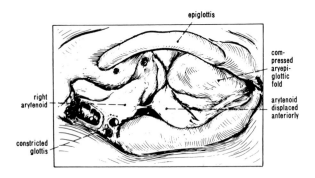

epiglottis

com-
pressed
aryepi-
glottic
fold

arytenoid
displaced
anteriorly

right
arytenoid

constricted
glottis

Figure 4–8   Sketch of laryngeal trauma showing anteroposterior laryngeal compression of
cartilages and soft tissues.

The glottic form most often results in dysphonia or aphonia, because in this type a thyroid cartilage fracture in the anterior commissure area displaces fragments of cartilage posteriorly, lacerating the vocal folds and causing edema (Fig. 4–8).

Trauma and vocal cord paralysis can occur from *laryngeal intubation* for ventilatory support, especially if the endotracheal tube is too large for the patient's airway (Fig. 4–9). Mucosal ulceration may lead to granuloma. Edema, mucosal laceration, and abrasion are temporary. Glottal strictures can result from untreated granulation. Dislocation of the arytenoid cartilages is said to result from careless laryngeal intubation, but the existence of such a lesion is very much in doubt. Dysphonia or aphonia are inevitable in such cases, depending upon the severity of the trauma. Posterior cricoarytenoid injury can result from nasogastric intubation and mimic recurrent laryngeal nerve palsy.

Prolonged endotracheal intubation can produce serious disorders of phonation due to traumatic irritation, edema, compressive effects, inflammation, ischemia, and loss of vocal fold mass. Scarring, granulomas, ulcerations, macerations, formation of membranes, fibrous tissue formation on the arytenoid cartilages, or within the interarytenoid space, cricoarytenoid subluxation, ankylosis, vocal fold paralysis, and subglottal stenosis can be produced by excessive endotracheal tube size, tube tip irritation, cuff pressure, and the natural curvature of the endotracheal tube. In a study of 17 patients, ages 17 to 85 years, who had been intubated for periods ranging from 10 hours to 4 weeks, Gallivan et al. (1989) found a total of 31 lesions in 16 of the 17 patients, 77 percent involving the vocal folds, 13 percent the arytenoid cartilages, and 10

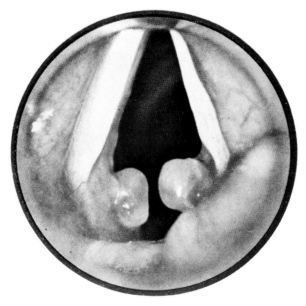

Figure   4–9   Postendotracheal   anesthesia
granulomas from trauma.

percent the interarytenoid notch and lumen between the vocal folds. Phonation, respiration, and coughing were compromised in these patients; voice impairment was virtually universal.

Endotracheal intubation can cause vocal fold paralysis (Ellis and Pallister, 1975; Hahn et al., 1970; Holley and Gildea, 1971; Yamashita et al., 1965). Lim et al. (1987), in a report of three patients who developed right vocal fold paralysis following endotracheal intubation during surgery unrelated to the neck, found severe hoarseness and the right vocal fold paralyzed in the paramedian position up to six weeks after surgery in two patients, and only slight voice improvement two months after intubation in a third patient. In all three patients, voice improvement was due to compensation by the unimpaired vocal fold. It is speculated that the cause of vocal cord paralysis occurs from pressure arising from an overinflated cuff of the endotracheal tube compressing the peripheral anterior branches of the recurrent laryngeal nerve.

Caustic substances swallowed by children and, often, adults who attempt suicide that cause grave damage to the larynx and esophagus are lye, ammonia, sodium hypochlorite (Chlorox), and orthophenylphenol (Lysol). Thermal traumas are caused by ingestion of hot liquids or solids or inhalation of hot gasses. Irradiation burns of the larynx occur as a side effect of the treatment of malignancies of the neck. Technically, vocal nodule and contact ulcer might be included, for they too are lesions secondary to trauma caused by vocal abuse; however, they will be discussed in a separate section.

Esophageal Reflux

Esophageal reflux, or gastroesophageal reflux, the regurgitation of hydrochloric acid from the stomach, has been implicated in vocal fold irritation, contact ulcers, and dysphonia. Inquiry into daytime and nocturnal acid reflux is an important component of the voice disorder history in patients with or without observed contact ulcer or contact ulcer granuloma. In a study of 32 patients suspected of having esophageal reflux, Koufman et al. (1988) found either intermittent or chronic dysphonia in 65.6 percent of the patients. In one subgroup of five patients who presented with chronic hoarseness, examinations revealed erythema and edema of the posterior larynx, laryngeal granulomas, and bouts of hoarseness related to reflux history.

Bowing

Bowing of the vocal folds is a term that describes an eliptical glottal shape during phonation due to failure of adequate anteroposterior tension of the vocal folds or to loss of tissue mass. Instead of the membranous portions of the folds adducting with straight vocal edges, they are curved. The intercartilaginous portions of the vocal folds are adducted; only the membranous portions fail to adduct. Causes of bowing are: (1) atrophy of the thyroarytenoid muscle owing to denervation; (2) bilateral cricothyroid muscle weakness due to superior laryngeal nerve lesions resulting in failure of anteroposterior stretching of the vocal folds; (3) loss of vocal fold tissue in the aging larynx; (4) iatrogenic lesions; (5) idiopathic.

Not all vocal fold bowing is organic; it can occur in patients with psychogenic voice disorders as well.

The associated dysphonia is *breathiness* and, in extreme cases, *aphonia* (Lejeune et al., 1983; Tucker, 1985; Koufman, 1986; Kahane, 1987). Bowing of the vocal folds has also been observed in the hypokinetic dysarthria of Parkinson's disease (Hanson et al., 1984) and in the flaccid dysphonia of myasthenia gravis (Neiman et al., 1975).

OBJECTIVE MEASUREMENT OF VOICE DISORDERS
DUE TO LARYNGEAL MASS LESIONS

Lesions that prevent the glottis from closing cause *breathiness* and *aphonia* having *high-* and *low-pitch* components. Severity is a further dimension of the voice disorder. As mentioned previously, despite efforts to perceptually classify abnormal voices into hoarse, harsh, breathy, strident, and similar types, too much patient variability exists to make these terms more than gross approximation at best. Although the skilled clinician can extract considerable information about

Figure 4–10   *Upper section, left to right.* Sequence of images from ultraspeed film of *normal* female larynx showing one cycle of phonation at 196 Hz. low intensity. Alternate film frames were omitted to conserve space. (*Lower section*) Graphic presentation of motion approximately at the antero-posterior midpoints of the membranous portions of the vocal folds. The upper curve indicates excursions of the right fold (*R*) in relation to an arbitrary median sagittal plane represented by the zero line. The motions of the left vocal fold (*L*) are below the line. Time is measured in film frames. The phase differences between the two vocal folds and their lateral shift while in contact often occur in the normal larynx. These laryngeal photographs present indirect, mirrored images. (*From* Moore, G.P.: Observations on laryngeal disease, laryngeal behavior and voice. Ann. Otol. Rhinol. Laryngol, 85:553–564, 1976.)

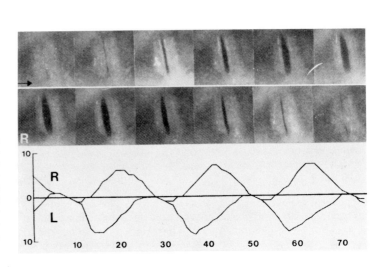

voice through listening, objective analyses need to be developed. Prediction of type, location, and extent of a vocal fold lesion on the basis of the acoustics of the voice may be just over the horizon.

The varieties of dysphonia associated with vocal fold pathologic states are the effects of jet noise caused by turbulent air passing through an aperture. Two kinds of airflow—laminar and turbulent—can be expressed as Reynold's number:

$$R = \frac{\text{Density} \times \text{Radius} \times \text{Velocity}}{\text{Viscosity}}$$

When R exceeds a critical value, the airstream becomes turbulent. Any obstacle to smooth airflow will intensify the turbulence, for example, a mass lesion of the vocal fold projecting into the glottic space. Rough vocal fold surfaces caused by inflammation similarly generate turbulence, and the degree of perceived hoarseness will depend on the ratio of the noise to the harmonic component (Isshiki et al., 1966).

High-Speed Motion Picture Analysis

In ultrahigh-speed motion picture analysis, the vocal folds are exposed with a laryngeal mirror and photographed with a high-speed camera. Then the excursion of the right and left vocal folds, the glottal transverse diameter, and the glottal area are computed and are displayed as a function of time. Physiologically normal vocal fold movements are shown in Figure 4–10. In this figure, during the opening phase the vocal folds move laterally, during the closing phase they move medially, and during the closed phase they are in contact with one another. The sequence of cycles is regular and uniform when pitch is held constant. In dysphonia, the duration of the cycle and the area of the glottis show random variations during a succession of cycles (Fig. 4–11). *Failure of complete glottic closure during the cycle is perceived as breathiness.* The many different voices heard in laryngeal disease are undoubtedly due to a multiplicity of cyclic variations. The cyclic behavior of the vocal folds depends upon the manner in which disease has interfered with their mass, configuration, and plasticity and upon infraglottal air pressure.

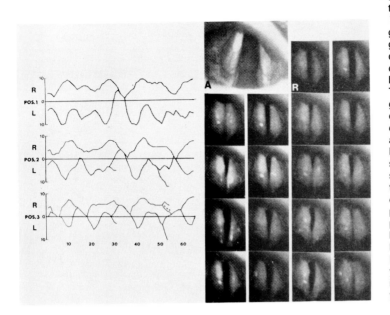

Figure 4–11 A male larynx with acute laryngitis and edema, particularly on the right vocal fold. The associated series of photographs from ultraspeed film begins at the upper left and reads downward progressively in each column. Alternate frames have been omitted to conserve space. The three sets of curves in the graph represent simultaneous vocal fold motions at three glottal locations: Position 2, approximately at the anterior-posterior midpoint; Position 1, halfway between Position 2 and the anterior commissure; and Position 3, halfway between Position 2 and the posterior commissure. The zero line approximates the median sagittal plane. Random, almost chaotic vibration associated with extreme hoarseness is evident. (*From* Moore, G.P.: Observations on laryngeal disease, laryngeal behavior and voice. Ann. Otol. Rhin, Laryngol., 85:553–564, 1976.)

Pitch Perturbation

Another method of quantifying normal and abnormal voice is to measure successive periods of each fundamental frequency cycle. The measure known as *pitch perturbation factor is the extent of rapid and abrupt change in adjacent periods of the fundamental frequency wave* (Iwata and von Leden, 1970).

Amplitude perturbations are also sensitive to laryngeal pathology. The pitch perturbation factor is determined by transcribing an audiosignal of a sustained vowel oscillographically, and measuring the period of successive waves according to the formula:

$$T_n = T_n - T_n + 1$$

where T_n is the duration of the period *n* in msec. and $T_n + 1$ is the duration of the period, *n+1*, in msec. Table 4-1 shows pitch perturbations in normal subjects. In this table, perturbations for normal male and female subjects show few changes in periods of adjacent cycles, with /ΔT/ ranging from − 0.6 msec. to + 0.5 msec. Figure 4–12 shows how the cumulative frequency rates of /ΔT/ calibrated for each 0.1 msec. period yield an ogive curve. The frequency rates of pitch perturbations /ΔT/ are 63.9 percent in 0.1 msec., 94.3 percent in 0.3 msec., and 98.1 percent in 0.5 msec. Whereas the pitch distributions in normal subjects show very small changes and yield a synchronous curve, pitch perturbations are significantly greater and more irregular in patients with laryngeal disease than in normals (Fig. 4–13).

Phonation Quotient

Airflow rate during phonation is another useful indicator of laryngeal dysfunction. Phonation quotient is *the ratio of vital capacity to maximum phonation time*.

$$\text{Phonation Quotient (PQ)} = \frac{\text{Vital Capacity}}{\text{Maximum Phonation Time}}$$

The PQ is obtained by sustaining the vowel /a/ as long as possible following deep inhalation. Airflow and air volume are measured by pneumotachography. Vital capacity is measured by means of a respirometer.

Table 4–1   The Distribution of Pitch Perturbations (or ΔT) for Normal Male and Female Subjects in Steady-State Portions of the Sustained Vowel*

ΔT	msec	FEMALE SUBJECTS		MALE SUBJECTS		BOTH SUBJECTS	
		Numbers	Frequency Rate (%)	Numbers	Frequency Rate (%)	Numbers	Frequency Rate (%)
+0.7 >	≧ +0.6						
+0.6 >	≧ +0.5	8	1.5			8	0.9
+0.5 >	≧ +0.4	1	0.2			1	0.1
+0.4 >	≧ +0.3	13	2.5	4	1.1	17	2.0
+0.3 >	≧ +0.2	31	5.9	15	4.3	46	6.7
+0.2 >	≧ +0.1	43	8.2	52	14.9	95	9.5
+0.1 >	> −0.1	349	66.9	207	59.5	556	63.9
−0.1 ≦	> −0.2	29	5.6	54	15.5	83	9.5
−0.2 ≦	> −0.3	29	5.6	12	3.5	41	4.7
−0.3 ≦	> −0.4	10	1.9	3	0.9	13	1.5
−0.4 ≦	> −0.5	1	0.2	1	0.3	2	0.2
−0.5 ≦	> −0.6	7	1.3			7	0.8
−0.6 ≦	> −0.7	1	0.2			1	0.1
Total periods		522		348		870	

*From Iwata, S., and von Leden, H.: Pitch perturbations in normal and pathologic voices. Folia Phoniatr., 22:413–424, 1970.

Mean Flow Rate and Maximum Phonation Time

Mean flow rate and maximum phonation time are additional measures of glottic efficiency. Recognizing that organic voice disorders are associated with increased air expenditure during phonation, Hirano et al. (1968) established normal standards of maximum phonation time and mean flow rate during sustained phonation. They found substantial evidence that phonation quotient is a reasonable clinical substitution for mean airflow rate (which is difficult to measure because it requires a pneumotachograph), and they found a significant negative correlation between maximum phonation time and mean airflow rate or the phonation quotient. Although maximum phonation time, flow rate, and phonation quotient signal laryngeal pathologic conditions, it must be stressed that they are not diagnostic of the type of the disease.

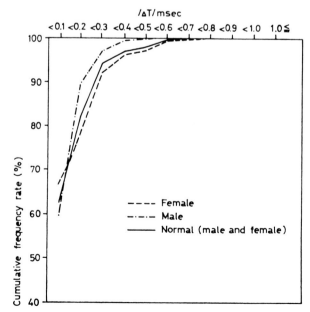

Figure 4–12   The ogive curve of pitch perturbations /ΔT/ for fundamental periods in normal subjects. The ordinate shows the cumulative frequency rate; the abscissa depicts the periods of /ΔT/ in msec. (*From* Iwata, S., and von Leden, H.: Pitch perturbations in normal and pathologic voices. Folia Phoniatr., 22:413–424, 1970.)

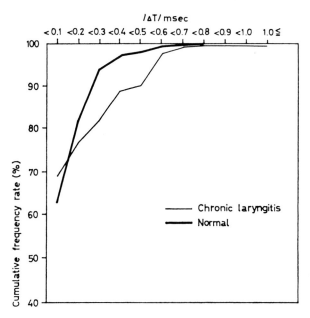

Figure 4–13 The ogive curves of /ΔT/ for fundamental periods in patients with chronic laryngitis. (*From* Iwata, S., and von Leden, H.: Pitch perturbations in normal and pathologic voices. Folia Phoniatr., 22:413–424, 1970.)

$$\text{Mean Flow Rate} = \frac{\text{Phonation Volume*}}{\text{Maximum Phonation Time}} \quad (1)$$

This equation states that the greater the volume of air expended, the faster the flow rate and the shorter the time required to complete the sustained phonation.

$$\text{Phonation Quotient} = \frac{\text{Vital Capacity}}{\text{Maximum Phonation Time}} \quad (2)$$

This equation states that the phonation quotient is a measure of the ratio of vital capacity to maximum phonation time. Thus, phonation quotient can be a measure of glottic efficiency just as mean flow rate is. A short maximum phonation time indicates a high-volume flow of air that would result in a high phonation quotient; the reverse is also true.

Acoustic Spectrography

The sound spectrograph is an electronic instrument that analyzes the speech signal by passing it through a series of filters and graphically represents its frequency, intensity, and durational characteristics on a paper printout. Either the subject speaks directly into a microphone or the speech signal is analyzed from magnetic tape. Figure 4–14 is a spectrogram of a normal subject's vowel prolongation, illustrating the highly periodic fundamental frequency, regular harmonic pattern in the formant frequency range, and absence of noise spectra. The sonogram of a patient with vocal

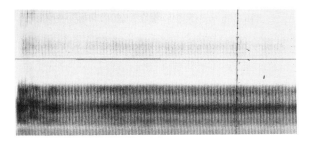

Figure 4–14 Sonogram of normal vowel /a/ prolongation showing regularity of fundamental and higher harmonics.

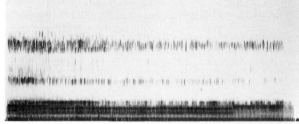

Figure 4–15 Sonogram of patient with vocal fold carcinoma on vowel prolongation showing irregularity and noise in higher harmonics on prolongation of the vowel /a/.

fold carcinoma (Fig. 4–15), in contrast to the normal subject, is characterized by (1) aperiodicity of the fundamental frequency, (2) noise components in the main formants of vowels, (3) loss of acoustic energy in the harmonic components of vowels, and (4) high-frequency noise components above 3 KHz. Such are the typical features in most vocal fold diseases. The noise components in laryngeal pathologic states are caused by turbulent airflow due to incomplete glottic closure and irregular movements of vocal folds.

Yanagihara (1967) had judges rate the degree of hoarseness produced by 167 patients with pathologic voices into slight, moderate, or severe. He then compared these listener ratings with the sonograms obtained from the same voice samples, classifying the sonograms into four severity types.

I. Voices judged perceptually to be slightly hoarse yielded sonograms in which irregular harmonic components were mixed with the noise components chiefly in the formant region of the vowels.

II. Voices judged perceptually to be moderately hoarse yielded sonograms in which the noise components in the second formants of /e/ and /i/ predominated over the harmonic components, and slight additional noise components appeared in the high-frequency region above 3 KHz in the vowels /e/ and /i/.

III. Voices judged to be severely hoarse produced second formants of /e/ and /i/ that were totally replaced by noise components and showed intensification of energy and expansion of range above 3 KHz.

IV. Voices judged to be severely hoarse produced sonograms in which the second formants of /a/, /e/, and /i/ were replaced by noise components, and even the first formants of all vowels lost their periodic components, which were replaced by noise components. High-frequency noise components were intensified.

The study, then, showed a direct relationship between the listener's perception of degree of hoarseness and the extent of disturbance seen in the spectrogram. As in previously described physical measures of abnormal voice, spectrographic analysis, even though able to identify dysphonia, has not yet been refined to the point of predicting the type or extent of laryngeal disease. It is unlikely that such lesion identification will take place, because similar structural, and therefore sound-producing, configurations can come from different types of lesions; trauma, infection, hypertrophy, neoplasia, and neurologic disease. Presently, the value of physical analysis of the voice is the addition of objective data to the overall diagnosis, in an intelligible form. The clinician wants to know, in comparison with normal, the mass, elasticity, and tension of the vibrating laryngeal components and how they have changed from previous analyses.

SUMMARY

1. Voice disorders caused by mass lesions in infants arise from congenital laryngeal malformations, neoplasms, inflammation, trauma, or malnutrition.

2. Voice disorders caused by mass lesions in children and adults stem from inflammation, neoplasms, endocrine disease, or trauma.

3. Objective measurements of vocal fold function in organic voice disorders include high-speed motion picture analysis, pitch perturbation factor, phonation quotient, mean flow rate and maximum phonation time, and acoustic spectrography.

4. Objective measurements cannot yet predict type and location of mass laryngeal lesions, but may assist in diagnosis and assessment of progress.

SUGGESTIONS FOR ADDITIONAL READING

Becker, W. (Ed.): Atlas of Otorhinolaryngology and Bronchoesophagology, Philadelphia, W.B. Saunders Co., 1969.
    Probably the best color photo atlas of laryngeal diseases.

Cohen, S.R., Thompson, J.W., Geller, K.A., and Birns, J.W.: Voice change in the pediatric patient: A differential diagnosis. Ann. Otol. Rhinol. Laryngol., 92:437–443, 1983.
  This article should be read for its extensive coverage of voice changes from organic disease in pediatric patients. Neurologic dysfunctions, congenital and chromosomal defects, tumors, infections, trauma, and metabolic and endocrine diseases are discussed and several tables are given containing many diseases within these general categories.
English, G.M.: Otolaryngology, New York, Harper & Row, 1976.
  This comprehensive, readable book can serve as a reference for greater depth of reading into the entire realm of organic laryngeal disease.
Lane, R.W., Weider, D.J., Steinem, C., and Marin-Padilla: Laryngomalacia. Arch. Otolaryngol., 110:546–551, 1984.
  An excellent review of a little known voice disorder in infants accompanied by a case study of surgical treatment of this condition.

REFERENCES

Bienenstock, H., and Lanyi, V.F.: Cricoarytenoid arthritis in a patient with ankylosing spondylitis. Arch. Otolaryngol., 103:738–739, 1977.
Damsté, P.H.: Voice change in adult women caused by virilizing agents. J. Speech Hear. Disord., 32:126–132, 1967.
Dumars, K.W., Jr.: Le cri du chat (crying cat) syndrome. Am. J. Dis. Child., 108:533–537, 1964.
Ellis, P.D.M., and Pallister, W.K.: Recurrent laryngeal nerve palsy and endotracheal intubation. J. Laryngol. Otol., 89:823–826, 1975.
English, G.M., (Ed.): Otolaryngology. New York, Harper & Row, 1976.
Gallivan, G.J., Dawson, J.A., and Robbins, L.D.: Videolaryngoscopy after endotracheal intubation: Implications for voice. J. Voice, 3:76–80, 1989.
Gould, W.J.: Vocal cords can speak of hormonal dysfunction. Consultant, 12:101–102, November, 1972.
Hahn, F.W., Martin, J.T., and Lillie, J.C.: Vocal cord paralysis with endotracheal intubation. Arch. Otolaryngol., 92:226–229, 1970.
Hanson, D.G., Gerratt, B.R., and Ward, P.H.: Cinegraphic observations of laryngeal function in Parkinson's disease. Laryngoscope, 94:348–353, 1984.
Hirano, N., Koike, Y., and von Leden, H.: Maximum phonation time and air usage during phonation, Folia Phoniatr., 20:185–201,1968
Holley, H.S., and Gildea, J.E.: Vocal cord paralysis after tracheal intubation. J.A.M.A., 215:281–284, 1971.
Isshiki, N., Yanagihara, N., and Morimoto, M.: Approach to the objective diagnosis of hoarseness. Folia Phoniatr., 18:393–400, 1966.
Iwata, S., and von Leden, H.: Pitch perturbations in normal and pathologic voices. Folia Phoniatr., 22:413–424, 1970.
Kahane, J.C.: Connective tissue changes in the larynx and their effects on voice. J. Voice, 1:27–30, 1987.
Koufman, J.A., Winer, G.J., Wu, W.C., and Castell, D.O.: Reflux laryngitis and its sequelae: The diagnostic role of ambulatory 24-hour pH monitoring. J. Voice, 2:1988, 78–89.
Koufman, J.A.: Laryngoplasty for vocal cord medialization: An alternative to Teflon. Laryngoscope, 96:726–731, 1986.
LeJeune, F.E., Jr., Guist, C.E., and Samuels, P.M.: Early experiences with vocal ligament tightening. Ann. Otol. Rhinol. Laryngol., 92:475–477, 1983.
Lejeune, J., et al.: Trois cas de délétion partielle du bras court d'un chromosome-5, C.R. Acad. Sci. Paris, 257:3098–3102, 1963.
Lester, B.M.: Spectrum analysis of the cry sounds of well-nourished and malnourished infants. Child Dev., 47:237–241, 1976.
Lim, E.K., Chia, K.S., and Ng, B.K.: Recurrent laryngeal nerve palsy following endotracheal intubation. Anaesth. Intens. Care, 15:342–345, 1987.
Mallard, A.R., and Daniloff, R.G.: Glottal cues for parent judgment of emotional aspects of infant vocalizations. J. Speech Hear. Res., 16:592–596, 1973.
Neiman, R.F., Mountjoy, J.R., and Allen, E.L.: Myasthenia gravis focal to the larynx. Arch. Otolaryngol., 101:569–570, 1975.
Novák, A.: The voice of children with Down's syndrome. In Hirschberg, J., Szépe, Gy., and Vass-Kovács, E. (Eds.): Papers in Interdisciplinary Speech Research, Budapest, Akadémiai Keadó, 1972, pp. 197–200.
Pearson, B.: Personal communication, 1979.
Smith, F.M.: Hoarseness—a symptom of premenstrual tension. Arch. Otolaryngol., 75:66–68, 1962.
Tucker, H.M.: Anterior commissure laryngoplasty for adjustment of vocal fold tension. Ann. Otol. Rhinol. Laryngol., 94:547–549, 1985.
Ward, P.H., et al.: The larynx in the cri du chat (cat cry) syndrome. Trans. Am. Acad. Ophthalmol. Otolaryngol., 72:90–102, 1968.
Wasz-Höckert, O., Lind, J., Vuorenkoski, V., Partenen, T., and Valanni, E., The Infant Cry. London, William Heinemann Medical Book, 1968.
Yamashita, T., Harada, Y., Ueda, N., Jashimo, J., and Kanebayasha, H.: Recurrent laryngeal nerve paralysis associated with endotracheal anesthesia. J. Otolaryngol. Soc. Jpn., 68:1452–1459, 1965.
Yanagihara, N.: Significance of harmonic changes and noise components in hoarseness. J. Speech Hear. Res., 10:531–541, 1967.

Chapter Five

INTRODUCTION

NEUROLOGIC VOICE DISORDERS IN INFANCY

NEUROLOGIC VOICE DISORDERS IN CHILDREN
AND ADULTS

Relatively Constant Neurologic Voice Disorders
Arrhythmically Fluctuating Neurologic Voice Disorders
Rhythmically Fluctuating Neurologic Voice Disorders
Paroxysmal Neurologic Voice Disorders
Neurologic Voice Disorders Due to Loss of
Volitional Phonation

ORGANIC VOICE DISORDERS: NEUROLOGIC DISEASE

INTRODUCTION

Highly integrated neurophysiologic control is necessary for normal phonation. The vocal folds must be adducted to the midline and kept there with balanced and bilaterally symmetrical adductor-abductor muscle tonus. Thyroarytenoid and cricothyroid muscle tension must be optimum. Glottal opening and closing has to be precisely timed, the folds adducted at the exact moment for onset of voiced consonants and vowels, and abducted for voiceless. Should they adduct too soon, voiceless sounds would be voiced; too late, voiced sounds would be voiceless. Yet they must not overadduct, for then they would obstruct the exhaled airstream and produce strained voice or voice arrest. Should they fail to adduct or suddenly abduct, voicing would become breathy or whispered. The extrinsic muscles of the larynx must be able to elevate and depress the larynx in the neck, otherwise pitch variation will be restricted. On the other hand, if fluctuations are excessive, pitch will change unexpectedly and inappropriately. Exhalatory airflow must be forced from the lungs under constant pressure from moment to moment, for a sudden increase or decrease in such pressure may adversely produce irregular pitch and loudness. Air must be forced from the lungs with adequate pressure, otherwise the voice will be insufficiently loud, and at other times air must escape under low pressure for low loudness levels.

When vascular, infectious, traumatic, neoplastic, and degenerative diseases damage regions of the nervous system that contain nerve cells responsible for phonation, abnormal voice is inevitable. Previous research has identified acoustically different dysarthrias and their associated dysphonias caused by damage to specific regions of the nervous system (Darley et al., 1969a,b). Flaccid, spastic, ataxic, hypokinetic, and hyperkinetic dysarthrias sound different because physiologically and anatomically dissimilar regions of the nervous system are damaged in each type, producing different muscular pathophysiology. Neurologic voice disorders exhibit the same relationship between anatomic location of lesion and acoustic effect as the dysarthrias. *In fact, neurologic voice disorders, technically, are dysarthrias; although they occur in isolation, most often they are imbedded in a more widespread complex of respiratory, resonatory, and articulatory dysarthric signs.* Dysphonia can be the first sign of neurologic disease, the remainder of the dysarthria following as the disease progresses. Such capricious and discrepant patterns of neurologic disease onset are common.

There are, then, as many types of neurologic voice disorders as there are dysarthrias:

1. Flaccid dysphonia
2. Spastic (pseudobulbar) dysphonia
3. Mixed flaccid-spastic (pseudobulbar) dysphonia
4. Hypokinetic (parkinsonian) dysphonia
5. Ataxic dysphonia
6. Choreic dysphonia
7. Dystonic dysphonia
8. Dysphonia of palatopharyngolaryngeal myoclonus
9. Dysphonia of organic (essential) tremor
10. Dysphonia of Gilles de la Tourette's syndrome
11. Apraxia of phonation

12. Akinetic mutism
13. Dysprosody of "pseudoforeign dialect"

These neurologic voice disorders tend toward either constancy or variability of their acoustic signals, depending upon whether or not the pathophysiology of the disease produces relatively steady or relatively fluctuating abnormal laryngeal or respiratory muscle movements. Neurologic voice disorders are subdivided into the following general categories, under which are subsumed specific neurologic dysphonias and aphonias:

1. Relatively constant neurologic voice disorders. Voice quality, loudness, or pitch deviations are relatively constant during contextual speech and vowel prolongation. Fluctuations may occur but are minor. This category includes flaccid, spastic (pseudobulbar), mixed flaccid-spastic, and hypokinetic (parkinsonian) dysphonias.

2. Arrhythmically fluctuating neurologic voice disorders. Abnormal muscular physiology produces unpredictable and irregular quality, loudness, and pitch fluctuations from moment to moment during contextual speech, which are especially prominent during vowel prolongation. Included are ataxic, choreic, and dystonic dysphonias.

3. Rhythmically fluctuating neurologic voice disorders. Abnormal voice parameters fluctuate relatively rhythmically from moment to moment and are particularly noticeable during vowel prolongation. In this group are included the dysphonias of palatopharyngolaryngeal myoclonus and organic (essential) voice tremor.

4. Paroxysmal neurologic voice disorders. Relatively infrequent, sudden bursts of aberrant voice are exemplified by Gilles de la Tourette's syndrome.

5. Neurologic voice disorders associated with loss of volitional phonation. The following neurologic voice disorders are not classifiable as dysarthrias but fall under the jurisdiction of: (1) apraxia of speech, including apraxia of phonation (no loss of muscle strength or coordination but loss of volitional control over laryngeal and respiratory movements); (2) akinetic mutism; and (3) dysprosody of pseudo-foreign dialect.

NEUROLOGIC VOICE DISORDERS IN INFANCY

Infant neurologic voice disorders cannot be classified according to the preceding scheme because there is limited knowledge of the relationship between abnormal voice and the neuroanatomic location of lesion in this age group. In general, however, newborn infants with central nervous system lesions of unspecified location cry in an excessively *high pitched, shrill, weak,* and *unsustained* voice. They require more intense and frequent pain stimuli in order to induce crying, and their cries are of abnormally short duration. For example, Karelitz and Fisichelli (1962) found that only 54 percent of neurologically impaired infants met the one-minute cry duration criterion, in comparison with 92 percent of normal infants. Such infants produced statistically significantly fewer total sounds. Some were *hypernasal* (Fisichelli, 1966). Cyanotic infants cried with *delayed latencies* (Karelitz and Fisichelli, 1962), had fundamental frequencies twice as high as normal infants, and *cried longer* than normal infants (Lind, 1965). The infants of drug-addicted mothers cried at abnormally high fundamental frequencies (Blinick et al., 1971).

Infants born with unilateral or bilateral vocal fold paralyses due to Xth (vagus) nerve lesions also cry abnormally. Such injury is caused by twisting the neck during breech presentations, infections, vascular diseases, and cranial malformations. The left recurrent laryngeal branch of the vagus is more frequently damaged than the right because of its longer course into the chest and, therefore, greater vulnerability to disease or damage from an enlarged heart, tumors, mediastinal cysts, and tracheobronchial tree malformations. The dysphonia may be solitary or one of several cranial nerve signs. The cries of infants with unilateral adductor vocal fold paralysis are either *weak* or *absent*. In bilateral abductor paralysis, the voice and cry may be *normal* due to the adequate approximation of the vocal folds, but such infants produce *inhalatory stridor* during crying because their vocal folds are too weak to be abducted during inhalation.

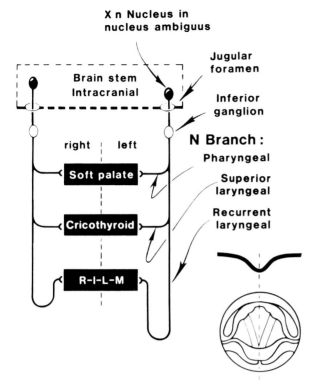

Figure 5–1 Pathway of the vagus nerve from brainstem to larynx. R-I-L-M: remaining intrinsic laryngeal muscles.

NEUROLOGIC VOICE DISORDERS IN CHILDREN AND ADULTS

Relatively Constant Neurologic Voice Disorders

FLACCID DYSPHONIA: XTH (VAGUS) NERVE LESIONS

Cell bodies of the vagus nerves, which supply the larynx and pharynx, are found deep within the reticular formation of the medulla in the *nucleus ambiguus.** A cluster of cells about 2 cm. long contains the cell bodies of cranial nerves IX, X, and XI. The vagus nerve emerges from the lateral surface of the medulla between the inferior cerebellar peduncle and the inferior olive. A series of discrete roots converge into a single trunk intracranially. Each vagus nerve trunk passes through paired openings, the *jugular foramina,* at the base of the skull, along with cranial nerves IX and XI (Fig. 5–1). Near its exit from the skull, each vagus nerve divides into three branches:

1. *Pharyngeal nerve.* The pharyngeal branch becomes identifiable as it emerges from the upper part of the *inferior (nodos) ganglion* of the vagus nerve and descends between the external and internal carotid arteries to the left of the middle pharyngeal constrictor muscles. At that point, it again divides into numerous filaments that join with branches from the sympathetic trunk and the glossopharyngeal and external laryngeal nerves to form the *pharyngeal plexus.* From there nerve fibers are distributed to the pharynx and to all the muscles of the *soft palate* except the tensor veli palatini, which is supplied by the motor division of the Vth cranial nerve.

---

*Experimental evidence in monkeys indicates that the superior one third of the nucleus ambiguus is responsible for the pharynx and esophagus; caudal to that is a center for cricothyroid muscle function; and caudal to that is a center for abductor laryngeal muscle function. The most caudal region is responsible for adductor muscle function.

2. *Superior laryngeal nerve*. This branch of the vagus nerve emerges from the inferior ganglion and descends alongside the pharynx, first posterior to the internal carotid artery and then medial to it. About 2 cm below the inferior ganglion, it divides into two additional branches, the internal and external laryngeal nerves.

   (a) *Internal laryngeal nerve*. This branch of the superior laryngeal nerve descends to the level of the thyrohyoid membrane and, piercing and entering it, further divides into two additional branches. Both contain afferent or sensory fibers from *mucous membrane* that

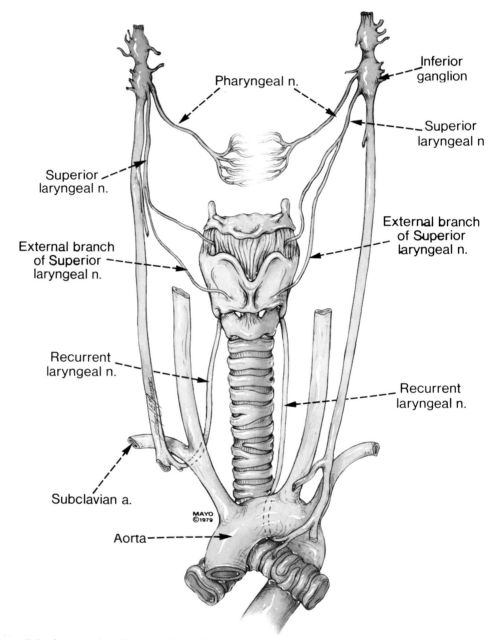

Figure 5–2 Asymmetric pathways of the left and right recurrent laryngeal nerves.

lines the larynx above the level of the vocal folds. They also contain fibers from muscle spindles and other stretch receptors in the larynx. The upper branch of the internal laryngeal nerve supplies the mucous membrane of the epiglottis, the vallecula, and the vestibule of the larynx. The lower branch supplies the mucous membrane of the aryepiglottic folds and the dorsum of the arytenoid cartilages.

    (b) *External laryngeal nerve*. This efferent or motor branch of the superior laryngeal nerve descends posterior to the sternothyroid muscle and innervates the *cricothyroid muscle*. It also branches to the inferior pharyngeal constrictor.

3. *Recurrent laryngeal nerve*. The term "recurrent" refers to the anatomic course of this nerve, which first descends to the lower neck and into the chest and then courses superiorly again. This nerve pair, unlike the rest that supply the larynx, is not bilaterally symmetrical (Fig. 5–2). The right recurrent laryngeal nerve arises from the vagal trunk in front of the *subclavian artery*. It loops under the artery from front to back and then ascends alongside the trachea behind the common carotid artery and, higher up, in or near the groove between the trachea and esophagus, entering the larynx behind the articulation between the inferior horn of the thyroid and the cricoid cartilage. In 70 to 80 percent of cases, the nerve divides into two or more branches before entering the larynx. The left recurrent laryngeal nerve splits off from the trunk of the vagus to the left of the *arch of the aorta,* winding under it from front to back. Ascending lateral to the trachea, it then pierces and enters the larynx, as on the right side. Both right and left recurrent laryngeal nerves supply *all the intrinsic muscles of the larynx except the cricothyroid*. They also supply sensory filaments to the mucous membrane lining the larynx below the level of the vocal folds, and they carry afferent fibers from stretch receptors of the intrinsic laryngeal muscles.

    The extrinsic laryngeal musculature is also implicated in lower motor neuron disease, although to a much lesser extent than the intrinsic muscles. Of the suprahyoid muscles, the anterior belly of the digastric is innervated by the mylohyoid branch of the inferior alveolar nerve; the posterior belly by the VIIth nerve; the stylohyoid by the VIIth nerve; the mylohyoid by the mylohyoid branch of the inferior alveolar nerve; and the geniohyoid by the first cervical spinal nerve (C_1) via the hypoglossal nerve. The infrahyoid muscles—the sternohyoid, sternothyroid, and omohyoid—are all innervated by the ansa cervicalis, and the thyrohyoid is innervated by fibers from C_1 via the hypoglossal nerve.

    The autonomic nerve supply to the larynx originates in the dorsal motor nuclei of the vagus as parasympathetic fibers that synapse in the inferior ganglion and accompany the somatic motor nerves to the larynx. Sympathetic nerve fibers enter the motor nerves through connections with the superior cervical ganglion. Autonomic nerve fibers have chiefly secretory and vasomotor functions and maintain muscle tonus.

Effects of Xth Nerve Lesions on Vocal Fold Movement and Phonation.   Lesions of the Xth nerve at any point along its pathway from the nucleus ambiguus in the brainstem to the musculature cause paresis (weakness) or paralysis (immobility) of laryngeal muscles as well as dysphonia or aphonia. The extent of weakness, the position of vocal fold fixation, the unilaterality or bilaterality of weakness, and the degree of voice impairment depend upon the location of the lesion along the pathway of the nerve and whether one or both nerves of the pair have been damaged. Refer to Figure 5–3 and Table 5–1 for the following discussion.

    1. *Intramedullary and extramedullary lesions affecting all branches of the vagus nerve to the larynx* (Fig. 5–3, I A,B). Lesions that damage vagal nuclei within the brainstem are called *intramedullary*. When the nerve trunk just outside the brainstem but still within the cranial cavity is damaged, the lesion is called *extramedullary*. If the lesion affects the nerve after it exits from the skull, it is called *extracranial*. Lesions at any of these three levels damage the vagus nerve *above the separation of its pharyngeal, superior laryngeal, and recurrent branches*. Therefore, *all muscles supplied by those branches of the vagus nerve below the level of the lesion will be weak or paralyzed*. Affected muscles, then, will be of three types: (1) those supplied by the pharyngeal branch of the vagus nerve. Consequently, the levator muscle of the soft palate, the levator veli

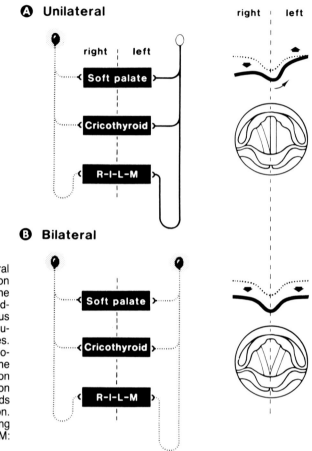

(A) Unilateral

right | left

right | left

Soft palate

Cricothyroid

R-I-L-M

(B) Bilateral

Soft palate

Cricothyroid

R-I-L-M

Figure 5–3 I Effects of unilateral and bilateral vagus nerve lesions at different locations on vocal fold and soft palate functions. Stipled line indicates lesion. (See Table 5–1 for corresponding information.) I A: Unilateral lesion of vagus nerve (nucleus), above origin of pharyngeal, superior laryngeal, and recurrent laryngeal nerves. The right vocal fold is fixed in an abducted position, whereas the left adducts to the midline on phonation. The soft palate is paralyzed on the right, is resting low, and pulls to the left on phonation. I B: Bilateral lesion. Both vocal folds are fixed in an abducted position on phonation. The soft palate is bilaterally paralyzed, is resting low, and does not move on phonation. R-I-L-M: remaining intrinsic laryngeal musculature.

palatini, will be weak or paralyzed on the same side as the lesion. (2) Because the superior laryngeal branch also lies below the level of the lesion, the cricothyroid muscle will be weak or paralyzed on the side of the lesion. (3) Because the recurrent laryngeal branch lies below the level of the lesion, the remaining intrinsic muscles of the larynx will be weak or paralyzed on the side of the lesion. The vocal folds will be paralyzed and fixed in the *abducted position* unilaterally or bilaterally. At rest and during phonation the soft palate will hang lower on the paralyzed than on the nonparalyzed side. On phonation, the nonparalyzed side will elevate, pulling the uvula and the midline of the soft palate toward the normal side. In bilateral lesions, the soft palate will rest at a lower than normal position and on phonation will elevate minimally or not at all bilaterally.

Unilateral lesions above the bifurcation of the pharyngeal branch of the vagus nerve causing unilateral vocal fold paralysis will produce severe *breathiness to whispered voice* and, in some instances, a *flutter or tremor* on vowel prolongation. There will be *reduced loudness and pitch* and possibly *falsetto pitch breaks.*

In bilateral vocal fold paralysis, the voice will be virtually *whispered,* owing to the wider glottal chink than is found in unilateral paralysis, and markedly *reduced loudness.* Unilateral soft palate paralysis will produce mild-to-moderate *hypernasality and nasal emission,* which will be much more severe if the paralysis is bilateral.

Associated signs will be a *weak, mushy, or absent glottal coup or cough,* dysphagia, and nasal regurgitation on swallowing liquids and solids. Pharyngeal paralysis results in a reduced or absent gag reflex and aspiration of secretions, which, if severe, may require tracheostomy.

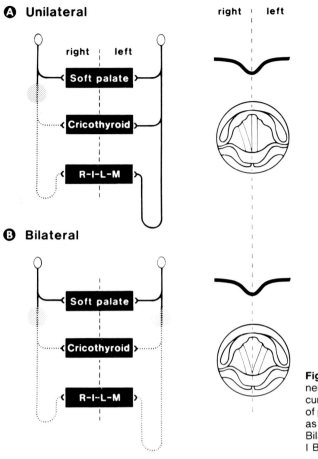

Ⓐ Unilateral

right | left

right | left

Soft palate

Cricothyroid

R-I-L-M

Ⓑ Bilateral

Soft palate

Cricothyroid

R-I-L-M

Figure 5–3 II A: Unilateral lesion of vagus nerve above origin of superior laryngeal and recurrent laryngeal nerves, but below bifurcation of pharyngeal nerve. Same effect on vocal folds as I A, but soft palate functions normally. II B: Bilateral lesion. Same effects on vocal folds as I B, but soft palate functions normally.

Diseases that cause Xth nerve lesions at this level are of several types: vascular, such as hemorrhage, thrombosis, and arteriovenous malformation; traumatic; primary or metastatic neoplastic; congenital defects of bone such as Arnold-Chiari malformation; inflammatory, such as poliomyelitis and Guillain-Barré syndrome; degenerative, such as amyotrophic lateral sclerosis; metabolic, exemplified by myasthenia gravis; toxic, such as metal (arsenic) or organic (botulism) poisoning; and others such as multiple sclerosis, diphtheria, and tetany.

2. *Extracranial lesions of the superior and recurrent laryngeal nerves but not the pharyngeal nerve* (Fig. 5–3, II A,B). Extracranial lesions high in the neck can spare the pharyngeal branch of the vagus but damage the nerve *above the origin of the superior and recurrent laryngeal nerves.* Because the pharyngeal nerve lies above the level of the lesion, the muscles of the soft palate and pharynx will be normal. However, because the superior and recurrent laryngeal branches lie below the level of the lesion, *the cricothyroid and remaining intrinsic muscles of the larynx will be paralyzed,* having the same effects on the vocal folds and voice as described in the previous section.

Causes of lesions below the bifurcation of the pharyngeal nerve but above the superior laryngeal include surgical trauma, infections, and idiopathic disease. The latter are discussed in greater detail later in this chapter.

3. *Extracranial lesions of the superior laryngeal nerve but not the pharyngeal and recurrent laryngeal nerves* (Fig. 5–3, III A,B). A lesion of the superior laryngeal nerve causes *weakness or paralysis of the cricothyroid muscle.* Because the pharyngeal and recurrent laryngeal branches are spared, the soft palate and remaining intrinsic laryngeal muscles are normal. On laryngoscopic

Table 5–1 Effect of Lesions of the Vagus Nerve on
Phonation and Resonation*

LEVEL OF LESION	EFFECT ON VOCAL FOLDS		EFFECT ON PHONATION	
	Unilateral Lesion	Bilateral Lesions	Unilateral Lesion	Bilateral Lesions
I. Above origin of pharyngeal, superior laryngeal, and recurrent laryngeal nerves	One vocal fold fixed in abducted position	Both vocal folds fixed in abducted position	Breathy, moderate, reduced loudness and pitch	Extremely breathy to whispered (aphonia)
II. Above origin of superior laryngeal and recurrent laryngeal nerves but below origin of pharyngeal nerve	Same as above	Same as above	Same as above	Same as above
III. Superior laryngeal nerve	Both vocal folds able to adduct, affected vocal fold shorter, asymmetric shift of epiglottis and anterior larynx toward intact side on phonation	Absence of tilt of thyroid on cricoid cartilage, inability to view full length of vocal folds because of epiglottic overhang, vocal folds bowed	Breathy, hoarse	Breathy, hoarse, reduced loudness, restricted pitch range
IV. Recurrent laryngeal nerve	One vocal fold fixed in paramedian position	Both vocal folds fixed in paramedian position	Breathy, hoarse, reduced loudness, diplophonia (not in all cases)	Breathy, hoarse, reduced loudness
V. Myoneural junction (myasthenia gravis)	Not applicable	Restriction of adductor-abductor movements	Not applicable	Breathy, hoarse, reduced loudness; symptoms worsen with sustained speaking

*Information in this table abstracted from: Rontal, M., and Rontal E.: Lesions of the vagus nerve: Diagnosis, treatment and rehabilitation. Laryngoscope, 87:72–86, 1977, and from Ward, P.H., Berci, G., and Calcaterra, J.C.: Superior laryngeal nerve paralysis: An often overlooked entity. Trans. Am. Acad. Ophthalmol. Otolaryngol., 84:78–89, 1977.

examination, the vocal folds appear deceptively normal. Consequently, dysphonia due to cricothyroid muscle weakness is often either missed or misdiagnosed as "functional." In unilateral cricothyroid paralysis, both vocal folds appear to adduct normally on phonation, but on closer scrutiny the vocal fold on the affected side *will appear shorter,* and an *asymmetric lateral shift of the epiglottis and anterior larynx toward the intact side* will be noted. In bilateral cricothyroid paralysis, there will be *an absence of tilt of the thyroid cartilage on the cricoid cartilage during phonation,* the vocal folds will *appear shorter than normal, the epiglottis will overhang and obscure the anterior portion of the vocal folds, and there will be bowing of the vocal folds* (Fig. 5–4). The soft palate will be normal because the pharyngeal branch of the vagus nerve has been spared. Unilateral cricothyroid muscle paralysis produces mild *breathiness or hoarseness,* normal or mildly *reduced loudness,* and mild *inability to alter pitch,* interfering with singing. In bilateral cricothyroid muscle paralysis, *breathiness and hoarseness* will be mild to moderate, *loudness will be reduced, and ability to alter pitch will be moderately to severely impaired,* causing serious

Table 5–1 Effect of Lesions of the Vagus Nerve on Phonation
and Resonation *Continued*

EFFECT ON SOFT PALATE		EFFECT ON NASAL RESONATION	ASSOCIATED SIGNS
UNILATERAL LESION	**BILATERAL LESIONS**		
One side low, immobile	Both sides low, immobile	Hypernasality, nasal emission	Glottal coup and cough absent, weak, or mushy; difficulty in swallowing; nasal regurgitation of food; aspiration of secretions; pharyngeal paralysis
None	None	None	Same as above, except no pharyngeal paralysis or difficulty in swallowing
None	None	None	None
None	None	None	Unilateral: Marginal airway, weak cough. Bilateral: Severe difficulty on inhaling for life purposes, inhalatory stridor, tracheostomy often necessary
Not applicable	Both sides low, immobile	Hypernasality, nasal emission; symptoms worsen with sustained speaking	Difficulty in swallowing, nasal regurgitation of food, inhalatory stridor, articulation defects

interference with singing. The cause of cricothyroid muscle paralysis is usually surgery or other trauma.

4. *Extracranial lesions of the recurrent laryngeal nerve but not the pharyngeal and superior laryngeal nerves* (Fig. 5–3, IV A,B). All muscles supplied by the recurrent laryngeal nerve are paralyzed, whereas those supplied by the remaining branches of the vagus, namely, the cricothyroid muscle and soft palate, are spared. The vocal folds are *fixed in the paramedian position unilaterally or bilaterally.* It is important to understand why the vocal folds are not paralyzed in the abducted position, as in the case of a lesion above the bifurcation of the superior laryngeal branch: *The intact cricothyroid muscle, still capable of stretching the vocal fold anteroposteriorly, acts as an adductor, thereby pulling the vocal fold closer to the midline.* Lesions above the level of the superior laryngeal nerve result in fixation of the vocal fold more laterally, in the abducted position (causing virtual aphonia), because the cricothyroid muscle as well as the remaining intrinsic muscles is paralyzed and unable to exert its adducting influence. In bilateral paralysis of the vocal folds due to

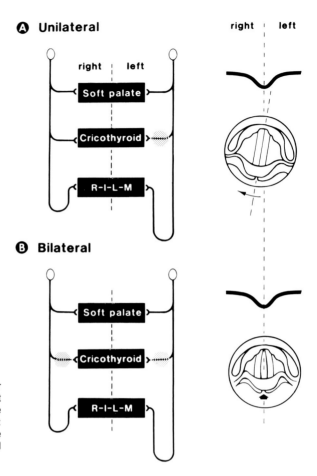

Figure 5–3 III A: Unilateral lesion of superior laryngeal nerve. Both vocal folds adduct, but the anterior larynx twists toward the intact side on phonation. The soft palate is normal. III B: Bilateral lesion. Both vocal folds adduct but are partially obscured by epiglottic overhang. Vocal folds are bowed. The soft palate is normal.

recurrent laryngeal nerve lesions only, *the vocal folds are adducted so close to the midline that phonation is virtually normal.* Paralysis of their abductors prevents widening of the glottis on inhalation, however, resulting in *inhalatory stridor* and compromising the airway. *Breathy-hoarse* quality, *reduced loudness,* and in some cases *diplophonia and falsetto pitch breaks* are heard in unilateral vocal fold paralysis from recurrent laryngeal nerve lesions.

Associated signs of unilateral vocal fold paralysis are a marginal airway and a weak cough or glottal coup. In bilateral paralysis, the airway is severely compromised, resulting in respiratory distress often requiring tracheostomy.

Conditions that cause recurrent laryngeal nerve lesions include trauma due to surgery, tumors of the nerve itself or impinging upon the nerve, vascular disease, infection, metabolic diseases, and idiopathic disorders.

Occasionally, inhalatory stridor can be mistaken for abductor vocal fold paralysis or an asthmatic attack when, in fact, these events, in all probability, are psychogenic (Patterson et al., 1974; Rogers and Stell, 1978; Cormier et al., 1981; Appelblatt and Baker, 1981; Kellman and Leopold, 1982; Rogers, 1980). Christopher et al. (1983) reported on five patients who had dramatic episodes of wheezing and who had been diagnosed as having uncontrolled asthma, symptoms that continued despite aggressive pharmacologic therapy. Laryngologic, psychiatric, and speech pathology studies, however, proved that these patients had a nonorganic disorder of the larynx that mimicked bronchial asthma. Indirect laryngoscopy disclosed that the asthmatic-like sounds were coming, not from the lungs, but from an unusual mode of glottic closure on inhalation and exhalation during tidal breathing. Psychiatric examinations indicated that all of the patients were unaware of their upper airway obstruction and thought that they were having bronchial asthmatic attacks. They were unable to reproduce the abnormal sound voluntarily. In all patients, treatment by a speech pathologist was effective and after 3 to 21 months' follow-up, these patients were asymptomatic.

A Unilateral

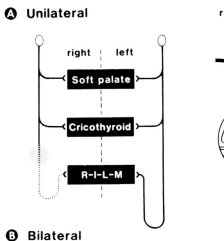

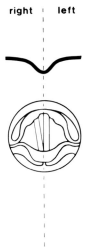

B Bilateral

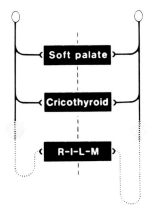

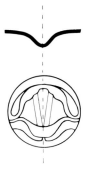

Figure 5–3   IV A: Unilateral lesion of recurrent laryngeal nerve. One vocal fold is fixed in a paramedian position on phonation, whereas the other adducts to the midline. The soft palate is normal. IV B: Bilateral lesion. Both vocal folds are fixed in a paramedian position on phonation. The soft palate is normal.

A Bilateral

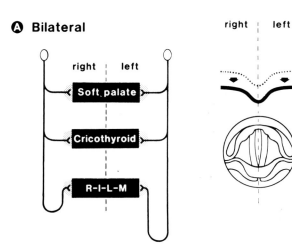

Figure 5–3   V A: Myoneural junction lesion (myasthenia gravis). There is bilateral paresis or paralysis of both adductor and abductor vocal fold movements on phonation and reduced or absent soft palate function.

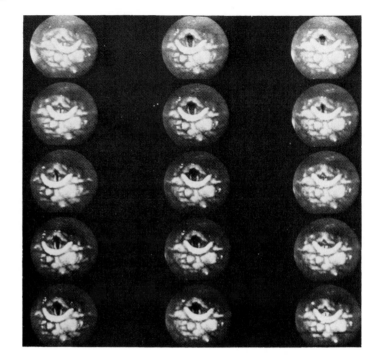

Figure 5–4 Frames from motion-picture photographs of vocal folds in bilateral cricothyroid muscle paralysis due to superior laryngeal nerve lesions. Absence of anterior tilt failing to lengthen and tense the vocal folds is noted by failure of anterior movement of the epiglottis, making it difficult to visualize the anterior commissure. Also visible is failure of complete vocal fold approximation on adduction due to bowing. (*From* Ward, P.H., Berci, G., and Calcaterra, T.C.: Superior laryngeal nerve paralysis: An often overlooked entity. Trans. Am. Acad. Ophthalmol. Otolaryngol., 84:78–89, 1977.)

What must be borne in mind, however, is that patients with *extrapyramidal movement disorders* also can produce laryngeal stridor at rest during tidal breathing because of adventitious adduction of the vocal folds as a component of the movement disorder. Moreover, sudden, paroxysmal inhalation often accompanies these stridorous inhalations.

5. *Myoneural junction disease: myasthenia gravis* (Fig. 5–3, V). The reduced availability of acetylcholine at the myoneural junction in myasthenia gravis causes progressive flaccid weakness or paralysis with strenuous muscular effort, as in prolonged voice use. Sometimes muscles supplied by the vagus nerve are the first to be affected by this disease. When it is confined to the larynx and soft palate, the signs often erroneously lead the examiner into nonorganic avenues of diagnostic thinking. Because myasthenia gravis causes bilateral weakness of the intrinsic laryngeal muscles, the *vocal folds adduct incompletely, sometimes bowing during phonation. Because abduction may be incomplete as well, inhalatory stridor occurs in more severe cases.* The soft palate elevates minimally or not at all on phonation, resulting in *hypernasality and nasal emission.* The voice of patients with myasthenia gravis is *breathy, sometimes hoarse, and flutter or tremorlike fluctuations* on vowel prolongation may be heard. *Loudness is usually reduced,* and there is a *restriction* of pitch range. All defects *become progressively worse with protracted speaking.*

Most often, myasthenia gravis produces the full complement of flaccid dysarthria: consonant imprecision due to associated tongue, lip, mandibular, and respiratory muscle weakness. The cough and glottal coup are weak or mushy, depending upon the severity of the disease at the time of examination. The etiology of myasthenia gravis has been described as a defect in the neurochemistry at the myoneural junction, specifically a failure of acetylcholine production. However, recent research gives evidence of an autoimmune mechanism responsible for the disorder.

6. *Disease of muscle.* The muscular dystrophies or myopathies can cause flaccid dysphonia. The three types of muscular dystrophies are the pseudohypertrophic (Duchenne), the limb-girdle, and the facioscapulohumeral (Landouzy-Dejerine). Their general features are a family history of disease, early age of onset, and atrophy or dystrophy of muscle. A heredofamilial type of myopathy is myotonic dystrophy, in which there is selective atrophy of muscles, including the speech musculature, resulting in flaccid dysarthria, including dysphonia. The masticatory and facial

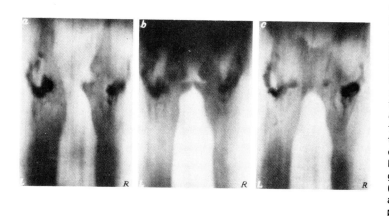

Figure 5–5 X-ray tomograms (posteroanterior) showing right vocal fold paralysis during quiet breathing, phonation, and effort closure. a: Quiet breathing. The paralyzed vocal fold projects into the airway. The smoothly contoured side is the normal side. b: Prolongation of the vowel /i/. The normal vocal fold adducts to meet the paralyzed one, giving a deceptively normal appearance, but there are asymmetric contours of the subglottic walls. c: Bearing down producing effort closure, illustrating the retained capacity for gross glottic closure activity. (*From* Ardran, G.M., Kemp, F.H., and Marland, P.M.: Laryngeal palsy. Br. J. Radiol., 27:201–209, 1954.)

muscles may be especially involved. The disease is progressive and appears for the first time in adulthood, between the ages of 20 and 30 years.

7. *Idiopathic vocal fold paralysis.* Some vocal fold paralyses defy diagnosis, that is, a specific etiology cannot be discovered despite thorough investigation. These are called "idiopathic" vocal fold paralyses.* Williams (1959) reviewed the records of patients with vocal fold paralysis over a six-year period; 66 of 181, or 36 percent, had an idiopathic disorder, consistent with the 33 percent found by New and Childrey (1932). The average duration was approximately 5½ months, after which spontaneous recovery occurred, although the dysphonia averaged one month longer than the vocal fold paralysis. The left vocal fold was paralyzed more often than the right. In the Williams study, the left vocal fold was paralyzed in 43 patients, or 65.2 percent, the right in 19, or 28.7 percent; and 4, or 6.1 percent, had bilateral paralyses. Blau and Kapadia (1972) consider idiopathic unilateral vocal fold paralysis to be one of the cranial mononeuropathies: A benign condition in which individual cranial nerve function is partially or totally impaired, the site of involvement undetermined, and the etiology unknown, and which has a high rate of spontaneous recovery within a period of nine months, as in the case of idiopathic Xth nerve interference.

Physiology of Flaccid Dysphonia. At the basis of the abnormally breathy and weak voice of flaccid vocal fold paralysis are an increased volume and velocity of air flow through the glottis and a failure of complete vocal fold vibration because of their flaccidity and improper position within the airway. The breathiness is produced by air turbulence as air flows through the glottis, which remains open throughout the glottic cycle. Posteroanterior tomograms of normal and paralyzed vocal folds are shown in Figure 5–5. In this figure, the tomogram labeled *a* is of a patient with right unilateral vocal fold paralysis in which the fold projects out into the glottis during quiet breathing. The following points are also notable.

1. The vocal fold on the normal left side is turned upward over the laryngeal ventricle, its free edge close to the lower surface of the ventricular fold. The laryngeal ventricle is barely visible.

2. On the paralyzed side, the vocal fold projects across the glottis, its edge close to the midline. The laryngeal ventricle is wide, and the ventricular fold is prominent and nearer to the midline than is the normal side.

3. The lateral wall of the subglottic space on the normal side is flattened or slightly convex, and on the paralyzed side, it is concave. The airway is consequently narrowed, and its central axis is deviated toward the normal side.

---

*As defined by *Dorland's Illustrated Medical Dictionary,* a morbid state of unknown causation or of spontaneous origin.

Figure 5–6 X-ray tomograms (posteroanterior) showing bilateral vocal fold paralysis during quiet breathing, phonation, and effort closure. a: Quiet breathing. Both vocal folds project into the airway. b: Prolongation of the vowel /i/. Incomplete adduction of true vocal folds and lack of demarcation between true and false folds are seen. c: Bearing down producing effort closure, illustrating the retained capacity for gross glottic closure activity. (*From* Ardran, G.M.,Kemp, F.H., and Marland, P.M.: Laryngeal palsy. Br. J. Radiol., 27:201–209, 1954.)

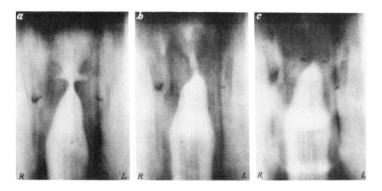

In *b*, the same patient is prolonging the vowel /i/. This illustration shows:

1. The normal vocal fold on the left approximates the paralyzed fold on the right and is aligned more horizontally with a thickened free edge.
2. On the paralyzed side, the vocal fold is tilted slightly upward, and its free edge is "tongue-shaped."
3. The laryngeal ventricle is larger on the paralyzed side.
4. The glottal slit appears to be displaced toward the paralyzed side.
5. The ventricular fold appears to be more prominent on the paralyzed side.

The tomogram *c* is of the patient during effort closure while bearing down. Despite the paralysis, effort closure is complete, demonstrating the compensatory ability of the sphincterlike closure mechanism, although in some patients the line of closure moves toward and beneath the vocal fold on the paralyzed side.

Posteroanterior tomograms of a patient with bilateral vocal fold paralysis are shown in Figure 5–6. Tomogram *a* illustrates quiet breathing, showing the vocal folds resting toward the midline, creating a narrower than normal glottis. On prolongation of the vowel /i/ (tomogram *b*), there is no demarcation between the true and false vocal folds, contrary to what is expected in the normal larynx. The axis of the vocal tract is asymmetric, and there is a wide glottal channel even during voice production. Tomogram *c* shows the same patient bearing down, again illustrating the reserve sphincter power of the larynx despite a bilateral vocal fold paralysis and inadequacy of phonation. In fact, all 15 patients examined by Ardran et al. (1954), despite their dysphonias and aphonia, were able to adduct the vocal folds during gross sphincteric effort closure.

Breathy voice quality and reduced loudness in unilateral and bilateral vocal fold paralysis, fewer syllables per exhalation, and more frequent inhalation during speech result from increased air flow through the glottis.

Hirano et al. (1968) obtained maximum phonation times, mean flow rates, and phonation quotients of patients who had vocal fold paralyses (Table 5–2). In 10 of 13 patients, maximum phonation time was shorter than normal, the product of excess expenditure of air. Mean flow rates in eight of the 13 patients were greater than normal, and in seven of 11 patients the phonation quotients were greater than normal. In three patients whose vocal folds had been injected with Teflon, clinical improvement was confirmed by an increase in maximum phonation time and a decrease in mean flow rate and phonation quotient. Ultraspeed motion picture studies of unilateral vocal fold paralyses show marked pitch and amplitude perturbations caused by the different rates of vibration of each vocal fold (Fig. 5–7).

Diplophonia, the simultaneous perception of two different pitches, is common in unilateral vocal fold paralysis. It is presumably caused by each vocal fold vibrating at a different frequency, owing

Table 5–2 Maximum Phonation Time, Mean Flow Rate and Phonation
Quotient in Cases of Vocal Cord Paralysis*

CASE	SEX	AGE (YR)	MAXIMUM PHONATION TIME (SEC)	MEAN FLOW RATE (CC/SEC)	PHONATION QUOTIENT (CC/SEC)	
43	M	39	14.4	205	331	Left, paramedian
44	M	45	3.9	382	1254	Left, intermediate, with atrophy
		45	18.7	125	261	After Teflon injection
45	M	59	5.8	484	559	Left, intermediate, with atrophy
		59	15.6	201	208	After Teflon injection
46	M	32	6.8	621	706	Left, intermediate, with atrophy
47	M	71	9.9	270	310	Left, intermediate
		71	24.1	117	128	After Teflon injection
48	M	78	21.6	99	141	Left, compensated
49	M	42	36.0	53	126	Right, compensated
50	F	29	7.6	280	*	Bilateral, paramedian
51	F	40	7.4	378	*	Bilateral, paramedian
52	F	67	18.8	92	160	Bilateral, paramedian
53	F	69	12.8	105	189	Bilateral, paramedian
54	F	64	8.1	309	316	Bilateral, paramedian
55	F	47	9.5	315	346	Right, intermediate
		47	20.6	145	160	Restricted abduction

*Respiratory tests inadequate.
*From Hirano, M., Koike, Y., and von Leden, H.: Maximum phonation time and air usage during phonation. Folia Phoniatr., 20:185–201, 1968.

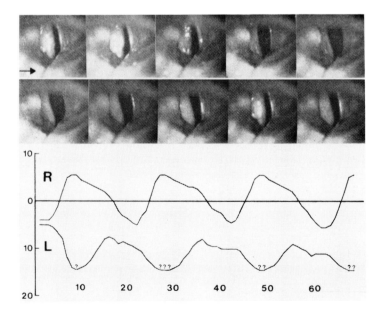

Figure 5–7 Frames from ultra-speed photography of unilateral vocal fold paralysis. Male larynx with paralysis of the left vocal fold. The sequence of photographs progresses from left to right in the top row followed by the same order in the second row. The graph illustrates the motions of the approximate anteroposterior midpoints of the glottal borders and demonstrates the absence of glottal closure, the crossing of an arbitrary median sagittal plane by the healthy vocal fold, the start of the lateral movements of the paralyzed vocal fold before the normal fold reaches its medial limit, and vibrations of both folds at the same frequency. (*From* Moore, G.P.: Observations on laryngeal disease, laryngeal behavior and voice. Ann. Otol. Rhinol. Laryngol., 85:553–564, 1976.)

to differences in their tensions. *Triplophonia,* three pitches being heard simultaneously, has also occurred.

Etiology of Vocal Fold Paralyses Producing Flaccid Dysphonia.   In a study of 633 cases of vocal fold paralysis, Huppler et al. (1955) found that the largest number, 272 patients, or 43 percent, were caused by thyroidectomy. The female to male ratio was 6:1, and in half the group, the vocal fold paralysis was bilateral. Cancer of the breast, thyroid gland, lung, tongue, mouth, pharynx, or larynx, as well as other primary and metastatic cancers of the neck, was the reason for surgery in these cases. Cardiovascular disease produced paralysis on the left side in all cases. The specific causes of heart disease were mitral stenosis, syphilitic aortitis and aneurysm, nonsyphilitic aneurysm, cardiomegaly, and congenital heart disease. Other causes of paralysis included specific neurologic diseases such as syringobulbia, poliomyelitis, and multiple sclerosis; trauma caused by automobile accidents, gunshot wounds, falls and blows to the neck, endotracheal intubation, bronchoscopy for an ingested foreign body; infections; tuberculosis; diphtheria; granuloma; and empyema. It is important to note that 184, or 29 percent, were idiopathic, as previously discussed.

> Vocal fold paralysis and flaccid dysphonia can occur as one of several signs in certain neurologic disease *syndromes.* In the *jugular foramen syndrome,* a lesion, usually a tumor, within or adjacent to the jugular foramen, compresses cranial nerves IX, X, and XI, causing ipsilateral weakness of the pharyngeal, laryngeal, trapezius and sternocleidomastoid muscles. Another syndrome is caused by posterior inferior cerebellar artery occlusion, producing infarction of the lateral medulla. Known as *Wallenberg's syndrome,* it is marked by dysarthria and dysphagia, ipsilateral impairment of pain and temperature sensation on the face, and contralateral loss of pain and temperature in the trunk and extremities. Because the nucleus ambiguus undergoes destruction, unilateral vocal fold paralysis and flaccid dysphonia occur. In general, any vascular or space-occupying lesion within the posterior fossa is capable of damaging one or both of the Xth nerve nuclei or their nerve trunks, causing unilateral or bilateral vocal fold paralysis and dysphonia.

Special Considerations in the Diagnosis of Flaccid Dysphonia: Myasthenia Gravis

   1. *Breathy voice and reduced loudness, even though the laryngologic examination is normal, ought to alert the clinician to the possibility of flaccid dysphonia due to lower motor neuron disease.*
   2. *Worsening of breathiness and weakness as a consequence of sustained effortful speaking ought to alert the clinician to the specific flaccid dysphonia of myasthenia gravis.* The fewer pathologic changes seen laryngologically, the more important is clinical listening. Bilateral, minimal weakness of the vocal folds is the most common reason for the failure to identify flaccid dysphonia laryngoscopically and is the reason such patients are often misdiagnosed as having functional or psychogenic voice disorders. It is important to remember that flaccid dysphonia can be the first sign of an encroaching neurologic disease of the peripheral nervous system. The dysphonia of myasthenia gravis is a classic example of a frequently misdiagnosed voice sign. Most of the time, it produces a complete dysarthria involving phonation, resonation, and articulation, and is not difficult to identify. (See Table 5–3 for a complete description of the dysarthria.) The changes of identification become considerably poorer when only one of the components of the peripheral speech mechanism is affected; the larynx is such a component. Several cases of monosymptomatic dysarthria in myasthenia gravis have been reported, as for example *hypernasality* (Wolski, 1967). Myasthenia gravis focal to the larynx producing *breathiness and weakness* without accompanying hypernasality or articulatory defect has also been reported (Neiman et al., 1975). In an article on early motor unit disease misdiagnosed as psychogenic dysphonia, Aronson (1971) reported the following case study.

*   *   *

> A 20-year-old secretary returned from vacation, and her parents noted that she had a weak voice. Two laryngologists and one internist diagnosed her voice change as "functional dysphonia." Yet psychiatric examination was unable to find a plausible psychologic explanation for her voice disorder. The following edited transcript of the intake interview shows the importance of history-taking in the diagnosis of voice disorders and how small clues can help the clinician think deductively about possible causes.

Clinician: When did all this speech business begin?

Patient: I was never one for speaking, because I was always quiet, but . . . I suppose this summer I've noticed, uh . . . well, its been called to my attention that I slur words.

C: What were you doing this summer when your voice disorder began?

P: Oh, I don't know. Like, I'd be sitting at the supper table and my words would seem all jumbled together. I think my parents were the first ones that called this to my attention. Ever since then I've caught myself.

C: Were you feeling well otherwise?

P: Yes. I had gone on vacation in May. I went down to the Bahamas about two weeks.

C: When you came back from vacation did you go right back to work?

P: Yes, like, I'd be on the phone a lot. My voice . . . first my throat, like my words wouldn't come out right . . . like they'd have to shove their way through.

C: Did you have any funny feelings in your throat?

P: Yeah, I've had difficulty swallowing. I mean, it doesn't hurt, or anything, it's just that it feels like a narrow passage . . . either when I am talking or swallowing.

C: Have you had any occasion to notice fluids coming through your nose as you swallowed?

P: Wait . . . like when I'm drinking like when it seems to go right up my nose?

C: Yes, how often?

P: Quite a bit of the time when I drink.

C: And that's something new?

P: Yes, it didn't happen before this summer. And, my mouth was always really dry. You know, like when you wake up in the morning? It feels like that all day.

C: Tell me, any emotional problems lately? Depressed at all? That kind of thing?

P: Hmm . . . Nothing exciting's happened, but I don't think I've been really depressed.

C: Your speech, you know, gives the impression of a certain lack of vitality. Not very vivacious. Are you that type of person?

P: No, when I was at college I was a cheerleader, and I was loud then.

C: You were loud then! (C. surprised at this description because of her extremely flat, lethargic effect.)

P: Yes, I mean, I could really belt it out, hours on end; but now, it's like I get tired inside, or something.

C: And that, again, has been true just since last summer?

P: Yes, I slowly noticed it.

C: How do you get along with your family at home?

P: Fine.

C: No problems especially around June? How about your love life? Anything developing there? Any disappointments?

P: I would like to get married next fall.

C: And, how long have you been going with this person?

P: About a year and a half.

C: Has this been a satisfactory relationship?

P: Uh huh.

C: I want to be sure that there isn't something that's really disappointing you, or . . . something that you're keeping back . . . because if there is, we'd like to know about it.

P: No. Truthfully, I can't say that there is any one thing that I've been depressed about.

C: When you say that there isn't any one thing, does that mean there are many things?

P: . . . No . . . (Long pause) . . . I don't know, I get nervous fast.

C: Tell me about that.

P: There's not much to say. I don't tolerate much. I know I should, but I just . . . I'm short-tempered . . . and, little things irritate me.

C: Like what, for example?

P: For example . . . like last week when I was here and we flew home and we flew over Chicago for an hour and a half . . . I was just madder than an old wet hen. And then they flew us back to Madison and we had to take the bus. (Laughs) I was just so nervous and uptight because of that. I was just so . . . I didn't want to talk to anybody.

C: Have you found this to be more apparent as of late? Or is this pretty much the way you've always been?

P: Hmm . . . I've always been kind of short-fused.

C: So this recent thing with the airline delay . . . your reaction didn't surprise you, particularly.

P: No, not really.

Physical examination of her peripheral speech musculature failed to disclose any obvious asymmetries or weakness of the lips, tongue, mandible, or soft palate at rest or during voluntary movement. Her general demeanor was introverted and expressionless, undoubtedly fostered by the low volume of her voice, its breathy quality, and the absence of pitch and inflectional

Table 5–3 Laryngeal-Phonatory Characteristics in the Flaccid Dysarthria of Myasthenia Gravis

FINDINGS	
Perceptual	
Phonation	Breathy voice quality, weak intensity. Deterioration of phonation during stressful counting or other prolonged speaking activities; reduced sharpness of cough after stressful speaking. Can exist in the absence of remaining signs of dysarthria
Resonation	Initially normal; hypernasality develops after stressful speaking
Articulation	Initially normal; articulatory imprecision develops after stressful speaking
Language	Normal
Physical	
Larynx	In milder cases, vocal folds may appear normal in structure and function despite dysphonia; absence of positive laryngologic findings does not exclude presence of milder degrees of bilateral adductor weakness of vocal folds. In more severe cases, folds may fail to adduct and abduct completely, bilaterally. Bowing may be present
Velopharynx	Initially normal; velopharyngeal insufficiency after stressful speaking. Hypoactive gag reflex
Tongue	Initially normal; tongue weakness after stressful speaking
Lips	Initially normal; lip weakness after stressful speaking; lateral smile
Teeth	Normal
Hard Palate	Normal
Mandible	Initially normal; mandibular muscle weakness after stressful speaking
General Medical	Patient may complain of general fatigue, particularly after exercise. Findings can be nonspecific, leading to erroneous diagnosis of functional illness
Other Neurologic Signs	
Peripheral Nervous System	Weakness of bulbar musculature; positive Tensilon test
Central Nervous System	Normal
Psychiatric/ Psychologic	Patient may complain of fatigue; loss of energy or loss of interest which may be erroneously diagnosed as signs of primary depression. Patients may become secondarily depressed, about lack of energy

variations. Her cough was possibly reduced in explosive power, but one could not be sure. *The test for fatigue of the motor speech mechanism in which the patient is asked to count rapidly and vigorously until told to stop revealed deterioration, not only of phonation in the direction of greater breathiness, but of palatopharyngeal and articulatory functions as well by the time the patient had reached the count of 90.* The number of syllables per exhalation began to drop because of air wastage at the glottis, and by the time the patient had reached 100 hypernasality and nasal emission had become apparent; one could feel vibration on the bridge of her nose during the production of non-nasal phonemes. By 150 her hypernasality and nasal emission had become clearly audible, and by 225 her articulation was markedly indistinct, the patient physically unable to continue.

The neurologic examination revealed mild but significant muscular weakness; there was a slightly greater width of the left palpebral fissure than the right, mild facial weakness on the left, mild diplopia on lateral gaze, bilateral weakness of the soft palate, and on repetition of the counting test of endurance, a similarly high degree of speech deterioration.

After speech deterioration due to prolonged counting, 0.2 ml. of edrophonium chloride (Tensilon) was administered intravenously. The patient had begun to count immediately after the injection, and approximately 30 seconds later audible improvement in her speech was noted, and according to the patient, it was approaching normal. Electromyography provided evidence of defective neuromuscular transmission in all muscles tested with repetitive electrical stimulation, and the diagnosis of flaccid dysphonia, and later dysarthria, due to myasthenia gravis was made.

* * *

A common clinical diagnostic trap is the interpretation of signs and symptoms as being psychogenic because the patient has a history of psychiatric illness. That the complaint can be organic in spite of such a history is illustrated in the following lesson learned by Ball and Lloyd (1971).

* * *

A slim, 16-year-old girl was admitted to the psychiatry ward following a series of arguments with her mother. She had been staying with an aunt who was a member of a religious sect in which "speaking with tongues" periodically occurred during times of religious ecstasy. Religion was continually held up to the patient as a way of salvation.

One day during an unusually emotional religious service, when the congregation was praying for the patient, she suddenly lost her voice. It returned spontaneously, but disappeared again on a similar occasion. She also complained of feeling tired and lacking energy. A few months later, she developed difficulty in swallowing food, suffered aspiration pneumonia, and had to be hospitalized. Physical examination, including neurologic studies, gave negative results, and the patient was placed under the care of a psychiatrist. It was his opinion that she was suffering from "hysteria," and a second psychiatrist described her as having a severe personality disturbance with schizoid features and as tending toward psychotic episodes.

In light of the previous negative physical findings, the disturbed family background, a schizophrenic mother, a premorbid history of shyness, and living with an aunt who placed great importance on "speech with tongues," a diagnostic formulation of hysterical aphonia, dysphagia, diplopia, and fatigue in a vulnerable personality would have been understandable. Instead, the patient was closely watched. Fatigability became obvious and confirmed the suspicion that the patient had an organic disease. Subsequently, myasthenia gravis was clearly demonstrated. Following treatment with pyridostigmine (Mestinon) and thymectomy, her condition improved. She became attractive and outgoing, developed a wide range of interests, and began working normally as a typist.

* * *

Equivocal and episodic physical signs in early myasthenia gravis are well known and are often precipitated by emotional stress, accounting for the disease's being commonly mistaken for a conversion reaction. This case illustrates the dangers of indiscriminate use of the "hysterical" diagnostic label, stresses the value of adequate neurologic training, and draws attention to the pitfalls resulting from reliance on preconceived ideas in diagnosis.

Occasionally, conversion dysphonia can masquerade as myasthenia gravis. Certain patients, because of knowledge of the disease gained through reading or contact with others who have had it, develop, on a conversion reaction basis, voice signs similar to those found in myasthenia gravis. By use of a control such as intravenous saline (the patient believing it to be Tensilon), the physician can establish whether, in fact, myasthenia gravis is present.

* * *

An 82-year-old former elementary school teacher was evaluated for a severely breathy dysphonia which had been diagnosed elsewhere as myasthenia gravis and for which she had been taking pyridostigmine (Mestinon). She was of the opinion that her dysphonia signified that she was being improperly treated for her disease. The neurologist began injecting *normal saline solution,* the patient believing that he was using Tensilon. As she began to count, by the time she had gotten to 10 her voice had become perceptively louder, and by 50 it had returned to normal. After informing the patient that she did not have myasthenia gravis, we found that her dysphonia was psychogenic and related to increasing irritation with her hard-of-hearing husband, with whom she found she could no longer communicate. Her voice disorder was eventually diagnosed properly as a conversion reaction.

* * *

Myasthenia gravis is a neuromuscular disease manifested by weakness and fatigability of striated muscles. Although its clinical features were isolated by the beginning of the 20th century, only recently has the mechanism of the weakness been identified: a reduction of available acetylcholine receptors at the neuromuscular junction caused by autoimmune mechanisms.

Muscle contraction is dependent upon stimulation of the motor endplate by the neurochemical transmitter acetylcholine, which is synthesized in the motor nerve terminals and is stored in vesicles. Each vesicle or "quantum" contains about 10,000 acetylcholine molecules. When a nerve impulse is transmitted down the axon of the lower motor neuron, the acetylcholine is released at specific sites opposite acetylcholine receptors on the postsynaptic membranes. When the acetylcholine combines with its receptors, a transient increase in membrane permeability to sodium and potassium ions results in muscle depolarization. This process is extremely swift, occurring in milliseconds, and is terminated by removal of acetylcholine by diffusion away from the myoneural junction and by the counteraction of acetylcholinesterase, which hydrolyzes the acetylcholine. The amplitude of depolarization is directly related to the number of acetylcholine molecules that stimulate receptor molecules. Any reduction of acetylcholine receptor interactions below a safety margin will result in failure of neuromuscular transmission, a principle necessary to the understanding of the decrement of muscle strength in myasthenia gravis.

SPASTIC (PSEUDOBULBAR) DYSPHONIA: PYRAMIDAL SYSTEM LESIONS

The remaining neurologic dysphonias are caused by supranuclear lesions, that is, lesions *above* the level of the Xth nerve nucleus and within the central nervous system (CNS). Not much is known about normal CNS control over the Xth nerve, although probably corticobulbar tracts synapse with vagus nerve nuclei in the same way as they do with the other cranial nerve nuclei. However, it is also likely that vagus nerve nuclei receive a disproportionately larger share of subcortical innervation to facilitate reflex laryngeal function, owing to its important life-sustaining responsibility. Such subcortical representation is substantiated by clinical and experimental evidence that phonation is preserved despite congenital absence of cerebral tissue and massive surgical, traumatic, infectious, or degenerative destruction of the cerebral hemispheres. What is singular about CNS control over the final common pathway to the larynx is the apparent extensive neural redundancy of the system in order to ensure the organism's survival, and the bilaterality of its laryngeal functions. The integration of the two sides of the larynx is such that under normal conditions, a discoordinated movement between the vocal folds has never been reported; what one side of the larynx does the other does simultaneously and equally, as if both right and left halves of the larynx were under the control of a single CNS center—unlike the unilateral control of the extremities and the lower facial musculature.

The Xth nerve nuclei are under the influence of both pyramidal and extrapyramidal systems. Voluntary control over the larynx is accomplished through the pyramidal system, sometimes

Laryngeal primary motor area of cerebral cortex

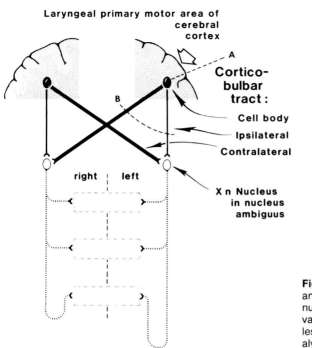

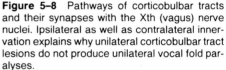

Cortico-bulbar tract:

— Cell body
— Ipsilateral
— Contralateral

X n Nucleus in nucleus ambiguus

right | left

Figure 5–8 Pathways of corticobulbar tracts and their synapses with the Xth (vagus) nerve nuclei. Ipsilateral as well as contralateral innervation explains why unilateral corticobulbar tract lesions do not produce unilateral vocal fold paralyses.

referred to as the "direct activating system," and neuroanatomically known as the *corticobulbar tracts*. Figure 5–8 schematizes the following.

1. The corticobulbar tracts begin in the *percentral gyri* of both cerebral hemispheres.

2. They descend as the *corona radiata*, become condensed in the *internal capsule*, and pass through the *cerebral peduncles*.

3. At the upper border of the *medulla*, some of the fibers cross over (decussate) to the other side of the brainstem, where they synapse with vagal nuclei in the nucleus ambiguus. The remainder synapse with vagal nuclei on the same (ipsilateral) side. *The implications of such bilateral corticobulbar innervation is that rarely, if ever, will a unilateral cortical or corticobulbar tract lesion cause unilateral vocal fold paralysis.* Such is not the case when the cell bodies or axons of the corticobulbar tracts are damaged *bilaterally.* Then, a characteristic and often severe dysphonia called *pseudobulbar* (spastic) dysphonia is heard, the voice having a *harsh, strained-strangled quality, abnormally low pitch, monopitch, monoloudness, and reduced loudness.* Rarely, however, does the dysphonia occur in the absence of its accompanying dysarthria. (See Table 5–4 for a summary of signs found in spastic [pseudobulbar] dysarthria.)

The strained-strangled, harsh voice quality is caused by hyperadduction of the true and false vocal folds, i.e., glottic constriction and resistance to the exhalatory airflow. Such spastic overadduction of the folds is undoubtedly due to the release of inhibition of excitatory nerve impulses transmitted to vagal nuclei.

Physiologic and acoustic studies of spastic (pseudobulbar) dysphonia are limited. Mean airflow rate is decreased in patients who phonate with hyperadduction of the vocal folds (von Leden, 1968), and fundamental frequency and frequency range are restricted (Kammermeier, 1969).

The pseudobulbar cry and laugh are seriously incapacitating signs associated with bilateral corticobulbar tract damage. This *reduced threshold for crying and laughter* has clinical diagnostic importance and needs to be recognized as one of the great social and psychologic burdens borne by patients with pseudobulbar palsy. According to Kreindler and Pruskauer-Apostol (1971):

1. Pseudobulbar laughter and crying seem to occur without adequate cause, often in response to nonspecific stimuli, although they are readily triggered by human interaction. The patient may be quiescent for a long period until addressed by another person, at which point spasmodic laughter or crying occurs after a short latency, somewhat in proportion to the amount of emotional loading of the question, statement, or situation.

2. There is an incongruity between the patient's inner emotional state and his external appearance of joy or melancholy; patients admit with embarrassment that they cry and laugh without experiencing the inner emotions usually associated with their outbursts.

3. The crying and laughter occur abruptly without the normal graded approach of a smile or frown prior to the full-blown laugh or cry. Because of this, such outbursts convey the impression of being stereotyped, automatic, and paroxysmal.

Table 5–4   Laryngeal-Phonatory Characteristics in
Pseudobulbar (Spastic) Dysarthria

FINDINGS	
Perceptual	
Phonation	Hoarseness or harshness having a strained-strangled quality. Pitch is abnormally low. Monopitch. Loudness is reduced. Monoloudness. Almost never occurs without accompanying signs of dysarthria. Inappropriate crying or laughter may be present
Resonation	Hypernasality
Articulation	Imprecise consonants; abnormally slow rate
Language	Normal, provided language areas are spared
Physical	
Larynx	Vocal folds appear normal in structure. Normal to hyperadduction of true and false vocal folds may occur bilaterally
Velopharynx	Bilateral velopharyngeal insufficiency. Hyperactive gag reflex
Tongue	Topographically normal. May be smaller, more contracted than normal. Tongue weakness. Slow alternate motion rate (AMR) on lateral movements and on /tʌ/ and /kʌ/ syllable repetitions
Lips	Weak, slow movements on AMR for /pʌ/
Teeth	Normal
Hard Palate	Normal
Mandible	Slow AMR
General Medical	Nonspecific
Other Neurologic Signs	
Peripheral Nervous System	*Normal*
Central Nervous System	Signs of spasticity
Psychiatric/ Psychologic	Nonspecific. Pseudobulbar crying and laughter may give erroneous impression of emotional lability and intellectual deterioration

4. The cry or laugh is impossible to interrupt or modify; it is virtually involuntary.

5. The degree of facial, thoracic, and abdominal muscle contraction visibly and incongruously exceeds accompanying phonatory signs of crying, laughter, or tears. *One acoustic characteristic of the cry is a long wail that rises in pitch, often reaching falsetto levels.* At times the crying will be produced with an unvoiced airstream, aptly described as "mute grimacing."

6. The patient may switch back and forth between crying and laughter without reason, giving the erroneous impression of emotional lability.

Such patients are subject to misinterpretation as being not only emotionally unstable but demented as well, a presumption not supported by a study of 60 patients who had pseudobulbar palsy. In this study, it was found that when intelligence test scores were adjusted for age and slowness of response caused by the spasticity, the patients performed as well as normal controls.

Lesions that produce pathologic laughter can be located in the corticobulbar tracts and beyond. Involuntary laughter has been reported in patients with tumors of the brainsteam and hypothalamus, caused by either stimulation of the floor of the third ventricle or infarction of the temporal lobe (Aschari and Colover, 1976; Haymaker and Kuhlenbeck, 1976). Other studies have implicated the internal capsule and surrounding basal ganglia.

Pseudobulbar palsy can result from any lesion of the corticobulbar tracts bilaterally; vascular and degenerative diseases involving the motor cortical areas bilaterally, vascular diseases and tumors of the internal capsule or brainstem, degenerative diseases involving the entire corticobulbar tract system, and infectious diseases.

MIXED FLACCID-SPASTIC (PSEUDOBULBAR) DYSPHONIA: XTH (VAGUS) NERVE AND PYRAMIDAL TRACT LESIONS

Dysphonias in mixed dysarthria produce the voice signs of each dysarthric component simultaneously. A common example is the mixed dysarthria in flaccid-spastic paralysis as exemplified by *amyotrophic lateral sclerosis* (ALS). A degenerative disease of bilateral corticobulbar tracts and lower motor neuron nuclei, spastic and flaccid paralysis and associated dysarthrias occur simultaneously, although the proportion of one over the other varies from patient to patient and within a given patient, depending upon the stage of the disease. Should the paralysis be predominantly spastic, hyperadduction of the true and false vocal folds will be seen, and the effect will be a primarily spastic or pseudobulbar dysphonia. If the disease expresses itself primarily as flaccid weakness, hypoadduction of one or both vocal folds will be seen on laryngologic examination, and the dysphonia will be predominantly flaccid. Pooling of saliva in the pyriform sinuses is common.

The dysphonia of mixed, flaccid-spastic dysarthria is typically a *harsh, strained-strangled sound* with degrees of *breathiness, reduced loudness, audible inhalation, and "wet hoarseness."* The "wet" or gurgly sounding voice is due to the accumulation of saliva in the pyriform sinuses and on the vocal folds resulting from the reduced frequency of swallowing. *Rapid tremor or flutter* on vowel prolongation, also noted in pure flaccid dysphonia, is common. Although the frequency of the flaccid "flutter" is yet to be quantified by research, we estimate that the range is from 9 to 12 Hz. Figure 5–9 is a comparison between the vowel prolongation of a normal subject and that of a patient with ALS. Note the considerable difference between the rapid undulations in the vowel prolongation of the patient with ALS and the relatively smooth output of the normal subject. (Table 5–5 is a summary of the mixed dysarthria of ALS.)

Carrow et al. (1974) analyzed and rated the dysarthrias of 79 patients, aged 20 to 65 years, who had motor neuron disease, including ALS. Speech samples were rated on a 1 to 7 scale of severity, 1 being normal and 7 severe (Table 5–6). Approximately 80 percent had harsh voice quality, 75 percent hypernasality, 65 percent breathy voice quality, 63 percent voice tremor, 60 percent strained-strangled quality, 41 percent audible inhalation, 38 percent excessively high pitch, and 8 percent excessively low pitch. It is apparent that dysphonia is a prominent and incapacitating characteristic of motor neuron disease.

The terms "motor neuron disease" and "amyotrophic lateral sclerosis" (ALS) are often used interchangeably, although it is preferable to use the term "ALS" only when pyramidal tract signs predominate. In patients in whom lower motor neuron signs are the most prominent, the term "progressive muscular atrophy" (PMA) is used. The peak incidence of motor neuron disease is in the fifth to seventh decades of life, with ALS occurring slightly later than PMA. The male to female sex ratio in ALS is 3:2, and in PMA it is 5:1. The disease presents with brainstem, i.e., bulbar, palsy in 30 percent of cases and progresses more rapidly than the spinal form, with death usually occurring within three years. Fasciculations are seen more often in ALS. Speech disturbance is considered to be the earliest sign in the bulbar type, according to Rose (1977), who states that the bilabial plosives are affected first owing to facial muscle weakness, the patient initially noticing difficulty in whistling. Palatal weakness causing hypernasality and nasal emission is usually, but not always, symmetric. The mandible droops, particularly in the pseudobulbar variety. The tongue is flaccid and atrophic, and it fasciculates.

The etiology of ALS is unknown. Theories include viral infection, the effect of malignancy, and, in the familial form, a genetic deficit of neuronal enzymes. An endemic form has been described in Guam among the Chamorro people, where the incidence is the highest in the world (57 percent). The most common causes of death are respiratory failure, pneumonia, and pulmonary infarction.

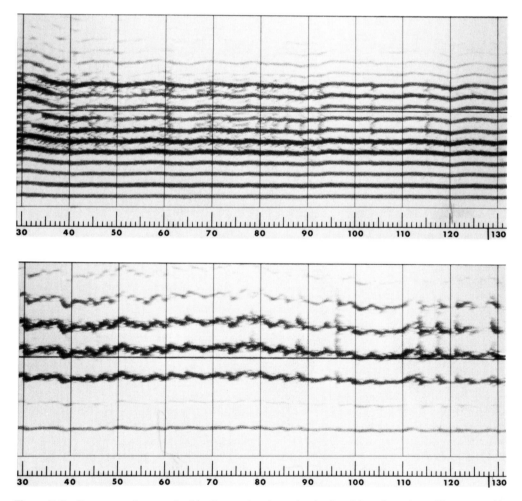

Figure 5–9   Sonogram of a normal subject's vowel prolongation (top) and that of a patient with amyotrophic lateral sclerosis (bottom). Note the relatively smooth tracing of the normal subject compared with the rapid undulations indicating the flaccid "flutter" of the patient with ALS. (50 mm = 1 sec.)

Table 5–5 Laryngeal-Phonatory Characteristics in the Mixed
Dysarthria of Amyotrophic Lateral Sclerosis*

FINDINGS	
Perceptual	
Phonation	Hoarseness or harshness having a strained-strangled quality; "wet" or "gurgly" component. Rapid tremor or "flutter" on vowel prolongation. Breathy if strong flaccid component; pitch is abnormally low. Monopitch. Loudness is reduced. Monoloudness. Inhalatory stridor if severe. Reduced sharpness of cough. Inappropriate crying or laughter may be present
Resonation	Hypernasality; nasal emission
Articulation	Imprecise consonants; abnormally slow rate
Language	Normal
Physical	
Larynx	Vocal folds appear normal in structure. If major component is spastic, vocal folds appear to adduct normally or may hyperadduct, along with false vocal folds. Adduction may be bilaterally symmetric, or one vocal fold may adduct less fully than the other. If there is a major flaccid component, vocal folds may adduct and abduct with less than normal excursions
Velopharynx	Bilateral velopharyngeal insufficiency, possibly asymmetric. Hyperactive gag reflex
Tongue	Topographically abnormal. Furrowed and reduced in size owing to atrophy. Fasciculations. Weakness. Slow AMR on lateral movements and on /tʌ/ and /kʌ/ syllable repetitions
Lips	Weak. Slow movements on AMR for /pʌ/
Teeth	Normal
Hard Palate	Normal
Mandible	Slow AMR
General Medical	Nonspecific
Other Neurologic Signs	
Peripheral Nervous System	Signs of flaccid paralysis
Central Nervous System	Signs of spasticity
Psychiatric/ Psychologic	Nonspecific. Pseudobulbar crying and laughter may give erroneous impression of emotional lability and intellectual deterioration

*Basically same as in any other nervous system disease affecting both pyramidal and lower motor neuron tracts bilaterally.

HYPOKINETIC (PARKINSONIAN) DYSPHONIA: BASAL GANGLIA LESIONS

The basal ganglia have both subcortical and cortical connections. This portion of the extrapyramidal system modulates nerve impulses to lower motor neurons. Damage to the substantia nigra in

Table 5–6   Abnormal Voice Dimensions in 79 Patients with Motor Neuron
Disease (ALS) Exhibiting Abnormal Voice Characteristics

DIMENSION	AFFECTED PERCENTAGE
Harsh Voice	79.95
Hypernasality	74.68
Breathy Voice	64.56
Voice Tremor	63.29
Strained-Strangled Voice	59.49
Audible Inspiration	40.51
High Pitch	37.97
Low Pitch	7.59

From Carrow, E., Rivera, V., Mauldin, M., and Shamblin, L. Deviant speech characteristics in motor neuron disease. Arch. Otolaryngol., 100:212–218, 1974.

the basal ganglia releases inhibition of nerve impulses to the lower motor neuron, causing rigidity and slowness of movements. When the speech muscles are affected, the dysarthria of parkinsonism, i.e., hypokinetic dysarthria, occurs (Table 5–7).

The dysphonia of parkinsonism consists of *reduced loudness and monopitch* (Darley et al., 1969a and b). In a study of 200 parkinsonian patients undertaken by Logemann et al. (1978), 178, or 89 percent, had signs of laryngeal dysfunction; 30, or ⅃5 percent, had *breathy voice quality;* 58, or 29 percent, had *roughness;* 90, or 45 percent, had *hoarseness;* and 27, or 13.5 percent, had *tremulousness* of voice. The characteristically monopitched voice arises from the rigidity and reduced range of motion of the intrinsic and extrinsic laryngeal muscles. Pitch change requires that the strap muscles elevate and lower the larynx, that the vocal folds be stretched and loosened by cricothyroid muscle contraction and relaxation, and that infraglottal air pressure be increased and reduced. If the laryngeal and respiratory musculature is rigid, as in parkinsonism, range of motion will be diminished. Controlled changes of infraglottal air pressure, necessary for the stress and emphasis of normal prosody, appear to be lacking in parkinsonian patients, whose respirations are not only shallow owing to the reduced range of motion of thoracic and abdominal muscle, but whose discrete chest pulses are diminished or absent, as well. The loss of variation in emphasis and stress in contextual speech is what gives the overall effect of flattening of prosody.

Clinicians need to be alert to *reduced loudness and breathy voice quality* as a sign of early hypokinetic dysarthria, even though remaining signs of the dysarthria and nonspeech signs of parkinsonism are not *apparent*. Such patients are frequently misdiagnosed as having "functional" dysphonia.

* * *

A year before coming to the Clinic, a 64-year-old minister had a coronary attack. He had been working exceptionally hard and had been under much stress trying to minister to a parish with insufficient funds. During the year following his attack, he noticed a diminution in the loudness of his voice and described it as "muffled." He revealed that, in his opinion, he might also have had a slight "stroke," because his left side seemed weak and his gait unsteady.

Laryngoscopic examination detected little in the way of laryngeal pathologic changes, the only finding being a slightly greater than normal space in the interarytenoid region of the glottis during phonation. A diagnosis of functional voice disorder was made.

On closer scrutiny, however, the patient's alternate motion rates on /p $\land$ /, /t $\land$ /, and /k $\land$ / appeared slightly accelerated and were produced with a less than full range of motion. The patient admitted to a slowing of his thinking during the year and a change in his handwriting.

Neurologic examination confirmed the presence of early parkinsonism. Although no single sign was convincing, when the speech, mild masking of facial expression, reduced arm swing, and cogwheeling of extremities were assembled, they argued strongly in favor of this neurologic diagnosis.

* * *

Table 5–7 Laryngeal-Phonatory Characteristics in the
Hypokinetic Dysarthria of Parkinsonism

FINDINGS	
Perceptual	
Phonation	Monopitch; reduced stress; monoloudness; reduced loudness; harsh voice quality; breathy voice quality. *Note:* Reduced loudness and breathiness in the absence of other neurologic signs can indicate early parkinsonism
Resonation	Normal
Articulation	Imprecise consonants; short rushes of speech; accelerated rate; stuttering-like repetitions of syllables, words, or phrases (palilalia)
Language	Usually normal. Language functions may be decreased as part of overall slowing of general intellectual processes
Physical	
Larynx	Vocal folds appear normal in structure. Adductor, abductor movements are bilaterally symmetric, but there may be incomplete closure of vocal folds, accounting for breathy voice quality
Velopharynx	Normal
Tongue	Topographically normal. Alternate motor rates (AMRs) for /tʌ/ and /kʌ/ sound rapid and are reduced in amplitude of movement
Lips	AMRs for /pʌ/ sound rapid and are reduced in amplitude of movement
Teeth	Normal
Hard Palate	Normal
Mandible	Reduced range of motion during articulation
General Medical	Nonspecific
Other Neurologic Signs	
Peripheral Nervous System	Normal
Central Nervous System	Signs of hypokinesia elsewhere in the body. *Note:* Hypokinetic dysarthria in *the form of dysphonia only can be the first sign of early parkinsonism*
Psychiatric/ Psychologic	Nonspecific. Masked facies may give the erroneous impression of flatness of affect or of depression

Motion picture studies of the vocal folds during phonation in 30 patients with Parkinson's disease disclosed a direct relationship between breathiness, and reduced loudness, and increasing amounts of glottic gap and bowing of the vocal folds (Hanson et al., 1984).

Physical measurements of respiration in hypokinetic dysarthria prove that such patients have shallow irregular breathing, pause between respirations, and experience periods of increased depth of respiration that alternate with periods of respiratory arrest. Postencephalitic parkinsonism patients have shallow respiration of twice the normal frequency; negligible differences between

Table 5–8   Laryngeal-Phonatory Characteristics in Ataxic Dysarthria

FINDINGS	
Perceptual	
Phonation	Frequently normal. Others have harsh voice quality, monopitch, monoloudness, excess and equal stress on ordinarily unstressed words or syllables, excess loudness, bursts of loudness, and coarse voice tremor
Resonation	Normal
Articulation	Imprecise consonants; irregular articulatory breakdown; distorted vowels; slow rate
Language	Normal
Physical	
Larynx	Vocal folds appear normal in structure and function
Velopharynx	Normal
Tongue	Topographically normal. Irregular and slow alternate motion rates (AMRs) on /tʌ/ and /kʌ/ and on lateral tongue movements
Lips	Irregular and slow AMRs for /pʌ/
Teeth	Normal
Hard Palate	Normal
Mandible	Normal
General Medical	Nonspecific. *Note*: Ataxic dysarthria may be a sign of moderate to severe hypothyroidism and drug and alcohol abuse
Other Neurologic Signs	
Peripheral Nervous System	Normal
Central Nervous System	Signs of ataxia
Psychiatric/ Psychologic	Nonspecific

vegetative, deep, and speech breathing; smaller than normal vital capacities; air wastage before speaking; and exhalations repeatedly interrupted by small inhalations (Darley et al., 1975).

Canter (1963) found that parkinsonism patients read orally at a median fundamental frequency of 129 Hz, which was statistically significantly higher than the median frequency of 102 Hz found in a control group of normal subjects. A similar increase in fundamental frequency was found by Kammermeier (1969). Schilling (cited by Darley et al., 1975), on the other hand, found pitch range to be considerably decreased. The results of studies of vocal intensity in parkinsonism are equivocal. Although they fail to prove that parkinsonian patients phonate at lower intensity levels, one's clinical impression is certainly that of reduced loudness. Perhaps one reason that controlled studies fail to prove quantitatively reduced loudness in parkinsonian patients is their paradoxic ability to produce louder voice on demand but not spontaneously.

Arrhythmically Fluctuating Neurologic Voice Disorders

ATAXIC DYSPHONIA: CEREBELLAR LESIONS

The cerebellum coordinates muscles and regulates skilled movements. Contained within the skull's posterior fossa, the cerebellum consists of an *anterior lobe, a posterior lobe,* and a *flocculonodular lobe.* It connects with the brainstem and structures above and below it by means of incoming and outgoing fibers that pass through the inferior, middle, and superior cerebellar peduncles to brainstem nuclei, the dentate nucleus, the thalamus, and the cerebral cortex. Of the many functions of the cerebellum, including equilibrium, posture, and gait, the posterior lobes are particularly

Table 5–9 Laryngeal-Phonatory Characteristics in the Hyperkinetic Dysarthria of Chorea

FINDINGS	
Perceptual	
Phonation	Intermittently harsh, strained-strangled voice quality; transient breathiness; distorted vowels; monopitch; excess loudness variations; monoloudness; excess, equal stress on ordinarily unstressed words or syllables; reduced stress; sudden forced inspiration/expiration
Resonation	Intermittent hypernasality
Articulation	Imprecise consonants; distorted vowels; prolonged intervals between syllables and words; variable rate; inappropriate silences; prolonged phonemes; short phrases; irregular articulatory breakdown
Language	Normal. Defective in patients who have undergone intellectual deterioration
Physical	
Larynx	Vocal folds appear normal in structure; intermittent hyperadduction
Velopharynx	Normal in appearance
Tongue	Topographically normal. Quick unpatterned movements at rest and during (AMRs) for /tʌ/, and /kʌ/, which are irregular
Lips	Quick unpatterned movements at rest and during AMRs for /pʌ/
Teeth	Normal
Hard Palate	Normal
Mandible	Quick asymmetric movements at rest and during speech
General Medical	Nonspecific
Other Neurologic Signs	
Peripheral Nervous System	Normal
Central Nervous System	Choreic movements elsewhere in the body
Psychiatric/ Psychologic	Intellectual and behavior changes associated with dementia, if present

concerned with voluntary movements. Lesions in this area result in a loss of muscle coordination, known as dyssynergia; a loss of the ability to measure range of motion, known as dysmetria; and tremor during voluntary movement, known as intention tremor. General movements are clumsy and uncoordinated (Daube et al., 1978).

Whether or not dysphonia is present may depend upon the severity of the ataxia. The dysphonia may take one of several forms: *sudden bursts of loudness, irregular increases in pitch and loudness* or *coarse voice tremor* (Table 5–8).

HYPERKINETIC (CHOREIC) DYSPHONIA: BASAL GANGLIA LESIONS

Quick, jerky, irregular, and unpredictable movements caused by lesions of the basal ganglia, probably the caudate nucleus, are found in Sydenham's chorea in children and Huntington's chorea, the hereditary type, in adults. In addition to the sudden uncontrolled movements of the lips, tongue, and mandible, movements of the respiratory and laryngeal musculature produce *irregular pitch fluctuations and voice arrests,* giving speech a jerky quality. In a study done by Darley et al., (1969a, b), the following phonatory aberrations were found: *sudden forced inspiration or expiration; harsh voice quality; excess loudness variations; strained-strangled phonation; mono-pitch; monoloudness; reduced stress; transient breathiness; and voice arrests.* (Table 5–9 summarizes the hyperkinetic dysarthria of chorea.)

HYPERKINETIC (DYSTONIC) DYSPHONIA: BASAL GANGLIA LESIONS

A slower form of hyperkinesia known as "dyskinesia" or "dystonia" is manifested by repetitive, slow, twisting, writhing, or flexing movements of the musculature. When only the speech musculature is affected, the terms "*orofacial dyskinesia*" or "*focal mouth dystonia*" are employed. In addition to vascular, degenerative, or mass lesions, this movement disorder can result from prolonged use of psychotropic and antiparkinsonian drugs. In cases caused by drug therapy, the dyskinesia does not appear until after prolonged use, and so the term "*tardive dyskinesia*" is used in reference to the late (tardy) appearance of the dyskinesia (Portnoy, 1979).

In addition to rounding, pursing, protruding, and lateralizing lip movements and tongue protrusion, rotation, and lateralization, similarly uncontrolled adductor and abductor laryngeal spasms cause *strained hoarseness* and *breathiness,* and sometimes paroxysmal *inhalatory stridor.* A form of dystonia involving the entire body is *dystonia musculorum deformans.* This disorder can produce profound laryngeal spasms that cause a highly strained or groaning dysphonia of a waxing and waning character.

Athetosis, also a slow hyperkinesia that is commonly seen in cerebral palsy, produces similar strained hoarseness and breathiness in addition to the writhing movements of the head, neck, torso, and extremities. In a study done by Darley et al. (1969a,b), patients who had dystonia gave evidence of *harsh, strained-strangled voice; excess loudness variations; voice arrests; short phrases; monopitch, monoloudness; reduced stress; inappropriate silences; and excess and equal stress on all syllables of words.* (Table 5–10 summarizes the hyperkinetic dysarthria of dystonia.)

Rhythmically Fluctuating Neurologic Voice Disorders

ORGANIC (ESSENTIAL) VOICE TREMOR

Voice tremor is a component of the essential tremor syndrome, called "benign heredofamilial tremor" when familial. *The voice tremor can be monosymptomatic* without evidence of tremor elsewhere in the body or can accompany the full syndrome of tremor of the upper limbs, head, face, or neck musculature. The rate ranges most often from 4 to 7 c./sec., and this tremor must be distinguished from those associated with parkinsonism, cerebellar disease, thyrotoxicosis, and anxiety. Normal humans have small tremor amplitudes of 6 to 12 c./sec. at rest and during intentional movements (Brumlik, 1962). Normal physiologic tremor has been reported in children at 5 or 6 c./sec. and in young adults at 10 c./sec., the change in rate taking place during puberty (Marshall, 1962). After about age 40 years, the tremor begins to decline from 10 to 6 c./sec.

Table 5–10 Laryngeal-Phonatory Characteristics in the
Hyperkinetic Dysarthria of Dystonia

FINDINGS	
Perceptual	
Phonation	Slow, continuous changes in strained-hoarse quality; breathiness; excess loudness variations; voice arrests; monopitch; monoloudness; reduced stress; excess and equal stress on ordinarily unstressed syllables and words
Resonation	Normal
Articulation	Imprecise consonants; distorted vowels; short phrases; inappropriate silences
Language	Normal. May be defective if dysarthria is associated with focal language disorders or diffuse intellectual disorders
Physical	
Larynx	Vocal folds appear normal in structure and function; intermittent hyperadduction
Velopharynx	Normal
Tongue	Topographically normal. Slow, unpatterned protusive, lateral, and rotatory movements at rest and during speech. AMR's on /tʌ/ and /kʌ/ are slow and highly irregular
Lips	Slow unpatterned lip rounding and spreading. Alternate motion rates for /pʌ/ are slow and highly irregular
Teeth	Normal
Hard Palate	Normal
Mandible	Slow unpatterned depression, lateralization, and elevation
General Medical	Nonspecific
Other Neurologic Signs	
Peripheral Nervous System	Normal
Central Nervous System	Signs of dystonia may be confined to larynx or may occur elsewhere in the body
Psychiatric/ Psychologic	Nonspecific. Intellectual and behavioral aberrations present if diffuse CNS disease is present

No uniform location of the lesion in the nervous system has been found in organic voice tremor. In his wide-sweeping review of the literature, Critchley (1949) documented many brainstem, caudate nucleus, and putamen locations; loss of cells in the cerebellum and dentate nuclei; and loss of cells within the triangle connecting the red nucleus, dentate nucleus, and inferior olive.

Essential tremor can produce three kinds of effects on voice:

1. If the alternating contractions of the adductors and abductors of the vocal folds are of equal strength, typical *organic voice tremor* will occur.

2. If the adductor movements are disproportionately stronger than abductor, the vocal folds will meet momentarily in the midline causing voice arrests, producing *adductor spastic dysphonia of essential tremor* (see Chapter 7).

3. If the abductor movements are disproportionately stronger than adductor, the vocal folds will over-abduct causing breathy air release, producing *abductor spastic dysphonia of essential tremor* (see Chapter 8).

The onset of organic voice tremor can be gradual or sudden. Brown and Simonson (1963) found that five of 27 patients had rapid onset of voice tremor: one while reciting the Lord's Prayer, a second while singing in church, and a third while talking at a board meeting. The other two noted abrupt onset of hoarseness and a strained feeling in the throat while talking, and, as these symptoms cleared, the voice tremor appeared. That these patients were older than the age of 50 years led the researchers to conclude that the rapid onset was due to occlusive vascular disease.

The voice of an individual with an organic tremor has a characteristically *quavering intonation* because of tremor of the laryngeal muscles, and often of the articulatory and respiratory muscles as well. Severe cases have a staccato abruptness of voice heard as *rhythmic voice arrests*. The tongue also moves in a rhythmic tremor both at rest and on protrusion.

Clinicians should remember that voice tremor can occur without associated tremors elsewhere in the body. Brown and Simonson (1963) found voice tremor to be the only tremor in six of 23 patients. For the entire group, the voice tremor ranged from 4 to 8 c./sec., although in 16 of the 23 cases, the tremor frequency was concentrated in the 5 to 6 c./sec. range.

The voice tremor in organic tremor is best demonstrated during vowel prolongation. The tremor can be smooth, or interrupted by the previously noted voice stoppages or vocal arrests. These voice arrests are caused by momentary obstruction of the exhaled airstream due to complete glottic closure simultaneous with the vertical movements of the larynx. The voice arrests come at the apex of each laryngeal oscillation.

A milder organic voice tremor can be masked during contextual speech. As Brown and Simonson noted in their study of 31 patients with this disorder, short-duration vowels were uttered without perceptible impairment, but the tremor became obvious during production of sounds of longer duration. It is of clinical importance to know that the severity of the tremor is greater during emotional stress and fatigue. Patients show little in the way of psychoneuroses, but many cases have occurred after acute emotional stress. (Table 5–11 is a summary of the dysarthria of organic voice tremor.)

PALATOPHARYNGOLARYNGEAL MYOCLONUS

Palatopharyngolaryngeal myoclonus refers to rhythmic or semi-rhythmic movements of the soft palate, pharyngeal walls, laryngeal musculature, eyeballs, diaphragm, and tongue. Technically, it is a slow form of tremor; myoclonus may be a misnomer. These signs may exist in isolation or in various combinations. When the soft palate is involved, abrupt, rhythmic, anteroposterior and vertical movements are present *during speech and at rest*. Pharyngeal muscle contractions can open and shut the eustachean tube, producing a bruit or clicking sound transmitted by the tympanic membrane and sometimes heard by others at a fair distance.

* * *

A 51-year-old male came to the clinic because of spasmodic blinking of the eyelids and right arm clumsiness following attacks of influenza. He noted a clicking sensation in his larynx that seemed to obstruct his breathing, and he complained of episodes of aphonia, breathy dysphonia, and a sensation of spasm in the larynx. At times he would gasp for air on inhalation. He had frequent contractions of the orbicularis oculi. He had slight bilateral sensory and motor paralysis of the pharyngeal muscles. Also, although he had some adductor weakness of the vocal folds, the outstanding feature noted on laryngoscopic examination was *constant,*

Table 5–11 Laryngeal-Phonatory Characteristics in the Hyperkinetic
Dysarthria of Organic (Essential) Tremor

FINDINGS	
Perceptual	
Phonation	Quavering or intermittent voice arrests during contextual speech. Rhythmic tremor and/or voice arrests on vowel prolongation ranging from approximately 4–7 c./sec. *Note:* In severe organic voice tremor, the voice arrests take the form of severe laryngospasm that may be mistaken for the syndrome of spastic (spasmodic) dysphonia. Patients with voice arrests may show a smoothing out of these arrests into ordinary tremor when sustaining a vowel at a high pitch level. Fluctuating strained-hoarseness along with tremor in more severe cases
Resonation	Normal
Articulation	Normal. May have irregular articulatory breakdowns reminiscent of ataxic dysarthria
Language	Normal
Physical	
Larynx	Vocal folds appear normal in structure. On vowel prolongation, adductor-abductor oscillations synchronous with voice tremor can be seen as well as pharyngeal wall movements. Tremor movements of larynx can be seen under skin of neck, with the larynx oscillating vertically. Voice arrests occur at the maximum laryngeal height of each oscillation
Velopharynx	Normal. Soft palate may move synchronously with laryngeal and pharyngeal tremor
Tongue	Topographically normal. On vowel prolongation, tremor movements of tongue may be seen synchronously with laryngeal tremor
Lips	Normal. May be tremorous
Teeth	Normal
Hard Palate	Normal
Mandible	Normal. May be tremorous
General Medical	Nonspecific
Other Neurologic Signs	
Peripheral Nervous System	Normal
Central Nervous System	Head and hand tremor, unilateral or bilateral, may be present. *Note:* Organic voice tremor may occur as an isolated sign, which is prone to misinterpretation as being psychogenic
Psychiatric/ Psychologic	Many patients report onset of voice, head, or hand tremor following an emotionally stressful life event. There is a danger of interpreting such events as proof that the tremor is psychogenic.

involuntary, rhythmic bilateral adductor movements of the vocal folds that occurred 60 to 80 times per minute and frequently interfered with inspiration by producing complete adduction before inhalation had been completed. He also had myoclonic twitching of the facial muscles synchronous with movements of the vocal folds. The pharyngeal muscles and soft palate did not participate in these movements. The disorder was diagnosed as postencephalitic myoclonic movements of the larynx and pharynx (Childrey and Parker, 1931).

*   *   *

Rhythmic adductor movements of the vocal folds, and gross upward and downward movements of the larynx, cause *momentary, rhythmic, phonatory interruptions.* However, because each myoclonic movement is brief, voice interruptions are rarely audible during contextual speech. They become apparent, however, during vowel prolongation, when one hears momentary voice arrests ranging among patients from 60 to 240 beats per minute. In rare instances the laryngeal myoclonus can be so severe that abrupt, strained voice arrests are produced.

It is easy to miss this disorder by failing to test for it by means of vowel prolongation, because the voice arrests are usually masked by contextual speech. Also, oral examination of the pharyngeal and palatal musculature *at rest* is imperative in order to detect the myoclonic movements. Scrutiny of the external surfaces of the neck is important in order to note subcutaneous laryngeal movements. Subjective signs of the syndrome are a clicking sensation in the larynx and a sensation of laryngeal spasm. Myoclonic movements can be unilateral or bilateral.

Although the syndrome is found in people of all ages, it is most common in those older than the age of 50, and it is most often of vascular origin. In an unpublished study of 28 Mayo Clinic patients, 13 had brainstem or cerebellar infarction, eight had a tumor of the cerebellum or fourth ventricle, five had head trauma producing posterior fossa damage, and two had degenerative CNS disease, including cerebellar atrophy in one. The site of the lesion varies, although the general region is the brainstem, specifically the dentate nucleus, inferior olive, superior cerebellar peduncle, red nucleus, and restiform body. Additional neurologic signs of a brainstem lesion can accompany palatopharyngolaryngeal myoclonus.

(Table 5–12 summarizes the dysarthria of palatopharyngolaryngeal myoclonus.)

Paroxysmal Neurologic Voice Disorders

GILLES DE LA TOURETTE'S SYNDROME

Georges Gilles de la Tourette (1885) first described the syndrome that bears his name in a report of nine patients with *multiple tics and involuntary vocalizations that included coprolalia and echolalia.* Isolating the movements and sounds in this unusual disorder is difficult because they blend into appropriate cultural, environmental, and psychologic contexts involving speech and throat clearing. A variety of involuntary movements have been observed: jumping, squatting, skipping, hitting, kicking; repetitive movements, for example, touching the floor; hesitating to pick up objects as if they were hot; and touching chin, lips, tongue, throat, and other people. Other complicated movements include startle reactions, esophageal spasm, and echopraxia.

Speech and nonspeech vocalizations include *grunts, barking, coughing, throat clearing, echolalia, and coprolalia,* the uncontrolled utterance of socially unacceptable language having to do with sexual and other bodily functions.

In a study done by Shapiro et al. (1973) of 34 patients, 27 male and seven female, the average age of onset was 7.4 years, ranging from 3 to 13 years. The age of onset is difficult to determine and is probably reported considerably later than the actual date.

According to Cohen et al. (1978), a neurologic basis for Gilles de la Tourette's syndrome is strongly supported by the high incidence of abnormal electroencephalographic and other neurologic findings and a history of difficult birth. Although only three of 15 patients studied by Golden (1977) had major personality problems, 11 of 15 had difficulties with school work, eight having learning disabilities. Only four of 15 had made a completely normal adjustment to school.

Table 5–12 Laryngeal-Phonatory Characteristics in the Hyperkinetic
Dysarthria of Palatopharyngolaryngeal Myoclonus

FINDINGS	
Perceptual	
Phonation	Momentary voice arrests during contextual speech if severe, but often undetectable under this condition. On vowel prolongation, momentary voice arrests occur rhythmically ranging from 60 to 240 beats per minute (1 to 4 c./sec). *Note*: Because often undetectable during contextual speech, vowel prolongation must be tested in all suspected cases
Resonation	Normal
Articulation	Normal. Patient may have articulatory defects of flaccid, spastic or ataxic dysarthria
Language	Normal
Physical	
Larynx*	Vocal folds adduct rhythmically and momentarily on vowel prolongation, synchronously with voice arrests. Myoclonic movements of larynx and pharynx can be seen observing the movements beneath the skin of the neck
Velopharynx*	Soft palate elevates and falls, and lateral pharyngeal walls adduct and abduct synchronously with laryngeal movements
Tongue	Normal. May enter into myoclonic movements in synchrony with above structures
Lips	Normal
Teeth	Normal
Hard Palate	Normal
Mandible	Normal
General Medical	Nonspecific
Other Neurologic Signs	
Peripheral Nervous System	Normal
Central Nervous System	Other signs of brainstem lesion may be present or absent
Psychiatric/ Psychologic	Normal

*In order to detect presence of this syndrome, observation of the oral musculature while patient is quiet and holding mouth open as steadily as possible is imperative; *myoclonic movements are present at rest as well as during phonation.*

A 17-year-old male wrote the following letter:

I think I have that Tourette's syndrome. It's crazy. All these years I have been trying to cure it myself, trying to control all those nervous mannerisms that drove me up the wall. Like stuttering, my eye twitching, coughing, shaking, whatever. I said, "How am I ever going to become a dancer or a lawyer if I can't get up in front of a crowd?" You know what this syndrome does? It prevents people from being comfortable, being themselves, so they just clam up and don't take that risk of being uncomfortable. They begin to reject themselves for what they are then. It's not like being fat or having crooked teeth, you can control those . . . But this is something you have absolutely no control over . . . There is nowhere to run, it is inside you, with you, and you can't leave it behind.

Patients with Gilles de la Tourette's syndrome respond well to haloperidol. Abuzzahab and Anderson (1974), in their review of drug treatment for the disease, found that 89 percent of patients improved and 67 percent maintained the improvement longer than six months, although there was no evidence that treatment alters the eventual outcome of the disease. (Table 5–13 is a summary of the dysarthria of Gilles de la Tourette's syndrome.)

Table 5–13 Laryngeal-Phonatory Characteristics in the Hyperkinetic Dysarthria of Gilles de la Tourette's Syndrome

FINDINGS

Perceptual (*Note:* The following vary among patients; not all are found in a given patient)

Phonation	Involuntary grunting, coughing, throat-clearing, barking, squealing, shrieking, screaming, gurgling, moaning
Resonation	Snorting, sniffing
Articulation	Whistling; clicking; lip-smacking; spitting; stuttering-like repetitions of sounds
Language	Echolalia; coprolalia

Physical

Larynx	Vocal folds appear normal in structure and function
Velopharynx	Normal
Tongue	Normal
Lips	Normal
Teeth	Normal
Hard Palate	Normal
Mandible	Normal

General Medical	Nonspecific

Other Neurologic Signs	
Peripheral Nervous System	Normal
Central Nervous System	Jerky bodily movements

Psychiatric/ Psychologic	Emotional, behavioral problems secondary to adverse social effects of above

Neurologic Voice Disorders Due to Loss of Volitional Phonation

APRAXIC APHONIA AND DYSPHONIA

Apraxia of phonation and respiration for speech along with apraxia of articulation results from lesions of Broca's area in the dominant cerebral hemisphere. More than one type of phonatory manifestation of apraxia of phonation and respiration occur: (1) No articulatory movements or laryngeal sound, voiced or unvoiced; (2) articulation produced with an unphonated airstream, i.e., whispered speech; (3) articulatory movements without accompanying exhalatory activity, patients

Table 5–14 Laryngeal-Phonatory Characteristics in Apraxia of Speech

FINDINGS

Perceptual

Phonation	Varies, from normal in some patients to mutism in others. Phonation may be impossible because of apparent loss of recall for integration of respiratory and laryngeal movements, resulting in trial-and-error efforts to phonate, but silent nevertheless. Aphonic (whispered) speech can occur. Inability to cough volitionally or clear throat
Resonation	Normal
Articulation	Phoneme omissions, substitutions, reversals, and additions; stuttering-like blocking
Language	May be relatively normal or aphasic

Physical

Larynx	Vocal folds appear normal in structure and function
Velopharynx	Normal
Tongue	Topographically normal. May have associated dysarthric signs. Trial-and-error nonspeech volitional movements (oral nonverbal apraxia)
Lips	Trial-and-error nonspeech volitional movements may be present. Sequential motor rates, the rapid sequencing of sounds from /pʌ/ to /tʌ/ to /kʌ/, may be mildly to severely impaired
Teeth	Normal
Hard Palate	Normal
Mandible	Normal
General Medical	Nonspecific
Other Neurologic Signs	
Peripheral Nervous System	Normal
Central Nervous System	A wide variety of dysarthric, apraxic, and other abnormal signs may coexist
Psychiatric/ Psychologic	Nonspecific

being unable to inhale or exhale voluntarily to command or in response to imitation even though they are able to do so reflexly for vital purposes. They are unable to cough volitionally, showing instead confusion and trial and error efforts, yet they are able to cough automatically. When asked to cough, they will sometimes say the word "cough" rather than produce the cough itself. (See Table 5–14 for a summary of laryngeal-phonatory signs in apraxia of speech.)

AKINETIC MUTISM

Deep and widespread cerebral and brainstem lesions can cause (1) muteness and failure to respond to questions or comments, yet (2) alertness and eye contact, but indifference to the examiner. These clinical behaviors have been noted in presenile and senile dementia (Alzheimer's and Pick's diseases), hydrocephalus, frontal lobe lesions, and brainstem trauma, and following seizures in children.

The akinetically mute patient sits with eyes open, performs no or few voluntary movements, is unresponsive, looks away from the examiner, may have sucking movements, and is mute. The mutism is relative, i.e., mute except when prodded, in which case the patient will speak, usually normally, if no associated dysarthria, apraxia, or aphasia is present. A spectrum of severity must be taken into consideration; a given patient may be mute all the time early in the recovery period, may be mute only some of the time later on, and may show only vestiges of mutism during advanced stages of recovery by nothing more unusual than prolonged latency of speech response. Akinetic mutism can result from anoxia, metabolic diseases, subdural hematomas with compressions, cerebrovascular accident, or tumors, and may be seen in advanced parkinsonism and following thalamotomy.

Cairns et al.'s (1941) original description of the akinetically mute patient follows (italics added):

> *The patient sleeps more than normally, but he is easily roused. In the fully developed state he makes no sound and lies inert, except that his eyes regard the observer steadily, or follow the movement of objects, and they may be diverted by sound. Despite his steady gaze, which seems to give promise of speech, the patient is quite mute, or he answers in whispered monosyllables . . . commands may be carried out in a feeble, slow and incomplete manner, but usually there are no movements of a voluntary character,* no restless movements, struggling, or evidence of negativism. Emotional movement also is almost in abeyance. A painful stimulus produces reflex withdrawal of the limb, and, if the stimulation is sustained, slow, feeble voluntary movement of the limbs may occur in an attempt to remove the source of stimulation, but usually without tears, noise, or other manifestations of pain or displeasure. The patient swallows readily, but has to be fed . . . fluctuations may occur in the intensity of this state. In its incomplete manifestations the patient may respond at times, though slowly and imperfectly by speech and voluntary movement . . . incontinence persists and there is little or no trace of spontaneous activity or speech.

Klee (1961), in his review of the literature, summarized the varied clinical behaviors of many patients with akinetic mutism:

> Patients remained in akinetic and mute states for periods ranging from weeks to months, then gradually began to follow movements in their vicinity with their eyes but without interest . . . consciousness clear, no disturbances of orientation, memory or powers of observation . . . always possible to make contact although required much patience . . . able to answer questions adequately but in monosyllables and apparently with difficulty . . . trance-like states . . . episodes during which the patient would, in the midst of household activities, suddenly become inert and unresponsive and as suddenly, about ten minutes later would resume where she had left off.

Daly and Love (1958) described a 14-year-old boy who had an astrocytoma of the upper part of the fourth ventricle, extending around the lower end of the aqueduct, with the ventricular system cephalic to the tumor being greatly dilated. After the operation, he developed a condition in which speech and movements were inhibited, although he could understand what happened around him and what was said to him. He began to speak 34 days after the operation, at first using only monosyllabic words or short sentences, and movements became gradually less inhibited during the latter part of a two-month observation.

Klee (1961) expands on the point that the degree of inhibition changes from one minute to the next, and that the duration of inhibition can be minutes to months:

> The patient may be almost totally immobile and mute or may have only a suggestion of hampering of speech and movement. In the most inhibited states, the appearance and movements of the eyes may be the only indication that the patient is conscious. If he speaks, it is often only after a long latent period, and then with monosyllabic words or short sentences, in a monotonous voice. Movements are slow, and they show a similar long latent period; the spontaneous activity may be less hampered than the voluntary. Variations in the degree of inhibition may occur from one minute to the next, and the inhibition may last for minutes or months. The patient's experience of the inhibition of speech seems to be that they know what they wish to say but that the words cannot be said aloud. They do not appear to have a clear idea of how inhibited they actually are.
>
> A summary of the lesions that have caused akinetic mutism follows: tumors of the third ventricle; hemangioma of the mesencephalon and in and around the third ventricle; basilar artery thrombosis; Wernicke's encephalopathy; encephalitis; and bullet wounds through the frontal lobes.

Frontal Lobe Dysphonia, Aphonia, and Mutism

Severe breathiness, aphonia, and mutism are common in patients who have had frontal lobe lesions, most commonly from traumatic head injuries, tumor, or vascular disease. It has been speculated that such disturbances in phonation are associated with affective or personality changes from damage to the limbic system and its cortical and subcortical connections, which are thought to be important in regulating affect and emotion and their vocal expression. These patients demonstrate generally reduced drive and apathy. In their review of a large number of studies of the effects of frontal lobe lesions on phonation, Sapir and Aronson (1985) concluded:

> These reports argue that damage or disturbance to the limbic system and its neocortical and subcortical connections has a profound effect on emotions and affect, vocal-facial expressions, and the conscious monitoring of these expressions. Specifically, such neural disturbances are said to be responsible for apathy, a "flat" affect and lack of drive, aphonic or hypophonic vocalisation . . . and poor insight into the inappropriateness of one's vocal and nonvocal behaviors.

Nevertheless, there always exists the potential for a patient who has a neurologic disease to develop a psychogenic voice disorder that can be misinterpreted as neurologic by association with the neurologic disorder. In four patients who had central and peripheral nervous system disease described by Sapir and Aronson (1987), their dysphonias turned out to be psychogenic because of time-related psychosocial problems. These experiences taught the authors the importance of not automatically assuming that all dysphonias associated with neurologic disease are neurologic, and that the clinician always needs to be sensitive to the possibility of a dysphonia triggered by the anxiety or depression over the neurologic disease itself or by personal and family problems generated by illness and hospitalization.

Dysprosody of Pseudoforeign Dialect

This chapter closes with a most unusual neurologic speech disorder, one that gathers within its purview pitch, inflectional, stress, and articulatory aberrations, leading the listener to conclude that the patient is speaking his or her native language with a foreign accent. On September 6, 1941, during an air raid over Oslo, Norway, a 30-year-old woman named Astrid L. was struck in the head by a shell fragment which took away her left frontal bone, exposing extruded, lacerated brain. Upon recovering consciousness in the hospital, she was hemiplegic on the right side, was aphasic, and had seizures. At first she could say only "yes" or "no," then she became agrammatic, and eventually she recovered full fluency. Unexpectedly, however, she sounded as if she were speaking her native Norwegian with a German accent. This strange development proved to be embarrassing for her, since her country was at war with Germany. She complained bitterly about being taken for German in the shops, where clerks refused to sell her merchandise. Yet she had never left Norway and had had no contact with the German language or with German-speaking people at any time in her life.

Table 5–15 Pseudoforeign Dialect

NUMBER OF CASES REPORTED, 1907–1978			
Mayo Clinic			13
Other			12
Total			25
	Number	Percentage	Age (yr)
Females	16	64	27–59
Males	9	36	29–71

That one could, as a result of head injury, seem to be speaking in a foreign accent is difficult for serious students of neurologic communicative disorders to accept. Dialects are traditionally considered to be learned behavior. The pronunciation of consonants and vowels, the stress patterns placed on syllables of words, and the pitch-inflectional patterns superimposed on syntax follow logical laws of learning. Astrid was decidedly an enigma to her neurologist, Monrad-Krohn (1947), who reported that she had undergone a complete change in the melody of her language. She overemphasized final pronouns, and her pitch would rise on such pronouns at places where they should fall. She failed to elide the final sounds of words with the initial sounds of succeeding words. *Dysprosody* was the term the neurologist used to describe aberrations of normal pitch and stress patterns such as this, analogous to what American phoneticians refer to as intonation and stress, what the French call *chanson de parler,* and what the Germans refer to as *sprach-melodie.*

Before Monrad-Krohn's report, in 1907 Pierre Marie had described a Frenchman who began to speak in an Alsatian dialect following a cerebrovascular accident. In 1919, Arnold Pick, reported a 29-year-old Czechoslovakian who began to speak in a Polish dialect, also following a cerebrovascular accident and right hemiparesis and aphasia. A search of the literature uncovered 25 such cases noted between 1907 and 1978, 13 from Mayo Clinic files; 12 from other sources (Table 5–15). Sixteen, or 64 percent, were females aged 27 to 59 years, and nine, or 36 percent were males aged 29 to 71 years. One patient had shifted from French to Alsatian, one from Czeck to Polish, one from Norwegian to German, three from British English to Welsh, and one from British English to French. From American English, four switched to German, two to Swedish, two to Norwegian, one to Spanish, two to "New England," one to Welsh, Scottish, or Irish, and three to Italian. Three were difficult to classify. It is interesting that 10 patients, or 40 percent of the group, had a shift to dialects that could be described etymologically as Germanic (German, Swedish, or Norwegian).

The onset of foreign dialect was associated with neurologic disease. Fourteen, or 56 percent, developed a dialect following cerebrovascular accident; six, or 24 percent, following head trauma; and in five, or 20 percent, the neurologic diagnosis was negative or equivocal. Six, or 24 percent, had histories of seizures following the cerebrovascular accident or trauma. An effort was made to determine the number of patients whose foreign dialect was embedded in or followed more classic dysarthria, apraxia, or aphasia. Seventeen, or 68 percent, had one or more of these neurologic speech and language signs in addition to the foreign dialect. In eight, or 32 percent, it was impossible to determine the presence of these associated signs. These unusual cases raise several questions.

1. Are these so-called dialectal changes truly dialectal, or do they only sound as if they are because the direction of defect is coincidentally the same as one finds in the learned behavior of a true dialect?
2. Is the dialect a primary component of the speech disorder, or is it a compensatory reactive change to a more primary one?
3. What specifically is happening at the phonemic, stress, and pitch-inflectional levels that gives the impression of foreign dialect?

4. Of the thousands of patients who develop speech changes due to cerebral disease, why have so few demonstrated this unusual dialectal change?

5. Are the pitch changes that partially characterize the dialect a signal that those regions of the brain that subtend musical production have been impaired?

6. What is the connection between the onset of foreign dialect and the high incidence of its occurrence during the recovery stages of dysarthria, apraxia, and aphasia?

If one were to submit the following speech characteristics to a specialist in neurologic communicative disorders without informing the clinician of the patient's history or clinical studies, into what classification of speech or language disorder would these signs best fit?

1. Distortions and prolongation of vowels and semivowels.
2. Consonants produced with slightly off-target tongue and lip placements, i.e., the sound is an allophonic deviation.
3. Substitution of one phoneme for another.
4. Blocking on initial consonants.
5. Equal stress placed on all syllables in words and sentences.
6. Prolongation of silent intervals between words.
7. Insertion of vowel sounds between words.
8. Inappropriate pitch patterns.
9. All the above produced inconsistently.

These composite features of patients with "foreign dialect" most closely resemble the patient who has apraxia of speech; they are characteristic of neither dysarthria nor aphasia. That is to say, they are similar to apraxia in a general sense. Obviously, there is something special about the "foreign dialect" patient's specific errors that distinguishes that person from the typical apraxic. Pitch inflectional patterns may be the factors responsible.

A search through the histories of such patients reveals a common denominator: the presence of severe dysarthria and apraxia of speech. Although some are also aphasic, in several no aphasia was present.

* * *

A 27-year-old female who had sudden onset of numbness in her right hand, right facial weakness, mild dysarthria, and no previous history of foreign language exposure, eventually developed an apraxia of speech. As the hours passed, her rate of spontaneous speech again became normal. However, she spoke with a foreign accent which several independent witnesses identified as German. The "r" sound was susceptible to mispronunciation and she hesitated slightly in an apparent search for either the right word or articulatory position, yet her speech was free, appropriate, and completely intelligible. There was no dysphasia, and when examined both one month later and seven weeks after onset, her speech had returned to normal in all respects. Her foreign accent had disappeared (Whitty, 1964).

* * *

A 31-year-old female, after awakening and relieving herself, became dizzy, couldn't get words out, and by the end of the day was able to say only one-syllable words, although she never had difficulty thinking of the right words. By the end of three weeks, she was talking in complete sentences, at first in a flat intonational pattern. As inflectional changes returned, they took on a Spanish-sounding accent. Another, a 46-year-old female with cerebral ischemia following clamping of the left common carotid artery and left cervical sympathectomy for left internal carotid artery aneurysm, had a "New England" dialect for the first time in her life, and an oral verbal apraxia in which she groped for tongue positions and initiated words incorrectly. She was also mildly aphasic.

* * *

Of 13 Mayo Clinic histories, eight, or 62 percent, had apraxia of speech as an antecedent to the onset of the "foreign dialect."

* * *

A 41-year-old woman developed a Germanic-sounding dialect following a gunshot wound in the right occipital and parietal bone, the bullet cutting through the brain and lodging just under the parietal bone. The patient had spent three years in Germany, where she had learned German while married to an Air Force pilot. She had hemiparesis, left homonymous hemianopsia, spasticity of the right leg, apraxia of the left leg, an ataxic gait, and an abnormal EEG indicating a focal abnormality with epileptogenic components, from the right posterior temporal regions predominantly. The evolution of her dialect began with complete absence of speech and a period of dysarthria and apraxia of speech which gradually disappeared, leaving the "foreign dialect" in its wake.

* * *

Broca's area is most frequently implicated in cases of sudden onset of foreign dialect. Very few dispute this localization except Cole (1971), who wrote about a patient who developed an Eastern European dialect following a brainstem lesion. While conceding that any brain lesion that disturbs the integration of motor speech is potentially capable of altering prosody, one critic of brainstem localization of this faculty, claimed himself to be enough of a romanticist to think that the subtle inflections and nuances of speech must ultimately come from the cerebral cortex. He reminded us that if Juliet had said "Romeo, Romeo, wherefore art thou Romeo?" in a monopitch, it is doubtful that Romeo would have done himself in for her; he didn't think Shakespeare wrote for the cerebellum.

SUMMARY

1. Neurologic voice disorders are components of dysarthria and are classified into the same subtypes as the dysarthrias, based on the location of the lesion in the nervous system and muscular pathophysiology.

2. Most neurologic voice disorders are acoustically distinctive, which contributes to their differential diagnosis.

3. Neonates and infants with neurologic disease cry abnormally.

4. Vocal fold paralyses due to Xth (vagus) nerve lesions and their effects on voice depend upon the location of the lesion along the nerve pathway from brainstem to muscle.

5. Ever present is the danger of misdiagnosis of neurologic dysphonia as being psychogenic, especially those resulting from mild neurologic diseases of the Xth nerve and from early bulbar myasthenia gravis.

6. Flaccid dysphonias caused by Xth nerve or myoneural junction disease are generally breathy and reduced in loudness due to vocal fold hypoadduction.

7. Spastic (pseudobulbar) dysphonia generally has a harsh, strained-strangled quality due to vocal fold hyperadduction.

8. Hypokinetic (parkinsonian) dysphonia is generally characterized by monopitch and reduced loudness resulting from the rigidity of muscles.

9. Ataxic dysphonia, when present in ataxic dysarthria, may be tremorous or may show sudden bursts of loudness due to reduced muscular feedback.

10. Choreic dysphonia consists of sudden alterations in pitch, loudness, and quality and, often voice arrests, resulting from uncontrolled jerking muscular movements.

11. Dystonic dysphonia consists of slower alterations in pitch, loudness, and quality and, often, voice arrests, resulting from slower, uncontrolled muscular movements.

12. Organic voice tremor can exist in isolation or as one of several tremors distributed throughout the body. The voice tremor, ranging from 5 to 12 c./sec., when severe, contains voice arrests resulting from hyperadduction of the vocal folds.

13. The rhythmic interruptions (60 to 240 beats per minute) on vowel prolongation in palatopharyngolaryngeal myoclonus are rarely heard during contextual speech.

14. In Gilles de la Tourette's syndrome, uncontrolled spontaneous coughing, grunting, throat clearing, and other aberrant laryngeal behaviors occur often, although not always.

15. Apraxia of speech can include apraxia of phonation, in which muteness or aphonia exist in place of volitional phonation, yet voice can be produced automatically, as in coughing or throat-clearing.

16. Muteness may be complete in severe cases of the akinetic mutism syndrome, and partial during later stages of recovery.

17. Aberrations in melody, stress patterns, and articulation in patients who have suffered CNS lesions can give the impression of a foreign dialect, called dysprosody of pseudo-foreign dialect.

SUGGESTIONS FOR ADDITIONAL READING

Adour, K.K., Schneider, G.D., and Hilsinger, R.L., Jr.: Acute superior laryngeal nerve palsy: Analysis of 78 cases. Otolaryngol. Head Neck Surg., 88:418–424, 1980.
This article should be read for a more detailed analysis of the laryngologic and voice signs and symptoms of lesions of the superior laryngeal nerve.

Faaborg-Andersen, K., and Munk Jensen, A.: Unilateral paralysis of the superior laryngeal nerve. Acta Otolaryngol, Stockh, 57:155–159, 1963.

Findley, L.J., and Gresty, M.A.: Head, facial, and voice tremor. Adv. Neurol. 49: 239–253, 1988.
This reference is an excellent review of the entire subject of tremor involving different parts of the body, their frequency characteristics, physical appearance, etiology, and management. It contains a well described section on tremor of the voice.

Gacek, R.R., Malmgren, L.T., and Lyon, M.J.: Localization of adductor and abductor motor nerve fibers to the larynx. Ann. Otol. Rhinol. Laryngol., 86:770–776, 1977.

Larson, C.R.: Brain mechanisms involved in the control of vocalization. J. Voice, 2:301–311, 1988.
Our understanding of *central nervous system control* over vocalization is considerably incomplete. This compact and lucid review of animal experiments and the effects of central nervous system lesions on phonation in humans identifies cortical and subcortical centers responsible for reflex and volitional vocalization.

Ward, P.H., Berci, G., and Calcaterra, T.C.: Superior laryngeal nerve paralysis: An often overlooked entity. Trans. Am. Acad. Ophthalmol. Otolaryngol., 84:78–89, 1977.
This article amplifies this chapter's discussion of the effects of vagus nerve lesions on vocal fold function.

REFERENCES

Abuzzahab, F.S., and Anderson, F.O.: Gilles de la Tourette's syndrome: Cross-cultural analysis and treatment outcomes. Clin. Neurol. Neurosurg., 1:66–74, 1974.

Appelblatt, N.H., and Baker, S.R.: Functional airway obstruction: A new syndrome. Arch. Otolaryngol., 107:305–306, 1981.

Aronson, A.E.: Early motor unit disease masquerading as psychogenic breathy dysphonia: A clinical case presentation. J. Speech Hear. Dis., 36:116–124, 1971.

Aschari, A.N., and Colover, J.: Posterior fossa tumors with pathological laughter. J.A.M.A., 235:1469–1471, 1976.

Ball, J.R.B., and Lloyd, J.H.: Myasthenia gravis as hysteria. Med. J. Aust. 1: 1018–1020, 1971.

Blau, J.N., and Kapadia, R.: Idiopathic palsy of the recurrent laryngeal nerve: A transient cranial mononeuropathy. Br. Med. J., 4:259–261, 1972.

Blinick, G., Tavolga, W.N., and Antopol, W.: Variations in birth cries of newborn infants from narcotic-addicted and normal mothers. Am. J. Obstet. Gynecol., 110:948–958, 1971.

Brown, J.R., and Simonson, J.: Organic voice tremor. Neurology (Minneap.), 13:520–525, 1963.

Brumlik, J.: On the nature of normal tremor. Neurology (Minneap.), 12:159, 1962.

Cairns, H., Oldfield, R.C., Pennybacker, J.B., and Whitteridge, D.: Akinetic mutism with an epidermoid cyst of the third ventricle. Brain, 64:273–290, 1941.

Canter, G.J.: Speech characteristics of patients with Parkinson's disease: I. Intensity, pitch, and duration. J. Speech Hear. Dis., 28:221–229, 1963.

Carrow, E., Rivera, V., Mauldin, M., and Shamblin, L.: Deviant speech characteristics in motor neuron disease. Arch. Otolaryngol., 100:212–218, 1974.

Childrey, J.H., and Parker, H.L.: Myoclonic movements of the larynx and pharynx. Arch. Otolaryngol., 14:139–148, 1931.

Christopher, K.L., Wood, R.P., Eckert, R.C., Blager, F.B., Raney, R.A., and Souhrada, J.F.: Vocal cord dysfunction presenting as asthma. N. Engl. J. Med., 308:1566–1570, 1983.

Cohen, D.J., Shaywitz, B.A., Caparulo, B., Young, G., and Bowers, M.D.: Chronic, multiple tics of Gilles de la Tourette's disease. Arch. Gen. Psychiatry, 35:245–250, 1978.

Cole, M.: Dysprosody due to posterior fossa lesions. Trans. Am. Neurol. Assoc., 96:151–154, 1971.

Cormier, Y.F., Camus, P., and Desmeules, M.J.: Nonorganic acute upper airway obstruction: Description and a diagnostic approach. Am. Rev. Respir. Dis., 121:147–150, 1981.

Critchley, M.: Observations on essential (heredofamilial) tremor. Brain, 72:113–139, 1949.

Daly, D.D., and Love, J.G.: Akinetic mutism. Neurology (Minneap.), 8:238–242, 1958.

Darley, F.L., Aronson, A.E., and Brown, J.R.: Differential diagnostic patterns of dysarthria. J. Speech Hear. Res., 12:246–269, 1969a.

Darley, F.L., Aronson, A.E., and Brown, J.R.: Clusters of deviant speech dimensions in the dysarthrias. J. Speech Hear. Res., 12:462–496, 1969b.

Darley, F.L., Aronson, A.E., and Brown, J.R.: Motor Speech Disorders. Philadelphia, W.B. Saunders Co., 1975.

Daube, J.R., Sandok, B.A., Reagan, T.J., and Westmoreland, B.F.: Medical Neurosciences. Boston, Little, Brown, and Co., 1978.

Fisichelli, V.R.: The phonetic content of the cries of normal infants and those with brain damage. J. Psychol., 64:119–126, 1966.

Gilles de la Tourette, G.: Etude sur une affection nerveuse caracterisée par de l'incoordination motrice, accompagnée d'echolalie et de coprolalie. Arch. Neurol. (Paris), 9:158–200, 1885.

Golden, G.S.; Tourette syndrome. Am. J. Dis. Child., 131:531–534, 1977.

Hanson, D.G., Gerratt, B.R., and Ward, P.H.: Cinegraphic observations of laryngeal function in Parkinson's disease. Laryngoscope, 94:348–353, 1984.

Haymaker, W., and Kuhlenbeck, H.: Pathologic laughter and crying. In Baker, A.B., and Baker, L.H. (Eds.): Clinical Neurology. Hagerstown, Md., Harper & Row, 1976.

Hirano, M., Koike, Y., and von Leden, H.: Maximum phonation time and air usage during phonation. Folia Phoniatr., 20:185–201, 1968.

Huppler, E.G., Schmidt, H.W., Devine, K.D., and Gage, R.P.: Causes of vocal cord paralysis. Proc. Staff Meet. Mayo Clinic, 30:518–521, 1955.

Kammermeier, M.A.: A Comparison of Phonatory Phenomena among Groups of Neurologically Impaired Speakers. Doctoral dissertation. Minneapolis, University of Minnesota, 1969.

Karelitz, S., and Fisichelli, V.R.: The cry thresholds of normal infants and those with brain damage. An aid in the early diagnosis of severe brain damage. J. Pediatr., 61:679–685, 1962.

Kellman, R.M., and Leopold, D.A.: Paradoxical vocal cord motion: An important cause of stridor. Laryngoscope, 92:58–60, 1982.

Klee, A.: Akinetic mutism: Review of the literature and report of a case. J. Nerv. Ment. Dis., 133:536–553, 1961.

Kreindler, A., and Pruskauer-Apostol, B.: Neurologic and psychopathologic aspects of compulsive crying and laughter in pseudo-bulbar palsy patients. Rev. Roum. Neurol., 8:125–139, 1971.

Lind, J.: The vocalization of a newborn brain-damaged child. Ann. Paediatr. Finn., 11:32–37, 1965.

Logemann, J.A., Fisher, H.B., Boshes, B., and Blonsky, E.R.; Frequency and concurrence of vocal tract dysfunctions in the speech of a large sample of parkinson patients. J. Speech Hear. Dis., 42:47–57, 1978.

Marshall, J.: Observations on essential tremor. J. Neurol. Neurosurg. Psychiatry, 25:122–125, 1962.

Monrad-Krohn, G.H.: Dysprosody or altered "melody of language." Brain, 70:405–415, 1947.

Neiman, R.F., Mountjoy, J.R., and Allen, E.L.: Myasthenia gravis focal to the larynx. Arch. Otolaryngol., 101:569–570, 1975.

New, G.B., and Childrey, J.H.: Paralysis of the vocal cords. Arch. Otolaryngol., 16:143, 1932.

Patterson, R., Schatz, M., and Horton, M.: Munchausen's stridor: Nonorganic laryngeal obstruction. Clin. Allergy, 4:307–310, 1974.

Portnoy, R.A.: Hyperkinetic dysarthria as an early indicator of impending tardive dyskinesia. J. Speech Hear. Dis., 44:214–219, 1979.

Rogers, J.H.: Functional inspiratory stridor in children. J. Laryngol. Otol., 94:669–670, 1980.

Rogers, J.H., and Stell, P.M.: Paradoxical movement of the vocal cords as a cause of stridor. J. Laryngol. Otol., 92:157–158, 1978.

Rose, F.C. (Ed.): Motor Neuron Disease. New York, Grune & Stratton, 1977.

Sapir, S., and Aronson, A.E.: Aphonia after closed head injury: Aetiologic considerations. Br. J. Disord. Commun., 20:289–296, 1985.

Sapir, S., and Aronson, A.E.: Coexisting psychogenic and neurogenic dysphonia: A source of diagnostic confusion. Br. J. Disord. Commun., 22:73–80, 1987.

Shapiro, A.K., Shapiro, E., and Wayne, H.L.: The symptomatology and diagnosis of Gilles de la Tourette's syndrome. J. Child Psychol. 12:702–723, 1973.

von Leden, H.: Objective measures of laryngeal function and phonation. Ann. N. Y. Acad. Sci., 155, Art. 1:56–67, 1968.

Whitty, C.W.M.: Cortical dysarthria and dysprosody of speech. J. Neurol. Neurosurg. Psychiatry, 27:507–510, 1964.

Williams, R.G.: Idiopathic recurrent laryngeal nerve paralysis. J. Laryngol. Otol., 73:161–166, 1959.

Wolski, W.: Hypernasality as the presenting symptom of myasthenia gravis. J. Speech Hear. Dis., 32:36–38, 1967.

Chapter Six

VOICE INDICATORS OF NORMAL PERSONALITY

VOICE AS AN INDICATOR OF DISCRETE EMOTIONS

VOICE AS AN INDICATOR OF PSYCHOPATHOLOGY

    Affective Disorders
    Schizophrenia

VOICE INDICATORS OF LIFE STRESS

PSYCHOGENIC VOICE DISORDERS

    Musculoskeletal Tension Disorders
    Conversion Voice Disorders
    Mutational Falsetto (Puberphonia)
    Childlike Speech in Adults

REBOUND PSYCHOLOGIC EFFECTS OF
VOICE DISORDERS

IATROGENIC VOICE REST

SUPPLEMENTARY STUDIES IN PSYCHOGENIC
VOICE DISORDERS

PSYCHOGENIC VOICE DISORDERS

Voice is more than a mechanical or acoustic phenomenon. It is a mirror of personality, a carrier of moods and emotions, a key to neurotic and psychotic tendencies.

—Brodnitz

VOICE INDICATORS OF NORMAL PERSONALITY

"Personality" encompasses those behaviors that distinguish each individual as being different from others, e.g., facial expression, gestures, posture, gait, intelligence, aggressiveness, confidence, attitudes, feelings, sensitivity, and emotional reactivity. How a person speaks—voice quality, pitch, loudness, stress patterns, rate, pause, articulation, vocabulary, syntax, and ideational content—qualifies as a trait of personality. However, attempts to show that voice reveals certain personality traits have been confounded by several semantic and methodologic obstacles:

1. Unsatisfactory definition of personality.
2. Questionable validity and reliability of personality tests.
3. Difficulty in defining voice variables.
4. Variations in research methodology, e.g., selection of subjects as to age, sex, and ethnic background; tests of personality and voice; parameters, methods, and units of measurement.

Nevertheless there has been no shortage of studies on the relationship between personality and voice. For instance, breathy voice has been associated with high neurotic tendency, anxiety, low dominance, and high introversion. Harsh/metallic voices correlate with high dominance and emotional instability; nasal whine reflects emotional instability and low dominance; and high loudness and low pitch are found with high dominance (Mallory and Miller, 1958; Moore, 1939). Hoarseness has been associated with reticence and self-consciousness. An increased speaking rate prompts testers to increase their ratings of competence. A decreased rate encourages them to evaluate the individual as being less competent, but more benevolent. Greater variations in fundamental frequency result in higher ratings of benevolence. Decreased variations in fundamental frequency reduce ratings of competence and benevolence. Increased mean fundamental frequency causes lower ratings of competence and benevolence (Brown et al., 1974; Williamson, 1945).

VOICE AS AN INDICATOR OF DISCRETE EMOTIONS

High pitch is associated with happiness, joy, confidence, anger, and fear (Davitz, 1964; Eldred and Price, 1958; Fairbanks and Pronovost, 1939; Huttar, 1968; Levin and Lord, 1975; Scherer et al., 1973; Sedláĉek and Sychra, 1973; Skinner, 1935; Williams and Stevens, 1969). Low pitch connotes indifference, contempt, boredom, grief, and sadness (Davitz, 1964; Eldred and Price, 1958; Fairbanks and Pronovost, 1939; Huttar, 1968; Sedláĉek and Sychra, 1973; Williams and Stevens, 1969). Wide pitch ranges are found during anger, fear, and contempt (Fairbanks and

117

Pronovost, 1939; Williams and Stevens, 1969). Narrow pitch ranges are associated with indifference, boredom, grief, and sadness (Fairbanks and Pronovost, 1939; Huttar, 1968; Williams and Stevens, 1969). Extensive pitch variability is associated with happiness, joy, anger, and fear (Fairbanks and Pronovost, 1939; Sedláĉek and Sychra, 1973). Diminished pitch variability is associated with indifference, grief, and sadness (Fairbanks and Pronovost, 1939). High loudness levels are associated with happiness, confidence, anger, contempt, and joy (Costanzo et al., 1969; Huttar, 1968; Williams and Stevens, 1969; Zuberbier, 1957). Low loudness levels are associated with boredom, grief, and sadness (Davitz, 1964; Eldred and Price, 1958; Huttar, 1968). Rapid rates are associated with happiness and joy, confidence, anger, fear, and indifference (Costanzo et al., 1969; Davitz, 1964; Eldred and Price, 1958; Fairbanks and Hoaglin, 1941; Huttar, 1968; Markel et al., 1973; Scherer, 1973). Slow rates are associated with contempt, boredom, grief, and sadness (Davitz, 1964; Eldred and Price, 1958; Markel et al., 1973; Fairbanks and Hoaglin, 1941; Huttar, 1968; Williams and Stevens, 1969).

VOICE AS AN INDICATOR OF PSYCHOPATHOLOGY

Affective Disorders

Affective disorders are psychiatric syndromes characterized by alterations in mood, such as depression, manic or hypomanic states, euphoria, and mood swings. A depressed outlook either may be lifelong or can occur for the first time in a usually cheerful person who unexpectedly becomes chronically sad, tearful, pessimistic, slow of thought, agitated, disinterested, unable to sleep and eat, and who senses a decline in feelings of self-worth. In one such group of 40 patients who demonstrated sadness, retardation of thought processes, anorexia, and insomnia, Newman and Mather (1938) said that their voices were dead or listless, and had narrow pitch range, infrequent pitch changes, slow rate, frequent pauses and hesitations, and reduced stress or emphasis patterns. In a second group that exhibited chronic gloom, self-pity, and dissatisfaction, speech patterns were different from the first; these had long gliding intonational or pitch changes over a wide pitch range, lively voices, normal rates but frequent pauses, harsh voice quality, and crisp articulation.

Monotonous downward inflectional patterns have been found in depressed patients (Moses, 1954). Whitman and Flicker (1966) found that pitch became higher and loudness lower in proportion to the degree of depression. In agitated depression, they found an increased articulatory rate as patients became more depressed. In a study done by Hargreaves and Starkweather (1964) in which acoustic spectrographic recordings were made during treatment of depression, as patients improved, their overall vocal intensity and their energy in the higher vowel formants increased. In 10 solidly depressed patients, five showed reduced loudness and diminished inflectional changes.

Patients in the manic phase of manic-depressive reactions produce a very different voice and articulation profile: press of speech; flight of ideas; vigorous articulation; clear, lively, and vital voice; wide pitch range; frequent gliding pitch changes; frequent emphasis and accent; and exaggerated pauses. As these patients become less manic, their pitch range narrows, emphasis patterns are reduced, pauses and hesitations begin to appear, and articulation becomes less vigorous (Newman and Mather, 1938).

Psychiatrists and psychologists have long acknowledged that they can tell much about their patients' emotional state and underlying psychodynamics by listening to their voices. The psychotherapist also uses the voice in ways that will create a more effective relationship with the patient. Reminding us that virtually all methods of psychotherapy involve two or more persons talking together, Bady (1985) wrote:

> Since I have been listening to my patients' voices I have also noted that changes in vocal quality accompany their progress. One patient achieved a lighter, less ponderous voice as he became more comfortable with his emotions. Another slowed down his rapid pace. A third achieved a less grating and more fluid tone.

In her own use of voice as a means of making her therapy more effective, the author further states:

> In my work I will intentionally use my voice along with my words. Sometimes I attempt through vocal tones to soothe an anxious, agitated patient. Other times I use my voice to stimulate a depressed and hopeless one. On still other occasions I talk to give the patient a human response and my words are less important than the vocal indication of my presence. Sometimes I remain silent in order to encourage separation from me. Occasionally my voice backfires on me, as when a patient notices my anger or my anxiety through the sound of my voice.

Noticeable differences between "peak" and "poor" therapy hours can be determined by an analysis of psychotherapists' voices. In one study the therapist's voice during peak therapy sessions was described as more open, lower in pitch, and of softer intensity, giving the impression of warmth, seriousness, relaxation, and closeness (Duncan et al., 1968).

Schizophrenia

In child schizophrenics, Goldfarb et al. (1956) described hypernasality; breathiness; hoarseness; glottalization; flat voice quality; insufficient or inappropriate volume and pitch changes; narrowed total pitch range; tendency toward excessively high pitch; inappropriate rate changes from phrase to phrase; prolongation of phonemes, syllables, and words; chanting quality; insufficient or inappropriate stress; hesitation after and repetitions of sounds or syllables; and flat, monotonous prosody. In another study, Goldfarb et al. (1972) noted the absence of a single specific clustering of these speech abnormalities in child schizophrenics, with the basic disturbance being loss of control and of regulation of speech.

In adolescent schizophrenia, Ostwald and Skolnikoff (1966) described a 15-year-old male's speech as having a nasal quality, articulatory imprecision or indistinctness, exaggerated intonational patterns, and a high and prolonged rise in pitch toward the ends of questions. As in childhood schizophrenia, there was excessive variability of rate and rhythm. Chevrie-Muller et al. (1971) found reduced pitch range, reduced rate, and increased pause time in female adolescent schizophrenics.

In an adult schizophrenic, melody or pitch patterns were found not to glide but to jump at intervals and without relationship to ideational content. Accent (emphasis or stress pattern) was inappropriate, and speech contained rhythmic monotonous repetitions of vocal patterns (Moses, 1954). Moskowitz (1951) described the speech of adult schizophrenics as monotonous, weak, flat, colorless, and gloomy. Saxman and Burk (1968) found significantly slower reading rates in adult schizophrenics than in normal subjects.

VOICE INDICATORS OF LIFE STRESS

Clinical and instrumental studies prove that otherwise normal voice perceptibly and measurably changes under emotional stress. A smooth, well-modulated voice signifies cortical control over the emotionally primitive, phylogenetically older nervous system. During subcortical emotional release, phonatory and respiratory control disintegrates. Massive automatic fight-or-flight reactions prepare the organism for increased physical work—fixing the upper extremities to the thoracic cage for combat, requiring firm adduction of the vocal folds and wide abduction to facilitate an increased volume and flow of oxygen in order to meet the body's increased metabolic demands. Such emergency physiologic states are incompatible with fine voice pitch, loudness, and quality control.

Most group studies to determine the effect of stress on voice have induced stress by either exposing subjects to threatening stimuli, asking them to lie, or requiring them to perform difficult tasks. These studies have been criticized, however, because the stresses did not represent real-life situations, and therefore their intensity may not have been sufficient to induce measurable emotional responses. Male-female differences were sometimes not taken into account, and subjects have been noted to mask their voice reactions to emotion. Despite these objections, the results of a cross-section of studies have established that *increased voice fundamental frequency (pitch) is directly related to increased stress.* Aviators and astronauts in distress show increased fundamental frequency proportional to the amount of stress experienced. Simonov and Frolov (1973), reporting on the effects of stress and fatigue on the voices of cosmonauts, found that increased heart rate correlated positively with increased intensity of the higher vowel formants. Voice pitch elevation corresponds directly with increased emotional tension in pilots, according to Khachatur'yants and Grimak (1972), Popov et al. (1971), and Williams and Stevens (1969).

Voice also indicates stress in patients prone to heart disease. Males with "type A" personality were found to be seven times more likely to develop coronary artery disease than "type B" personalities (Friedman and Rosenman, 1959). The type A personality has such traits as excessive drive, ambition, aggressiveness, impatience, and a habitual sense of time urgency when challenged by the environment. Subsequently, Rosenman et al. (1964) discovered that type A personalities had similar voice and speech patterns; explosive semiviolent accentuations in prosody that carried a "certain aggressive timbre" but that appeared only when that person was interested in or excited about the subject under discussion. The type B personality spoke in an "unruffled, rather smooth manner without explosive or aggressive accents."

These observations were made at the time by clinical description only, but in a study done by Friedman et al. (1969), they were measured in the following manner. The voice was amplified, converted into direct current, and fed into a resistor-capacitor network with an output modulation that consisted of a 60 Hz signal. The purpose of this apparatus was to permit identification of both the loudness with which the patient modulated the voice and the duration of the loudness burst. In order to induce exhibition—the eagerness to win or excell at a challenging activity and to release latent hostility—a two-paragraph diatribe was composed in which an officer exhorts his troops prior to battle. The subject was asked first to look over the paragraph in preparation for reading it into the microphone. Even prior to the experiment itself, the type A subjects blurted out the identical question, "Do you want me to read this with expression?," whereas no type B subject ever asked that question. Nineteen type A male volunteers free of clinical coronary artery disease and 18 type B male volunteers also free of coronary artery disease were tested. Of the 16 type B subjects tested, almost all had few or no vocal escalations exceeding 2.5 cm. in wave height. Their average noise-free period (45 seconds) was approximately the same as the average total time (46 seconds), resulting in an average index of 1.06, the ratio of the total reading time to noise-free time. The majority of type A subjects, 14 of 19, exhibited a number of vocal escalations exceeding 2.5 cm. in wave height. Consequently, their average noise-free period of 30 seconds was significantly less, $p < 0.001$, than in type B subjects. Their average index, 1.50, was also significantly greater, $p < 0.001$, than that of the type B subjects. From this study, the authors concluded that voice analysis successfully segregated the majority of type A from type B personalities.

PSYCHOGENIC VOICE DISORDERS

In the literature and in the clinic, the terms "functional," "psychogenic," "psychosomatic," and "nonorganic" are used synonymously in reference to a group of voice disorders that exist in the absence of organic laryngeal pathology. The label "functional" appears most often. However, from a survey of clinicians' usage, Perelló (1962) found no less than eight interpretations of "functional voice disorder": (1) No apparent alteration in structure detected by laryngoscopic examination; (2) negative laryngoscopic examination but positive stroboscopic examination; (3) dysphonia disproportionately severe when compared with existing anatomic lesions or inflammations; (4) disorder of nervous origin with variable symptoms and conducive to the formation of organic lesions; (5) disorder reversible (as opposed to organic disorders, which are usually irreversible); (6) function is altered (the disorder disappears when the organ is used correctly); (7) incorrect motor utilization (therefore, it is a dysfunction); and (8) desire to mask ignorance of exact cause.

Objection to the term "functional" mainly has to do with its ambiguity and lack of precision, especially in light of the following realities. (1) There is more than one functional voice disorder.

(2) They not only sound different but also occur for different reasons and, therefore, should be considered as separate subtypes. (3) Most subtypes can be traced to emotional or psychologic causes. More accurate, then, is the term "psychogenic voice disorders." *A psychogenic voice disorder is broadly synonymous with a functional one but has the advantage of stating positively, based on an exploration of its causes, that the voice disorder is a manifestation of one or more types of psychologic disequilibrium, such as anxiety, depression, conversion reaction, or personality disorder, that interfere with normal volitional control over phonation.*

Why do only certain persons react to environmental stress and interpersonal conflict by developing an abnormal voice? Why is it that others who have emotional reactions to stress and conflict never have voice problems? Why is it that still others express their personal problems through some organ system other than the larynx? No satisfactory answers to these questions have been found. Perhaps each person is predisposed by personality or physiologic makeup to hyperreact through a particular neuromuscular or visceral system. Those who are prone to develop voice disorders might be called *laryngoresponders* to designate their predisposition to developing laryngeal and voice disorders as their unique avenue for the expression of emotional distress.

If everyone who was unable to express emotion developed an abnormal voice, not just certain predisposed persons, clinics would be overwhelmed by patients with psychogenic voice disorders. The distinguished director and writer, Elia Kazan (1988), gives a casebook description of what it is like not to be able to express one's feelings openly. To anyone's knowledge, he never developed a psychogenic voice disorder, but if he had, the following thoughts would have fit the disorder perfectly.

> When someone works in the arts, he works from craft, not emotion. . . . I'd done play after play that I had no true feeling for, and I'd again and again suppressed the feelings I did have, choked them off, my hands pressing at my throat, stifling the scream that, if it could be heard, would be my true voice.
> Speak now, I said to myself, release your true feelings before it's too late. Be yourself. Take your place in the world. You are not a cosmic orphan. You have no reason to be timid. Respond as you feel. Awkwardly, crudely, vulgarly—but respond. Leave your throat open. You can have anything the world has to offer, but the thing you need most and perhaps want most is to be yourself. . . . Admit rejection, admit pain, admit frustration, admit pettiness, even that; admit shame, admit outrage, admit anything and everything that happens to you, respond with your true, uncalculated response, your emotions.
> Work on it. Stir up the lump whenever you can. Raise your voice.

Musculoskeletal Tension Disorders

In the physically healthy individual, states of tension come about in two ways: (1) from *exogenous sources,* such as overwork, tense working conditions, professional worries, unhappy family life, or unfavorable situations of occupational placement; and (2) *endogenous sources,* such as peculiarities of personality structure that tend to induce tension (e.g., perfectionism, compulsive attitudes, overambitious drives, lack of adaptability through inflexible rigidity, or uncontrolled outbursts of anger). Under such conditions, tensions may build up without appropriate release. States of increased tension eventually lead to *augmented nervous irritability.* As a result of this continuously increasing state of neural reaction, the musculature is incited to higher tonus, in excess of the actual demands made on it (Luchsinger and Arnold, 1965, p. 15).

One cardinal principle in clinical voice disorders is that: *The extrinsic and intrinsic laryngeal muscles are exquisitely sensitive to emotional stress, and their hypercontraction is the common denominator behind the dysphonia and aphonia in virtually all psychogenic voice disorders.* The responsible factors are anxiety, anger, irritability, impatience, frustration, and depression. On laryngoscopic examination, the vocal folds either are normal, are mildly inflamed, fail to adduct completely, hyperadduct, or are slightly bowed. *In general, however, the extent of visible pathology is incongruously minor or absent in comparison with the severity of abnormal voice.*

Musculoskeletal tension can by detected manually by the clinician and can be sensed by the patient. The tension produces *elevation of the larynx and hyoid bone.* The clinician tests for such tension by encircling the larynx with the thumb and middle finger in the region of the thyrohyoid space, feeling to determine whether the space has been narrowed by laryngeal elevation. (See Chapter 13.) The larynx and hyoid bone resist being manually moved laterally or vertically. When the larynx and hyoid bone are pressed and kneaded in the areas indicated, the patient will respond with *discomfort or pain,* sometimes quite severe, depending upon the degree and duration of the muscle tension. The pain will be either unilateral or bilateral, although more often it is unilateral. The normal larynx does not respond in this manner, so that discomfort and pain with normal-appearing vocal folds are most often diagnostic of laryngeal musculoskeletal tension. If the larynx is pulled down after the sensitive areas are kneaded, and if decreased hoarseness and breathiness and increased volume follow, such is proof that musculoskeletal tension was responsible for the dysphonia. This test is also the main component of the therapy for these disorders.

In the section on conversion aphonia, it is stated that patients who whisper as a sign of a conversion reaction also exhibit extreme musculoskeletal tension, with the larynx suspended high in the neck and the entire hyoid-laryngeal sling remarkably stiff. The aphonic does not whisper because of passivity of the musculature; on the contrary, the musculature is under supercontraction. This fact was demonstrated in the laboratory by Tarrasch (1946), who recorded electromyographic potentials from the sternocleidomastoid and thyrohyoid muscles bilaterally during quiet respiration and attempts to phonate. She found considerable spasticity of the musculature in aphonic patients. Van den Berg (1962) cites Faaborg-Andersen's electromyographic study of the intrinsic muscles of the larynx in normal subjects who whispered voluntarily. Even under such artificial conditions, increased electrical activity was found in the adductor laryngeal muscles. Similarly, in an x-ray tomographic study done by Zaliouk and Izkovitch (1958), a patient with conversion aphonia showed spasticity of the supraglottic larynx.

Not only does laryngeal musculoskeletal tension produce discomfort or pain when the examiner applies pressure in the regions described, but patients also volunteer information about spontaneous pain radiating to the ear, sternum, and mid-chest. They feel as if a foreign body were stuck in the throat, and report difficulty in swallowing, constriction, and swelling or compression in the pharyngolaryngeal area. Takahashi et al. (1971) reported on 652 cases of a disagreeable sensation in the pharyngolaryngeal region and found a high incidence of neurotic tendencies in this group. Some had carcinophobia after a close friend or relative had died of the disease. They concluded that dysphoric affective states play an important part in producing these sensations. The relationship between dysphonia, musculoskeletal tension, and environmental stress is illuminated in the following case study.

* * *

A 37-year-old single female, a registered nurse, noted a "cracking" of her voice five months prior to coming to the Clinic, at first only a few times a week but becoming more frequent, so that by the end of three weeks she had become continuously hoarse. She consulted her family doctor, who thought that her dysphonia was due to postnasal drip and prescribed cough syrup, and, later, ampicillin without benefit. She was next examined by an otolaryngologist, who noted irritation of her vocal folds but did not offer a diagnosis or treatment. Two months after onset, her voice returned to normal while she was on vacation in Mexico, but it worsened upon reentry to the United States. She went back to her family doctor, who prescribed Valium and Decadron, which were also ineffective, and attempted to treat her disorder as if it were myasthenia gravis by prescribing Mestinon, which also was of no benefit.

Indirect laryngoscopy showed normal vocal folds, and neurologic examination failed to disclose any evidence of myasthenia gravis or other neurologic disease. Her general medical examination was normal.

Her voice was *continuously strained, hoarse, and produced with above-normal physical effort.* On vowel prolongation, she produced a clear voice at a higher pitch level. Her cough and glottal coup were normally sharp, indicating good vocal fold adduction. *She reacted with discomfort and pain, grimacing in response to pressure over the posterior region of the hyoid bone bilaterally. Her larynx, at rest and on phonation, was positioned high in her neck, close to the hyoid bone. Her voice improved momentarily when the larynx was moved downward by the examiner during vowel prolongation.* Asked if her dysphonia could be a reaction to emotional stress, and asked to describe any upsetting events that might have occurred surrounding the onset and development of her dysphonia, she became momentarily silent, frowning, as if taken off-guard by the question. After a few moments' reflection, she smiled and, as if it were occurring to her for the first time, said that in fact, she had been struggling with a distressing situation. Shortly before her dysphonia, a local newspaper editorial had appeared that was critical of the costs of the patient's position as a public health nurse and that argued for the elimination of her job. A bitter conflict broke out between her department and the editor, with accusations flying in both directions. Caught in the middle, the patient grew increasingly angry over the unfairness of the allegations, yet had no means of responding to them.

As she disclosed this information, her frustration and anger became apparent. Her face flushed, and although on the verge of tears, she continued to talk. *During the next few minutes, her voice spontaneously returned to normal.* She was gratified and surprised at this sudden and unexpected improvement. She said she had suspected that her voice disorder had something to do with the conflict at home *but had not appreciated its importance until the question had been put to her directly.* She ought to have suspected the connection, she said, when her voice had begun to improve following a resolution of her job problem shortly before coming to the Clinic.

*   *   *

Consultation with several specialists before arriving at a diagnosis and treatment of the disorder is typical in patients who have musculoskeletal tension dysphonia. Undramatic and indistinguishable from hoarseness due to other causes, musculoskeletal tension dysphonia is treated erroneously as if it were laryngitis. Diagnostically important in the cited case were the strained voice, tightness, hoarseness, history of voice return while on vacation, and pain in response to pressure in the region of the larynx. The diagnosis was confirmed when the voice returned spontaneously as the patient ventilated her feelings. Loosening of her character armor, physical relaxation, abandoning of defenses, and freeing of affective expression through weeping or laughter are diagnostic and therapeutic in such cases.

VOCAL ABUSE IN CHILDREN

The consequences of hyperadduction of the vocal folds are three kinds of secondary laryngeal pathologic states: (1) inflammation, (2) vocal nodules, and (3) contact ulcers. There is a tendency to think of these as vocal abuse disorders because they are associated with strenuous speaking, singing, yelling, screaming, coughing, and throat-clearing. But abuse or misuse is not the *primary* etiology, however. Rather, it is an intermediate link in the chain of causes that begins with an *emotionally determined impetus to vocalize aggressively.* The effect of such behavior is to produce traumatic lesions, leading many clinicians to categorize vocal nodule or contact ulcer as organic voice disorders. But, from a *fundamental etiologic* point of view, they are probably better characterized as psychosomatic, because the lesions were the result of abnormal speaking behavior, more often than not motivated by personality or emotional factors.

The effects of vocal abuse exist on a severity continuum. School-age children who abuse their voices will have either normal-appearing vocal folds, inflammation without discrete lesions, or discrete lesions. Senturia and Wilson (1968) reported on 32,500 children aged 5 to 18 years and found that 1962 (6 percent) had abnormal voices. Of that abnormal group, 338 aged 6 to 11 years were given voice, hearing, psychometric, and laryngologic examinations. The males predominated over females by a ratio of 2:1. Of these voice-defective children, 147 were given laryngoscopic examinations, and 47.5 percent were found to have varying degrees of redness or edema or both, in the region of the arytenoid cartilages. The complete larynx could not be viewed on indirect laryngoscopy in all 147 children, but the entire vocal folds could be visualized in 92. Of those 92 children with abnormal voice, 63 had discrete lesions such as nodules, hyperplasia, and diffuse or localized edema. The predominance of lesions in males compared with females was almost 3:1 in children having discrete vocal fold lesions, and more than 2:1 in those not having discrete lesions.

The voice signs within this group of 92 children consisted of *whispering, breathiness, and stridency.*

The amount and type of classroom voice utilization of children diagnosed as having hoarse voices was compared with that of children who had normal voices by Barker and Wilson (1967). The length and loudness of utterances were tabulated for 14 children in the control group (normal voice) and for 14 in an experimental group (hoarse voice). The researchers found that the children with normal voices produced an average of 20.92 vocalizations in a 2-hour period, compared with 61.50 vocalizations by the children with hoarse voices within that same time period. The difference between the two groups was significant beyond the 0.01 level. Of interest is the observation that the children with the abnormal voices were more active within the classroom during unstructured periods than were the children with normal voices.

The theme of personality aggressiveness, hyperactivity, emotional reactivity, and family problems in dysphonic children with and without discrete vocal fold lesions touched upon in this study is of considerable importance in understanding the factors responsible for vocal abuse. In the aforementioned study done by Barker and Wilson, social workers investigated the family structure of both the voice-defective and the normal children. Of 153 who were classified as having abnormal voices, 65 percent came from homes in which there was excessive family conflict whereas 35 percent came from homes in which there was considered to be none. Of 97 children whose voices were normal, only 35 percent, came from conflict-ridden homes, i.e., almost twice as many children with abnormal voices came from home environments that were considered pathologic.

Cheerleading can be a cause of vocal abuse. Many studies have proved that the result can be chronic dysphonia with or without vocal fold damage. Jensen (1964), for example, found that 12 percent of 377 cheerleaders were dysphonic. Andrews and Shank (1983) found that 37 percent of 102 high school cheerleaders had a history of voice problems. Reich et al. (1986) surveyed 146 female cheerleaders ranging in age from 15.5 to 18.6 years and found that, at one time or another, 32 percent had experienced acute aphonia and 86 percent complained of dysphonia. The average number of times that these students became aphonic during a given season was 4.2 and dysphonic, 7.3.

VOCAL NODULES IN CHILDREN

Vocal nodules in children are associated with vocal misuse or abuse. The nodule is a small, white or grayish protuberance on the free margin of the vocal fold at the junction of the anterior and middle third (Fig. 4–4a). It is a tissue reaction to frictional trauma between the folds, a growth of hyperkeratotic epithelium with underlying fibrosis. The nodules may begin with a submucous hemorrhage and may develop from the fibrosis of an organizing hematoma. In the very early stages of vocal abuse, there may be nothing more than a localized capillary hemorrhage, swelling of the vocal fold edges, and redness of the folds. Later, fibrosis and the fully developed, roughly semicircular, grayish or white nodule forms.

> Vocal nodules represent a degeneration of the lamina propria with fibrosis and edema. Acute vocal nodules are morphologically different from chronic. In the acute phase, the squamous epithelium is normal but covers an edematous stroma with thin-walled blood vessels, loose fibrous tissue, and lymphocytes. In the chronic phase, the nodules possess a thickened epithelium and demonstrate acanthosis, keratosis, and fibrosis with minimal edema of the underlying connective tissue.
>
> Three stages of vocal nodule formation have been described: (1) a local accumulation of fluid in the subepithelial layer of the vocal folds; (2) an organized inflammatory response with accumulation of protein and increased vascularity; (3) further organization of the lesion with fibrosis and possibly keratosis of the epithelium (Arnold, 1962). They vary in size from no larger than a pinhead to as large as a split pea. Early nodules may appear red, gelatinous, and floppy, whereas chronic nodules are typically white and conical or hemispherical and appear hard and fixed to the underlying mass of the mucosa (Vaughn, 1982).

The nodule is located at the junction of the anterior and middle third of the vocal fold because the maximum point of trauma at this relatively anterior position is produced by phonation at higher pitch levels, as in screaming or singing. After the nodule has been formed, the resultant dysphonia has a *breathy, husky,* or *foggy* quality, with a tendency toward *low pitch.* The dysphonia results from the loading by the nodules of the vocal folds. As they project into the glottis, they cause airstream turbulence. The breathy or husky quality is the effect of failure of vocal fold closure in the region of the nodules.

Children who develop vocal nodules differ in personality and family history from those who do not. Nemec (1961) observed that children with hyperfunctional dysphonia, including vocal nodules, were more aggressive and less mature and had more difficulty in managing stressful situations than children with normal voice. Mosby (1967) studied 25 children, 16 with vocal nodules and nine with other types of dysphonia, by means of a battery of psychologic tests. He found a high incidence of neurotic personality conflict, over-repressed aggression, feelings of inadequacy, poor relationships with parents, and severe dependency needs. Wilson and Lamb (1973), in a study of 12 children with vocal nodules and 12 with normal voices, concluded that children with vocal nodules had personalities that included marked aggressiveness, lack of control, or passive, over-controlled adjustment to aggression. By administering the California Test of Personality, Glassel (1972) compared 15 children, aged 7 to 11 years, who had vocal nodules with 15 who had normal voices. He found that the children with nodules scored significantly poorer on all measures of personality adjustment; they had reduced feelings of belonging, a reduced sense of personal worth, withdrawal tendencies, and antisocial feelings. However, not all children with nodules were vociferous according to the popular stereotype, although they manifested the same degree of neurotic tendency as those who were. In a study of 77 children with vocal nodules, Toohill (1975) found that the parents of 62 described them as screamers, incessant talkers, or loud talkers. Sixty-six were described as having one or more of the following personality traits; aggressiveness, hyperactivity, nervousness, tenseness, frustration, or emotional disturbance.

Further evidence of psychoneurotic tendencies in children who develop vocal nodules comes out of a study by Green (1989). She had the mothers of 30 children with vocal nodules and 30 control mothers rate their children's behavior on a standardized checklist of abnormal behaviors called the Walker Problem Behavior Identification Checklist. The children with vocal nodules, 22 of whom were male and 8 were female, ranging in age from 3 to 12 years, received a substantially higher percentage of abnormal ratings than the control group. More than 60 percent of the children with vocal nodules were rated as positive on the following traits: (1) temper tantrums when the child can't get his way; (2) argues and wants to have the last word; (3) doesn't obey until threatened; (4) complains of others' unfairness. Also rated high was the tendency toward overactivity and restlessness and the need for approval for tasks attempted. Not more than 20 percent of the children with normal voices received ratings for these behaviors. From this study, the author concluded that:

> The concept of the development of vocal nodules in children has traditionally conjured a fixed mental picture of vocal abuse in a vociferous child. . . . The present research suggests that such a focus is too simplistic and that the people working with children with vocal nodules may need to consider a multiplicity of etiological and management variables.

Vocal nodules have been found in association with velopharyngeal insufficiency. The need for higher intraoral pressures and for increased loudness causes overdriving of the vocal folds. (See Chapter 9, Nasal Resonatory Disorders, for a more detailed discussion.)

VOCAL NODULES IN ADULTS

The etiology and pathology of vocal nodules in adults are basically the same as in children, with minor variations. Whereas the incidence of vocal nodules is higher in male children than in females, this trend is reversed in adults. Singing as a primary or contributory cause is strong in adulthood. Adult females with nodules have some of the same personality characteristics and daily habits as children who develop nodules. They are talkative, socially aggressive, and tense, and have acute or chronic interpersonal problems that generate tension, anxiety, anger, or depression. Even when the nodule appears to be the sole result of abuse from singing or other strenuous vocal activity, it is often found that these were not the only factors responsible for the vocal abuse; these patients had also entered a period of their lives in which concomitant emotional stress had surfaced.

* * *

A 63-year-old married female was referred by the Department of Otolaryngology with a diagnosis of bilateral small vocal nodules. She had begun to complain of hoarseness eight years previously whenever she had to use her voice strenuously, such as over background noise or during animated conversation. She had been seen by laryngologists and speech clinicians who had made the diagnosis of vocal abuse and given "exercises," which were ineffective. Aside from her voice difficulties, her health had been good, although she complained of general fatigue with prolonged voice use.

On examination, her voice was nearly normal; there was a slight hoarseness consistent with the size of the nodules observed by the otolaryngologist. Complete motor speech examination failed to disclose any evidence of dysarthria, and the remainder of the examination of the speech structures failed to disclose any other defects.

While giving the social-psychologic history, the patient said she believed that her husband was responsible for her voice problems. She described him as a voluble speaker, loud and animated. The patient, during most of her married life, had to raise her voice in order to compete with his during discussions, not only when they had company but also when they were alone together. "He dominates the conversation . . . that's his personality . . . his nature . . . you're never going to change that . . . he is a shouter and I am a quiet talker." Despite this marriage-long contrast in their personalities, her voice troubles first began when she became interested in activist politics and needed to express her opinions in a more forthright manner. She volunteered that she believed she had gotten into the habit of using her voice excessively and with a great deal of tension as a reaction to her husband's vocal manner. "Now, even when I have to talk to a group, I tense up." When her voice was bad, she complained of shooting pains from her larynx to her ears, and on examination she had pain in response to pressure over the hyoid region and thyroid cartilage.

Joint discussion with the patient and her husband confirmed her testimony; he proudly confessed to being "vociferous, aggressive, dominating," more concerned with his own opinion than hers. He described her as a "sounding board" and not nearly as concerned with her opinions as with his own. "I know it's selfish and cruel . . . she's a very tranquil individual and I am not . . . I'm the second last angry man!" She said to him, "You are a monopolizer of conversations . . . my main complaint is when there are other people in the conversation . . . he interrupts them . . . won't let them finish. He'd rather talk than do anything else. Unfortunately, it becomes a monologue."

* * *

What emerges from this examination is not only a basic difference in how these two individuals communicate, but an even deeper disagreement as to what ought to be said and what is best left unsaid. Not only is the psychogenic etiology of this woman's vocal nodules substantiated by an in-depth interview, but the results of that interview also point to the requirement for more than symptomatic voice therapy.

The balance between vocal abuse and emotional stress is different in each patient with vocal nodules. Whereas in the previous study, emotional and personality factors were prominent, vocal abuse is more apparent in the following, although the patient is not free of stress.

* * *

A 39-year-old farm wife and mother of three boys had sung most of her adult life for weddings, funerals, and baptisms. One year before coming to the Clinic, she had hoarseness occurring intermittently but did not consult anyone until seven months later. Examination showed a thickening of the mucosa of the left vocal fold and a small blood clot on the posterior third of that fold. Laryngologic examination during the current consultation showed clear evidence of bilateral vocal nodules at the junction of the anterior and middle third of the vocal folds.

The patient was a pleasant, energetic, healthy housewife and mother of a highly musical family. In addition to her heavy singing schedule, her daily talking habits were prodigious; teaching, singing, talking, using her voice all day long with her children and her neighbors, and speaking on the telephone.

* * *

Special cases of vocal nodules in adults occur in the culture of the pop singer, whose voice usage is often one of extreme abuse with or without coexisting fatigue and emotional stress. Greene (1972) had these interesting comments about this subgroup in Britain.

Pop singers claim an immensely important role in entertainment . . . although professors of singing in the classical style do not recognize their vocalization indeed as singing. The senior coach of the Covent Garden Opera Company has said he would not consider them seriously as candidates for the course . . . Their members are legion and they give pleasure to millions. They are largely untrained, having muscial sense and personality and pleasing voices but some, it must be admitted, have little natural vocal endowment. For many it is a short life but a lucrative one and when the voice is lost through vocal abuse they drop out of "show biz."

The vocal gymnastics and tricks peculiar to each singer, the double notes, acute pitch changes, the scoops and swirls have to be executed against the deafening competition of amplified music . . . Despite the use of a hand microphone they must still "belt it out" at the top of their voices . . . The sound-pressure levels created by the bands and rock and roll groups are so great that they exceed the safety levels for avoidance of hearing impairment.

The common run of cabaret and pop-group singers perform for many hours on end starting at midnight and going on into the early hours. When not singing they are smoking and talking in a dry, hot and polluted atmosphere. It is not surprising that chronic laryngitis and vocal nodes are common.

* * *

A 19-year-old nightclub singer complained of intermittent hoarseness for three to six months. She was a backup vocalist in an eight-piece brass band and sang six days a week. Laryngologic examination revealed moderate-sized vocal nodules bilaterally at the junction of the anterior and middle third of her vocal folds.

In addition to the close relationship between singing and dysphonia—the patient complaining of less voice trouble when on vacation—she disclosed recent life stresses concerning problems with a boyfriend in the band. At the same time, she began to examine her career goals, summing up her feelings over the past six months by saying, "I'm feeling a lot of emotional stress I've never felt before . . . just seems like everything is coming down at once . . ." She admitted to being depressed during the time of her voice and personal problems.

* * *

CONTACT ULCER

The second vocal abuse—musculoskeletal tension—emotional stress voice disorder having secondary traumatic tissue reaction is contact ulcer or contact ulcer granuloma. Instead of epithelial tissue developing, as in vocal nodule, a contact ulcer is an erosion of the mucosa (Fig. 4–4b). Occurring unilaterally or bilaterally, the ulcers are found at the junction of the middle and posterior third of the vocal folds, the intercartilaginous region, at the tips of the vocal processes of the arytenoid cartilages. The hard cartilaginous undersurfaces of the vocal processes strike the mucosa of the opposite vocal fold, causing hyperemia, the formation of granulation tissue, and, finally, an ulcer crater with its raised, inflamed margins.

Contact ulcer is a disorder primarily of adult males in their forties; adult females are affected rarely, and children virtually never. Male susceptibility may be due to their tendency to adopt a low-pitched voice, moving the locus of force of vocal fold contact posteriorly. Ulcerations in the region of the arytenoid cartilages can also result from trauma due to laryngeal intubation.

Clinical and research studies point to certain common characteristics among adult males who develop contact ulcer (Peacher, 1947; Peacher and Hollinger, 1947).

1.   Hypertonic laryngeal musculature as a component of generalized musculoskeletal tension

2. Habitual use of an excessively low voice pitch level
3. Explosive speech stress patterns
4. Sharp, abrupt glottal attack (coup de glotte)
5. Restricted pitch variability
6. Phonation using excessively high infraglottal pressure with bursts of intensity

Some patients with contact ulcer complain of discomfort or pain coming from deep within the neck radiating to the lateral neck area or ear, a tickle in the throat, an urge to clear the throat, a lump in the throat, and an aching or dryness. The classic profile of the contact ulcer patient is a male in his forties who uses his voice intensively in his daily life and is either a lawyer, teacher, minister, actor, or salesman. In personality, he is tense and hard-driving and is often under chronic stress. Cigarette smoking, alcohol consumption, exposure to air pollutants, and extremes of air temperature and humidity are contributory factors. Musculoskeletal tension secondary to emotional stress is a predisposing factor responsible for the mechanically damaging hyperadduction of the vocal folds, and some believe that autonomic nervous system effects are responsible for vasoconstriction of the laryngeal mucosa, reducing blood supply to that region and thereby increasing its susceptibility to trauma.

The dysphonia of the patient with a contact ulcer is characteristically *low pitched, hoarse,* and *grating.* Not only does chronic vocal abuse produce contact ulcer, but sudden traumatic yelling or shouting can also precipitate it. It often occurs following laryngitis, particularly when the patient has continued to abuse the voice during the throat infection. The following studies are typical of contact ulcer patients.

* * *

A 43-year-old steel plant supervisor had an 11-month history of laryngitis, during which he developed a contact ulcer. His dysphonia had become chronic four months after he had begun working in the machine shop of his plant, during which time he used his voice constantly, having to raise it to high loudness levels in order to be heard over the environmental noise. This environment was also dusty, hot, and dry in the summer and cold and damp in the winter. Moreover, he sang in a male chorus, and he complained of long working hours and general fatigue. On examination, his voice was hoarse and low in pitch with some acoustic evidence of breathy air escape.

A 41-year-old professor of English literature had a five-year history of episodic hoarseness in association with lecturing, which became worse during resumption of a regular teaching schedule and assumption of new duties as a curriculum supervisor. Indirect laryngoscopy showed a contact ulcer granuloma on the posterior third of the left vocal fold. His voice was hoarse and excessively low in pitch and gave indications of breathy air escape. He described his style of lecturing as "animated" and "forceful," with a tendency to use an unnaturally low pitch. He perfectionistically prepared his lectures and delivered them under conditions of anxiety and tension. He found that his voice would tire toward the end of each lecture, and he would feel muscular tension in his neck and pain in his throat, sometimes expanding into headache.

A 48-year-old automobile plant manager gave a two-month history of hoarseness with upper respiratory infection. Indirect laryngoscopy showed bilateral contact ulcer granulomas at the bases of both vocal folds. His voice was hoarse with excessively low pitch. Vocal abuse and emotional stress coincided with manufacturing problems, his dysphonia developing shortly after spending six hours a day in the shop talking over noise levels approaching 100 decibels. Much of his speaking had to do with reprimanding employees for inefficiency, and at the same time, he was regularly involved in public speaking in civic organizations.

* * *

VENTRICULAR DYSPHONIA

Closely allied to musculoskeletal voice disorders is ventricular dysphonia, or dysphonia plicae ventricularis, characterized by a continuously *strained, harsh,* or *hoarse low-pitched* voice described as rattling, rumbling, cracking, and tickerlike. To some, it gives the impression of phonating during strangulation, and to others it has a groaning, animal quality suggesting exertion of extreme effort. The voice disorder derives its name from the fact that voice is produced by vibration of the false or ventricular vocal folds rather than the true folds. Its etiology is unclear. Because it has been noted to occur in muscularly tense people, it is probably best classified as a musculoskeletal tension disorder. *It is important to note that many patients who have organic disease of their true vocal folds which are incapable of producing adequate sound, compensate by using their ventricular folds instead.*

Conversion Voice Disorders

This group of psychogenic voice disorders originates from the psychoneurosis known as a *conversion reaction.* A conversion reaction is any loss of voluntary control over normal striated muscle or over the general or special senses as a consequence of environmental stress or interpersonal conflict. The criteria for conversion reactions are that they:

1. Are specific physical symptoms or syndromes that cannot be traced to any anatomic or physiologic disease.

2. Are unconscious simulations of illness, which the patient is convinced is of organic origin.

3. Serve the psychologic purpose of enabling the patient to avoid awareness of emotional conflict, stress, or personal failure that would be emotionally intolerable if faced directly.

4. Can occur in any sensory or voluntary motor system.

Examples of sensory conversions are loss of general sensation in response to touch, pressure, or pain, or impairment of the special senses of vision or hearing. Motor conversions take such forms as weakness, incoordination, complete loss of movement control ("paralysis"), or unusual or bizarre movements anywhere in the body.

The word "conversion" was first used by Freud to explain a mechanism by which an unbearable idea is rendered innocuous by having its energy transmuted into some bodily form of expression, i.e., conversion is a theoretical conception of a clinical finding. Sensory or motor loss in the absence of organic disease is a defense mechanism against a threat from the environment. Somehow the psychic energy generated by that threat is transmuted or converted into a somatic sign, and, as in conversion voice disorders, the somatic sign is symbolically related to certain specifics about the threat or conflict that created it.

The idea that psychic energy can be transformed into physical or "organic" dysfunction is difficult to grasp. Freud's theory of "libidinal" conversion to physical dysfunction has been the subject of much criticism because of its metaphorical quality. It becomes more acceptable, however, if modernized to mean *symbolization* of the conflict or unbearable idea. In their contemporary interpretation of the meaning of conversion reaction, Ziegler and Imboden (1962) wrote the following clarifying explanation:

> We have found it useful to consider the patient with a conversion symptom as someone enacting the role of a person with "organic" illness, symbolically communicating his distress—dysphoric affect and/or unacceptable fantasy—by means of somatic symptoms. In our conceptual model, this somatic mode of communication does not serve to "discharge" pent-up emotion but, rather like any other language, it is useful as an instrument in negotiating interpersonal transactions. Through the conversion reaction, the fact that the patient is in distress is formulated to himself and communicated to others in the egosyntonic terms of "physical illness," and the patient thereby distracts himself (with varying degrees of success) from the more immediate perception of his dysphoric affect. Human beings may communicate their feelings and ideas to themselves and others in a variety of modes such as ordinary consensual language, sign language, dreams, autistic verbal symbols of schizophrenia, or autistic somatic symbols of conversion reaction. Conversion may be viewed as operating, in this way, like other psychological processes. . . . In many conversion reactions seen clinically the message of emotional distress is communicated primarily in nonverbal ways (to the patient himself as well as the others in his transactional field) in terms of somatic symptoms which are, in effect, an analogic code . . . The patient unconsciously chooses particular

symptoms according to his conception of illness, as derived from his own past experiences with illness or from his observation of others . . . His particular symptoms will then simulate physical illness in a relatively expert or relatively crude manner, depending upon the degree of congruity between his imagery of illness and that of the observer . . . Within this context of unconsciously simulated illness, specific symptoms may develop or receive prominence because they are especially suited to the symbolic representation of specific fantasies, affects, and motivational conflicts.

Sometimes "hysteria" is used in place of conversion reaction, e.g., "hysterical voice disorder," "hysterical aphonia," or "hysterical dysphonia," in which case hysteria and conversion are used interchangeably and synonymously. Technically, this failure to differentiate the two terms is incorrect. *Conversion* refers to somatization of an emotional conflict, as elaborated previously, whereas *hysteria* refers to a personality type or behavior pattern. Criteria for hysteria are: (1) An immature or egocentric person who has a propensity to develop subjective complaints involving various parts of the body, prompting that person to consult many physicians and to submit to a succession of operations. (2) In the case of a female, one who is seductive or flirtatious, sometimes hostile or manipulative, and who accents or highlights her sexuality by her manner, voice, dress, and gait, thus revealing an insecurity in this sphere. (3) A suggestable, dependent, shallow person, dramatic and theatrical in manner and labile in affect, who takes cues from what seems to be expected according to the environment and who plays a series of superficial roles in relating to other people. Many individuals satisfy one or more of these criteria for hysterical personality but do not have a conversion reaction. Conversely, many patients with conversion reaction bear none of the personality or behavior traits of the hysterical personality.

A conversion voice disorder (1) exists despite normal structure and function of the vocal folds, (2) is created by anxiety, stress, depression, or interpersonal conflict, (3) has symbolic significance for that conflict, and (4) enables the patient to avoid facing the interpersonal conflict directly and extricates the person from the uncomfortable situation. The onset of the voice disorder is almost always associated with emotional conflict. For many years, the misconception abounded that the only voice sign of conversion was whispering or aphonia. However, *conversion voice disorders come in many forms:* muteness, aphonia, and less dramatic forms of dysphonia, such as breathiness, hoarseness, falsetto pitch breaks, and continuous falsetto. The multiplicity of voice signs of conversion reaction has been substantiated by Aronson et al. (1966), who found identical criteria for conversion reactions in patients whose problems ranged from muteness to varying degrees and types of dysphonia.

CONVERSION MUTENESS

The most extreme and incapacitating conversion voice disorder is muteness or mutism, in which the patient neither whispers nor articulates, or may articulate without exhalation. Entering the room with notebook and pencil, they write their questions and answers, and although unaware of what they are revealing, involuntarily cough, showing their normal vocal fold adduction. The patient will also cough sharply on request without being aware of the incongruity between their normal cough and manifest inability to phonate. Patients who present with one form of conversion voice disorder very likely have experienced other forms.

Common findings in such patients are chronic stress, primary and secondary gain, indifference to their symptom, other manifestations of conversion, poor sex identification, suppressed anger, immaturity and dependency, neurotic life adjustment, and mild to moderate depression. Different as these individuals are from one another, a common denominator runs through their histories: *(1) A breakdown in communication with someone important to that person. (2) A conflict between wanting but not allowing oneself to express anger, fear, or remorse verbally. (3) Fear or shame standing in the way of expressing feelings via conventional speech and language.*

* * *

A 44-year-old female presented with no use of speech structures for communication. All her responses were written. Her history was one of struggle and deprivation from birth. She was the youngest of ten, her family being burdened by five other children from her father's former marriage. By the time she was 20, her father then dead and most of the children gone, she had been saddled with the responsibility of caring for her aging mother and two older sisters. She lived a Cinderella-like existence, doing the household chores and being dominated by her sisters, who rarely allowed her out of the house. Under these circumstances, at age 23, she had her first conversion symptom, a "paralysis" of the right arm lasting two weeks. Three years later, she became severely depressed and unable to work for several months. Then, at age 27, her mother, "the only person who ever loved me," died. Shortly thereafter, she developed a "paralysis" of both legs and became an invalid for one and a half years. Physical therapy effected a "dramatic cure." Her doctors, who knew of her hostile and dependent relationship with her sisters, urged her to get out on her own. Six years later, at age 35, she married a 27-year-old man with a son from a previous marriage. She had made an adjustment to life. Financial worries and behavior problems in the son were followed by episodes of dysphonia. During the winter prior to the present interview, she had many episodes of intermittently phonated-whispered voice. Her present episode had begun nine months before with a period of whispered speech lasting seven months and finally giving way to muteness and writing notes.

* * *

CONVERSION APHONIA

Conversion aphonia refers to involuntary whispering despite a basically normal larynx. Indirect laryngoscopic examination indicates normal or partial adduction of the vocal folds on vowel production or coughing. Even without laryngoscopic examination, normalcy of the vocal folds can be heard as the patient coughs and makes other glottal sounds unassociated with speech. Similar to dysphonia associated with musculoskeletal tension, the larynx in conversion aphonia is often elevated in the neck along with the hyoid bone and the entire laryngeal-hyoid sling is rigid and is difficult to move manually in any direction.

Within the category of aphonia falls a considerable variety of whispers: pure or noiseless; harsh, sharp, or piercing; intermittent high-pitched squeaks and squeals; moments of normal voice. The sharpness of the whispering indicates that the intrinsic laryngeal muscles are in a state of hypercontraction, even though the vocal folds are prevented from approximating.

Approximately 80 percent of patients with conversion aphonia are female. Many have had previous episodes of aphonia or dysphonia that have spontaneously cleared. Onset can be sudden, within seconds or minutes, or over a period of hours, beginning with hoarseness that turns into aphonia. Conversion aphonias and dysphonias are often triggered by colds or flu and associated laryngitis. Upon recovery from the upper respiratory infection, the dysphonia remains, worsening to aphonia. Often, onset is associated with fatigue or exhaustion. Discomfort, pain, and tightness in the larynx, and upper and lower neck and chest regions are common in the conversion group, as they are in the musculoskeletal tension group. *As in conversion muteness, aphonic patients give histories including either acute or chronic emotional stress, symbolic significance of the voice loss, primary and secondary gain, a tendency toward indifference to the incapacitating effects of the voice, and conversion reactions in other regions of the body at different times in their lives.* Additional findings are emotional immaturity, neurotic life adjustment, and mild to moderate depression.

Although the following studies are of patients with conversion aphonia, they could apply equally to patients who are mute or to those who are dysphonic.

* * *

A 14-year-old girl's parents were separated and involved in divorce litigation. She had markedly ambivalent feelings toward her father. Her latest episode of aphonia occurred an hour after a violent argument with him on the telephone over her request for Christmas money.

A 58-year-old housewife learned of her brother's death. En route to his funeral, she received word that her sister-in-law had died. She awoke the next morning with aphonia that continued for the next two years.

A 31-year-old secretary and mother of three had been carrying on an extramarital affair for nine years and was fearful that this relationship would be discovered. During the past year, she had been having disagreements with her employer, and her fear of being fired was the only factor that kept her from "telling him off." Her aphonia occurred shortly after her boyfriend lost his job and moved to a new location, preventing her from communicating with him; she had begun to consider breaking off their relationship.

A 26-year-old police officer was not happy in his work but would not tell anyone of his feelings, particularly his parents, for fear of disappointing them, as they had encouraged him to enter police work. He had always been quiet, unaggressive, and reluctant to lose his temper. He had had previous episodes of aphonia and dysphonia which had cleared spontaneously, but this most recent one failed to improve over a three- to four-week period. The main reason for his dislike of being a policeman was an inability to exert authority—a fear that he would say the wrong thing or reap dislike or disapproval from those he tried to reprimand. He would find himself becoming nervous and upset when having to give a motorist a ticket; if the motorist argued with him, he would shake and get mixed up. He had no idea that his voice losses were related to his attitudes toward his work until after symptomatic voice therapy and discussion with a psychiatrist, when he began to realize that his voice loss was an attempt to change jobs. He finally came to realize that he must tell his family about his feelings and return to his previous job, which was that of a dyer in a textile mill, where he could be alone with his thoughts.

*   *   *

We are reminded of an important personality characteristic of patients with conversion voice disorders: their difficulty in dealing maturely and openly with feelings of anger. The following exchange illustrates the point:

*   *   *

C: You would say, then, that you are not very good at telling people how you feel.
P: Certainly not. I look calm to everybody, but I'm not. When something bothers me I get it right here (motions to her throat) and I just tighten up.
C: You're not the type that can talk back and let off steam.
P: (Smiles) With my voice the way it is? Why, that's impossible.

*   *   *

Here is a more detailed case study of a 33-year-old, married woman who went to her otolaryngologist after becoming aphonic. The case illustrates the sheer depth and complexity of human problems that can underlie voice loss, the importance of not approaching aphonias and dysphonias as voice disorders only, and *the importance of delving into the psychosocial history in order to obtain the underlying etiology of the voice disorder.*

*   *   *

Otolaryngology: This 33-year-old woman has a history of recurrent sinusitis. Earlier this year, she noted sore throat and sinus drainage. She has been unable to speak normally for a week, along with difficult and painful swallowing, reduced appetite, tinnitus, and dizziness when she blows her nose. Her vocal folds are inflamed on examination. *Impression:* Severe upper respiratory infections with bronchitis and laryngitis. Her dysphonia seems out of proportion to the physical findings. She has a good cough. *Psychogenic aphonia.* See Speech Pathology.

Speech Pathology: History. This 33-year-old, married female with two boys aged 4 and 9 years was referred from the Department of Otolaryngology because of suspected psychogenic aphonia. She says she lost her voice 13 days ago. She awoke with a "scratchy" voice, which disappeared within an hour, and she has been whispering ever since. She had one similar voice loss for two days when she was 16 years old.

Examination: The patient was aphonic on examination. However, her cough and coup de glotte were normally sharp. She had +2 musculoskeletal tension and discomfort in the thyrohyoid region in response to palpation.

Diagnostic-therapeutic musculoskeletal tension reduction in the laryngeal-hyoid region *produced completely normal voice within 15 minutes.*

The psychosocial history portion of the examination disclosed serious and chronic emotional problems, which the patient described with considerable crying.

1. She has been desperately unhappy living in a small town where she feels completely isolated with no one to talk to.

2. She feels overburdened having to care for her two children, the youngest of which is exceptionally active and difficult to control.

3. She and her husband fight a great deal over material possessions and about one another's parents. They rarely go out together. He often leaves her alone when he goes hunting and fishing.

4. She complains bitterly about her husband's parents, who dislike her intensely and don't talk to her when they see her in public.

5. She is estranged from her own parents, whom she describes as eccentric and crude. (It is important to note that she lost her voice on the day of an impending visit from her parents.)

6. She cries most intensely while describing her sister's suicide five years ago. She has never spoken to anyone about her feelings concerning her sister's death.

7. She is embarrassed and fearful that her husband will continue to criticize her as being like her sister, and she expresses misgivings as to whether or not she might have the capacity to commit the same act.

Impression: Psychogenic aphonia, probably conversion disorder.

Recommendation: (1) Normal voice followed symptomatic voice therapy, as noted. (2) Discussed with patient and husband the importance of psychiatric consultation. They agreed.

Psychiatrist: This 33-year-old, married mother of two sons was referred for psychiatric consultation by Speech Pathology.

She described developing her difficulty with her voice the day she received news that her father had invited himself and her mother to stay with her and her husband for an indefinite time while her husband went on a hunting trip. Throughout the initial part of the interview, the patient repeatedly returned to her father's physical and verbal abuse and his critical and demeaning nature throughout her entire life. On more recent visits, he has become sexually inappropriate toward her. She describes several other recent sources of life stress and perceives herself to be irritable and unhappy during the past five years, since her younger sister's death by suicide. Since then, she has been more argumentative and difficult to get along with. Other complaints are social and emotional isolation, finding it difficult to make friends and to get babysitters for her two children. She has a poor relationship with her in-laws, whom she perceives as mean to her and judgmental and unsupportive of her throughout her marriage, particularly after the birth of her first child, who had a congenital leg deformity. Recently, she impulsively and angrily confronted them. When they responded defensively in anger, she saw this as confirming their lack of caring and their meanness.

She is frustrated within her marriage, perceiving that her husband's work prevents him from spending sufficient time at home, and she feels isolated, unhappy, and unsupported.

Her family history is positive for suicide in her younger sister, who was diagnosed as schizophrenic and who spent considerable time in and out of psychiatric institutions. She has an alcoholic brother and paternal grandfather, and her maternal grandfather committed suicide during the Depression.

She believes that her upbringing was unhappy—that her father was abusive and uncaring and her mother passive and dominated. Her father treated the girls in the family with disrespect, was demeaning and at times physically abusive. He valued only his sons. She is angry with her mother, who did not defend her and her sisters from this behavior. She was particularly close to her younger sister when they were growing up and they served as support and confidant for each other. In her midteen years her sister became extremely troubled and got involved with a bad crowd at school and with drugs. Her behavior continued to deteriorate, and her sister was disowned by the rest of the family, while the patient repeatedly tried to rescue her and help her. This situation continued for a number of years until this young woman committed suicide. The patient relates having had to deal with funeral home arrangements and visitations and that no one else in the family attended or was supportive. She expresses feelings of guilt and a sense that she should or could have done more despite her repeated attempts to help, although her efforts were undone or rebuffed by her sister.

The mental status examination disclosed the patient to be neatly and stylishly dressed and groomed, appearing younger than her chronologic age. The initial part of the interview consisted of a dramatic litany of many individuals in her life who had or have been "treating me mean." She became tearful while discussing her sister's death and her guilt, remorse, and feelings of isolation. She was able to acknowledge an underlying sense of low self-esteem. At the end of the interview, she was less distraught, more sad, and more comfortable than at the beginning. She acknowledged that she needed to continue to talk with someone. There was no evidence of a thought disorder or gross cognitive impairment. *Her voice remained normal throughout the entire interview.*

Impression: (1) Adjustment disorder with mixed emotional features. (2) Dysthymic disorder. (3) Histrionic personality traits. (4) Secondary marital discord. (5) Conversation aphonia (by history; voice normal on examination).

Recommendation: This patient needs psychotherapy. I will look into different treatment options that would be available for her.

* * *

CONVERSION DYSPHONIA

Varying degrees and types of hoarseness—with and without a strained-harsh quality, high-pitched falsetto breaks, breathiness, intermittent whispering with moments of breathy and normal voice, and other variants too numerous, diverse, and indescribable to mention—occur for the same psychodynamic reasons as muteness and aphonia. A study undertaken by Aronson et al. (1966) comparing mute and aphonic patients with those having varying forms of dysphonia, done in order to determine similarities and differences in the etiology of their voice signs, showed that this dysphonic group was not essentially different in terms of case history, personality, and clinical criteria for conversion reaction from mute or aphonic patients (Table 6-1).

An important finding among all these patients, regardless of voice type, is that despite the psychoneurotic explanation for their voice signs, *few have incapacitating* psychiatric disturbances. In many ways, they have adjusted to their anxiety or depression. Many are willing to continue as they are rather than submit to any therapy. Others are earnest in their desire for a better voice.

PSYCHOGENIC ADDUCTOR SPASTIC DYSPHONIA

As we shall see in the next chapter, certain patients who have an intermittently strained voice, or complete voice arrests from hyperadduction of the vocal folds during contextual speech, *descriptively* called adductor spastic dysphonia, have excess laryngeal musculoskeletal tension caused by *psychologic stress.* Some of these patients have conversion reaction, in which the adductor spastic dysphonia is produced by the same mechanisms that produce conversion muteness and conversion aphonia.

In other patients, the adductor spastic dysphonia is a sign of a *neurologic disorder*, and that is the reason why proper differential diagnosis between the psychogenic and neurologic types of spastic dysphonia is so important. Following is a case study of a young man who developed psychogenic adductor spastic dysphonia, which in all probability was a conversion reaction.

* * *

History: A 29-year-old, single male office worker was referred by Otolaryngology for the evaluation of dysphonia. The patient had complained for several years of an abnormally strained voice. However, laryngologic examination failed to demonstrate any structural lesions or weakness of the vocal folds. He was referred to Speech Pathology for further investigation of the cause of the voice disorder and for therapy.

Examination: This patient has a moderate to severe *adductor spastic dysphonia* consisting of intermittent waxing and waning of strained hoarseness and moments of complete voice arrests due to adductor laryngospasms. Vowel prolongation is clear some of the time but

Table 6–1 Psychiatric Characteristics of 27 Patients with "Functional" Voice Disorders*

Psychiatric Factor	GROUP I (MUTE)	GROUP II (CONTINUALLY WHISPERED)											GROUP III (INTERMITTENTLY) WHISPERED-PHONATED)							GROUP IV (CONTINUALLY PHONATED)								Total +	Total −
	1	2	3	4	5	6	7	8	21	22	23	24	9	10	11	12	13	25	26	14	15	16	17	18	19	20	27	+	−
Acute stress	−	−	+	+	+	−	+	+	+	−	−	−	−	+	−	+	−	−	−	−	−	−	+	−	−	+	−	10	17
Chronic stress	+	+	+	−	−	−	−	−	+	+	−	+	−	+	+	+	+	+	+	−	−	−	+	−	−	−	+	13	14
Conflict symbolism	−	+	+	+	+	+	−	−	−	+	−	−	−	+	−	+	−	+	−	−	−	−	+	+	−	+	+	15	12
Primary gain	−	+	+	+	+	−	+	−	−	−	−	+	−	+	−	+	−	−	+	−	−	−	+	+	−	+	+	13	14
Secondary gain	+	+	+	+	−	+	+	+	−	+	+	−	+	−	+	−	+	−	+	+	−	−	+	−	+	−	+	17	10
Indifference	+	+	+	+	−	+	+	+	+	+	+	−	−	−	+	−	−	+	−	−	+	−	+	−	+	+	+	17	10
Clinical hysteria	+	−	−	−	−	+	+	−	+	+	+	−	+	−	+	+	−	−	−	−	−	−	+	+	−	−	+	12	15
Other conversions	+	−	−	−	−	+	+	−	+	−	−	+	+	−	−	−	−	−	+	−	−	−	+	+	−	−	−	8	19
Somatic complaints	−	−	−	−	−	−	−	−	+	+	+	+	−	−	−	−	+	+	−	−	−	−	+	+	−	−	−	7	20
MMPI conversion†	+	−	−	−	−	+	+	−	+	−	+	−	+	−	+	−	−	−	+	−	−	−	+	−	−	−	+	9	18
Marital discord	−	−	−	−	+	−	−	+	−	+	−	−	+	+	−	+	+	−	+	−	−	+	−	+	−	−	−	10	17
Poor sex identification	+	+	+	+	+	+	+	+	+	+	−	−	+	+	+	+	−	−	−	−	−	+	−	+	+	−	+	18	9
Anger	+	+	+	+	+	+	+	+	+	+	+	+	−	+	+	+	+	+	+	−	+	+	+	+	+	+	+	25	2
Immature-dependent	+	+	+	+	−	+	+	−	+	−	−	+	−	+	+	+	−	+	+	−	+	−	+	+	+	+	+	18	9
Neurotic life adjustment	+	−	+	+	−	+	−	+	−	+	+	+	−	−	+	+	+	+	+	−	−	+	−	+	+	−	−	16	11
Mild to moderate depression	−	+	+	−	−	−	+	+	−	−	−	−	+	−	−	−	+	+	−	−	−	−	−	−	−	−	−	7	20

*From Aronson, A.E., Peterson, H.W. Jr., and Litin, E.M.: Psychiatric symptomatology in functional dysphonia and aphonia. J. Speech Hear. Disord, 31:115–127, 1966.
†Minnesota Multiphasic Personality Inventory.

interrupted by varying degrees of strained hoarseness. The remainder of the oral-physical and speech examinations failed to disclose evidence of motor-speech disorder.

The psychosocial history background to the voice disorder is highly positive. The patient's voice problems began four years ago as *whispered speech,* which lasted three years, except for a 10-month interval during which his voice returned to normal. When the abnormal voice reappeared, it had the intermittently strained voice quality identical to his voice on examination. He has no family history of voice disorder or neurologic disease, including tremor.

The patient is a college graduate who majored in business administration. He is unmarried and lives with his parents. He admits to several problems in his emotional and personal life.

1. He has a history of "fears" that he has difficulty describing. They emerge in the form of nightmares and sudden unpredictable terrors triggered by everyday incidents. For example, he developed a "great fear" a few years ago upon viewing a wax figure in a museum that made him feel as if he were "losing control." For this, and other reasons, the patient has been undergoing psychiatric treatment.

2. The patient expresses considerable ambivalence about living with his parents. He enjoys the comforts of familiar surroundings, being waited on by his parents. At the same time, he is irritated with himself and with them because of his dependency. He does not wish to hurt his parents' feelings, but he is chronically irritated by his father's continuous, perfectionistic criticism of his habits—how he conducts his life, reminding him to straighten his tie and to get his hair cut, and refusing to allow him to use the family car. His mother, whom he describes as frequently irritable, badgers him to get married, which he would very much like to do, but he has always had difficulty establishing compatible relationships with women. He describes his mother as "nagging" and his father as "intolerant."

The patient moved out of his parents' home for nine months, during which *his spastic dysphonia disappeared.* He lived in an apartment, by himself, a few blocks from his parents, but he felt the need to visit them every night. He then moved back into his parents' apartment, whereupon *his spastic dysphonia promptly returned.*

During a discussion with the patient and his parents, they corroborated their son's description of the family relationships, his father saying, "He is afraid to get out on his own. He is overdependent upon us."

The patient, for his part, and with some irritation, rejected the interpretation that his voice disorder had anything to do with his ambivalence about living at home, although later he reluctantly admitted that there might be some connection. Nevertheless, he continued to ask questions revealing that he was looking for an organic explanation for his spastic voice.

Impression: Psychogenic adductor spastic dysphonia, possibly *conversion disorder.* His initial voice problem sounds like he had *conversion aphonia,* and now he has an *adductor spastic dysphonia.* Both the aphonia and the spastic dysphonia disappeared for long periods, only to return. Organic (neurologic) forms of spastic dysphonia do not remit to this extent.

The conflict in which this patient is trapped has to do with his need for his parents' support; however, for this he has had to accept being cast in the role of an adolescent by his parents' continuation of their lifelong overconcern and overcriticism of him. He is unable to separate from his parents and is chronically angry at their overcontrol, but he is unable to vent his anger at them for fear of disturbing them and upsetting the domiciliary arrangements that he enjoys. His spastic dysphonia may be seen as a somatic manifestation of his inability to express his true feelings to his parents.

Recommendations: During an extensive and frank discussion with the patient and his parents, during which the probable underlying dynamics of the voice disorder were discussed, it was re-emphasized that the voice disorder was not caused by organic illness and it was strongly suggested that the patient return to his psychiatrist for more intensive psychotherapy with the objective of helping him to become more self-reliant and less dependent on his parents for emotional and physical support. A full report will be sent to the patient's psychiatrist.

*   *   *

Mutational Falsetto (Puberphonia)

Failure to change from the higher pitched voice of preadolescence to the lower pitched voice of adolescence and adulthood is called "mutational falsetto." In males, the voice may move upward in pitch during puberty, giving the impression of a female voice. This high-pitched falsetto type is *weak, thin, breathy, hoarse, and monopitched, giving the overall impression of immaturity, effeminacy, and passiveness.* In some males and females, the change in voice pitch may have begun but failed to descend completely, stopping somewhere between the pubescent and the adolescent voice. The pitch is lower than the falsetto type but retains a similar weakness, thinness, hoarseness, and monopitch.

Mutational falsetto is not due to any anatomic immaturity of the larynx or vocal folds. The larynx is anatomically and physiologically capable of producing a normal low-pitched voice.

The etiology of mutational falsetto is probably psychogenic, but its dynamics have not been investigated in detail. The individual and family background cannot be depicted other than superficially. The prevailing opinion is that the pubescent or adolescent, if male, acquired a stronger feminine than masculine attachment and self-identification, and a neurotic need to resist the normal transition into adulthood. Variations along these themes include embarrassment about an excessively low-pitched voice developing earlier than the patient's contemporaries, forcing the pubescent male to retain the high-pitched voice, or the unconscious or conscious need to maintain a higher pitched singing voice because of the rewards attendant upon that skill.

Psychologic immaturity may not be the only cause of this disorder. Other factors are: (1) Delayed maturation in endocrine disorders that retards laryngeal development, perpetuating a high-pitched voice which then becomes difficult to abandon because of its longer-than-normal persistence into adolescence, even after the larynx has attained normal size. (2) Severe hearing loss preventing the individual from perceiving his or her voice during adolescent voice change. (3) Weakness or incoordination of the vocal folds or of respiration because of neurologic disease during puberty. (4) General debilitating illness during puberty, which not only may delay overall growth during puberty but, because of the physical restrictions of being bedfast, may reduce the range of respiratory excursions and, consequently, tidal air volumes, preventing the development of adequate infraglottal air pressure necessary for full vocal fold displacement.

The following laryngeal-respiratory postures and movements are bases for the high-pitched mutational falsetto voice (Fig. 6-1).

1. The larynx is elevated high in the neck.

2. The body of the larynx is tilted downward, apparently having the effect of maintaining the vocal folds in a lax state.

3. With the vocal folds in a flabby state, they are stretched thin by contraction of the cricothyroid muscles.

4. The vocal folds are thus in a state of reduced mass and offer little resistance to infraglottal air pressure.

5. Respiration for speech production is shallow, and on exhalation infraglottal air pressure is held to a minimum, so that only the medial edges of the vocal folds vibrate and do so at an elevated fundamental frequency.

Mutational falsetto is found in patients of all ages, some as young as 14 or 15 years and brought by their parents, and others volunteering themselves for help later in life after a long struggle with this social and psychologic handicap. Almost all those seeking help for the first (or tenth) time in their 50s or 60s testify that their voices have broken into deeper or lower pitch levels during shouting or lifting. Characteristically, they fail to recognize the message of normalcy that these downward pitch breaks reveal. The falsetto voice is the only one they know. Producing a sharp glottal attack with or without the examiner exerting downward force on the larynx during phonation elicits the low-pitched voice. The psychologic penalties of mutational falsetto are great, labeling the male bearer as feminine. Use of the telephone is particularly embarrassing, since callers misinterpret the male with falsetto as being female. Teasing of young males in school and rejection for employment are additional problems.

Clinicians often miss the diagnosis of mutational falsetto because of unfamiliarity with the syndrome. Yet it is one of the easiest and most rewarding disorders to treat. Familiarity with the distinctive sound of mutational falsetto and the method of testing for it should be mandatory in the training of all speech pathologists and laryngologists.

Transsexualism

Changing one's anatomy in order to assume the opposite sexual role is called "transsexualism." The majority of such changes are from male to female. Such individuals need, in addition to an altered physical appearance, speech that conforms to the chosen sexual identity. The effects on the larynx of the administration of female hormones for the enhancement of female characteristics are apparently minimal. The successful elevation of fundamental frequency in transsexuals as a consequence of voice therapy has been reported by Bralley et al. (1978). These researchers were able to elevate fundamental frequency in one patient from 145 to 165 Hz after seven therapy sessions. Kalra (1977) was able to change the fundamental frequency of a male-to-female transsexual from a mean of 168 to 196 Hz after four therapy sessions. These patients reported satisfaction with their increased fundamental frequencies, although as it turned out, voice pitch was not the only method of effecting changes: Altered phoneme production, inflectional patterns, and even vocabulary contributed to the total impression of femininity.

Childlike Speech in Adults

Adults, adolescents, and children are seen in clinical practice who present with childlike speech patterns. The effect of a mature person speaking like a child is created by a combination of

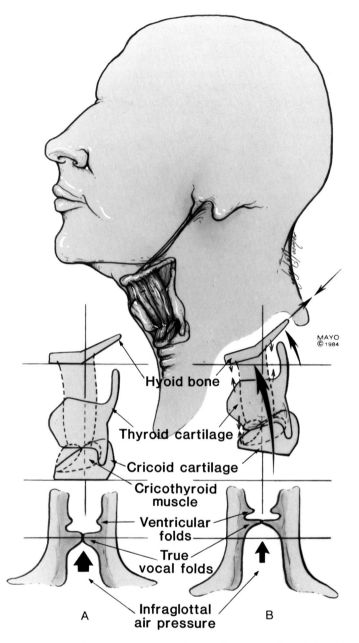

MAYO
© 1984

Hyoid bone

Thyroid cartilage

Cricoid cartilage

Cricothyroid
muscle

Ventricular
folds

True
vocal folds

A   Infraglottal   B
          air pressure

Figure 6-1   Comparison of Normal Laryngeal Position with that of mutational falsetto. A = Normal phonation. Note relatively low position of larynx, ample thyrohyoid space, blunt edges of vocal folds and high infraglottal pressure. B = Mutational falsetto. Note relatively high position of larynx, narrowed thyrohyoid space, thin edges of vocal folds and low infraglottal pressure.

phonatory, resonatory, and articulatory modifications. However, in addition to the speech patterns that simulate those of a child, the impression of immaturity is augmented by facial expressions, gestures, and postures that convey dependency and passiveness. The aberrant speech patterns usually consist of: (1) *elevation of habitual pitch;* (2) *exaggerated and ingratiating inflexional patterns;* (3) *articulation with reduced mouth opening;* (4) *open facial expression with raising of eyebrows;* (5) *cherubic smiling;* and (6) *demure head movements, bodily postures, and gestures.*

Regressive speech serves the purpose of relieving the person from the responsibility of relating to others on an adult plane. It says, in effect, that the person does not wish to be regarded as an adult with the responsibilities for mutual interaction that an adult relationship entails. The following case study illustrates one variation on the theme of childlike speech in adults.

*   *   *

Speech Pathology: This is a 26-year-old, divorced woman with two young children who is a student in a junior college. She was referred by the school counselor, who was concerned about the patient's speech because of its implications for her future ability to succeed academically, socially, and vocationally. She feels self-conscious about her speech and is afraid to start conversations.

On examination, she had a high-pitched voice produced with childlike inflectional patterns. She articulated with small, smiling mouth postures and spoke with her head cocked to one side, using supplicating, ingratiating gestures as she did so.

Prior otolaryngologic examination established that her larynx was of normal size. On phonatory examination, she was able to lower her pitch considerably when instructed to do so but was unable to sustain a low-pitched voice during conversational speech.

Symptomatic voice therapy was administered during seven voice therapy sessions over a period of one month during which the patient was able to lower her pitch and eliminate many of her childlike mannerisms. Having accomplished this change in her external means of communication, she began to express the need for greater independence and complained that she found it difficult to use the more adult speech patterns that she had learned in social relationships because of the persistence of her childlike and dependent self-image.

Psychiatric consultation with the possibility of psychotherapy was recommended, to which the patient acquiesced somewhat reluctantly but realized that changing her speech alone would not solve all of her interpersonal and self-image problems. A psychiatric consultation was arranged.

Psychiatry: This patient was seen in psychiatric consultation because of her unusual voice and speech mannerisms, which would appear to be associated with her basic personality and self-concept. Her entire demeanor, including her gestures, posture, manner of speech, and tone of voice, come across as a very small, dependent, and naive child.

Her history suggests that she has always been a very passive and dependent person. As she talks about her current situation and past problems, she does not give any indication that she recognizes that she may have played a part in them. All of the difficulties in her life, as she sees them, are due to unavoidable circumstances or to "not nice" people.

She, herself, does not actually complain about her voice. She indicates that a counselor who is working with her said that it would be better if she had "a more assertive voice." She says that some people act like they think she has a nice voice, while others seem surprised by it. In her very childlike way she indicates that she always has been very shy with people and that she doesn't speak up very often. She says that she can talk to "nice people" but doesn't like to talk to people who are not nice, saying that "some people are rude." These terms "nice" and "not nice" seem to be almost her only adjectives in describing others.

The patient never liked school, didn't see much point to it, and didn't see why she should have to go to school. She felt that "a lot of the kids were not nice and some were rude." She had considerable difficulty academically.

Regarding her voice, she comments that before she was 13 years old her voice was both lower in pitch and louder, but, even then, she said she was shy and would rarely speak up. She rather passively accepted others' opinions that maybe her voice is a problem.

It is my impression that this patient's voice is simply the most obvious component of the overall manner in which she presents herself. Her speech is the external sign of an hysterical personality structure in which she envisions herself in the role of a tiny, passive, dependent child who almost, but not quite, speaks "baby talk" and who is upset by people who are "not nice," people who might challenge her playing of this role. At this time, she does not express any insight or concern about her personality problems or her own pattern of behaving or relating.

Psychotherapy summary: Throughout several months of weekly therapy, this patient continued to speak in a very high-pitched, infantile voice. There were moments when this type of speech would improve throughout the hour, but it was quite unusual for this to happen. During initial therapy sessions, the patient presented herself as someone who is very rigid and moralistic. She would come regularly to therapy; however, she became upset when a session had to be canceled and refused to come or call. She seemed to handle very poorly any absences or fluctuations on the part of the psychiatrist. She seemed relatively uninvested in the therapy and saw to it that the sessions remained superficial. She was quite resistant toward efforts to enable her to gain insight into her interpersonal problems and into the deeper issues causing her childlike demeanor. Any expression of painful affect was usually met by fleeing from the therapy session. She was extremely sensitive to any change in schedule, which was followed by weeks of nonattendance. Finally, she failed to return even after contact with her by telephone. She does not seem capable of handling insight-oriented psychotherapy and does not seem to have the ego strength to tolerate a transferential relationship.

* * *

REBOUND PSYCHOLOGIC EFFECTS OF VOICE DISORDERS

To possess a voice disorder, whether psychogenic or organic, is to experience demoralization. Voice is part of the person. Self-alienation occurs when our voices are no longer "us." Once the patient learns that the voice disorder is not a threat to health, an adverse secondary psychologic reaction sets in triggered by the patient's rejection of his or her own voice and by the reactions of listeners. "What is the matter with your voice? . . . You should do something about your voice!" Change in facial expression of listeners upon hearing the abnormal voice is detected easily by the patient. It is only a brief time from the onset of the disorder until the patient begins to dread meeting others, aquaintances and strangers alike. The individual with a defective voice elects to speak less and less often in order to avoid such reactions. We observe the depressing effects of voice disorders in well-adjusted patients with organic voice disorders as well as in those whose disorders are psychogenic. In addition to their primary psychologic discomfort, patients with psychogenic voice disorders have amplification of their already unhappy state because of self and listener rejection of the voice.

If the patient's voice disorder is severe enough to interfere with intelligibility, the situation can be even worse. It is difficult to understand these individuals in noisy and even quiet environments, so that their voice disorders seriously interfere with their professional, business, and social lives. Consequently, the effect of the voice disorder on others and on the patient becomes circular and escalating: The patient's frustration and anger elevate musculoskeletal tension, and whatever primary organic or psychogenic voice disorder existed up to that point is worsened to an even greater degree of severity. It is axiomatic that emotional stress exacerbates virtually all voice disorders, whether organic or psychogenic. Those who are privileged to care for individuals who have moderate to severe voice disorders will become convinced that the anger, frustration, anxiety, depression, and discouragement that these patients experience from the social effects of the disorder itself is tantamount to an illness requiring as much attention as the voice per se.

IATROGENIC VOICE REST

They told me not to talk too much. I feel, if I'm all right, why are they asking me to keep quiet? Now that they told me not to talk, I'm worried. Never to scream? Never to sing? They also told me not to cough. I've been holding my voice back. The aggravation is sitting right here (points to neck and chest). I can't let it out.

Any illness induced by the actions of the clinician is called *iatrogenic*. Voice disorders can be caused or worsened by the actions of the clinician. The patient who undergoes surgery on the vocal folds or on those regions of the neck or chest that may result in paralysis of the vocal folds may experience dysphonia, either temporarily or permanently. What cannot be predicted in such cases is the extent of the patient's suggestibility upon recovery from surgery. Upon hearing the abnormal voice, the patient may become anxious or depressed and may develop a musculoskeletal tension or even a conversion voice disorder superimposed upon the organic one. Psychogenic voice disorders following laryngeal surgery have occurred because of unconscious hostility toward the surgeon.

A second, and perhaps more common iatrogenic voice disorder begins with the ill-advised prescription of voice rest. With the exception of a few surgical procedures requiring voice rest (and even then only brief rest is required), *to advise patients with organic, and particularly psychogenic, voice disorders to whisper or remain mute for days or weeks is the worst advice that can be given a patient with a voice disorder*. The larynx and voice are exceptionally suggestible and responsive to anxiety. When a clinician suggests voice rest, a seed of doubt is planted about that patient's basic ability to phonate. The common result is a secondary psychogenic voice disorder. An added complication of voice rest is that failure to use the vocal folds causes flaccidity of nonuse, creating still another dysphonia in addition to that already present. How the idea of voice rest originated as a "therapy" is not clear. One suspects that it is the choice of clinicians who, knowing little about the care of the patient with a voice disorder, reason by analogy that inasmuch as rest is good for many things, it ought to be good for the voice too. The following testimony is from a speech clinician who herself was placed on voice rest.

> It all seemed so simple . . . a nodule on the right vocal band would be removed under general anesthesia and one or two weeks of vocal rest would be advised. The Christmas season appeared the quietest time in terms of diminished teaching responsibilities with the hope that the hoarseness I exhibited for several months would be diminished.
>
> Optimistically, I entered the hospital situation, even having them obligingly do the blood work and allow me to go "out to dinner." Lovely hotel, food lacked style! The surgery was uneventful, occurring early in the morning and I returned home that evening, drowsy but well. Flowers arrived and solicitous calls came constantly. It all seemed a lark! I was perfectly in control of the situation. Clinically, it would be an interesting situation for someone in the field of Speech Pathology. What followed was a nightmare of psychologic trauma.
>
> As director of a large speech and language center, it seemed only reasonable that I could return to work immediately. My family, who at first seemed delighted with a silent mother and wife, quickly began to realize that this same person would need them to answer her phone calls, make calls, and generally accomplish those things which require voice. This, in itself, would have been no problem. What I didn't plan on was the feeling of isolation. The ungodly sense of being a spectator to the world! We read about this psychologic phenomenon; we talk about it when we teach. Until one experiences the detachment and the profound loneliness, one cannot readily understand what the words vocal silence really mean.
>
> Few people enjoy talking to someone who can give only a "yes" or "no" return. Cryptic notes, written on magic slate, soon lose their readability, as well as their interest. My husband as well as my colleagues appeared annoyed at the frequent taps on their shoulders or the snapping of my fingers: two methods I used to focus attention on my slate.
>
> As an individual who has worked long years at creating dialogue in my household, my family showed deep resentment toward the monologue situation. Mother could not talk about her feelings. Her body was fine, why didn't she talk? My disability became almost a personal affront and inconvenience. Even my dearest friends soon tired of calling and waiting for phone taps: one equaled yes, two equaled no, and multiple taps meant goodbye. The burden of conversation on the part of the speaker became more problematical than anticipated. How difficult it must be for the parent who receives little or no response from their child!
>
> Peoples' responses generally ranged from humor to a singing or gestural response which assumed that I could not hear or speak. One bright-eyed stranger asked me if I were a mute.
>
> The frustration of not being in control was devastating. One constantly needs someone else, and locked within you are all the reactions and impressions that for years you have learned to share and enjoy. The very antithesis of one's basic personality was operating.

As I write this I am still silent . . . eagerly awaiting the end of this journey. My need to write this is based on my need to communicate and to assist those of us who work with aphasia, vocal problems, and other speech and language problems, to attempt to gain some insight into the psychological and emotional aspects of the problems involved. My entire approach to therapy has altered as a result of this experience. Never again will I read, hear, or advise "vocal rest" with the same lack of understanding or empathy (Fiedler, 1977).

The following study illustrates a repeated finding in the practice of voice disorders: When patients become dysphonic or aphonic, either unconsciously, or voluntarily, as in vocal rest, they seem to lose their sense or feel for volitional phonation. It is an experience that teaches the clinician that the patient has undergone some sort of loss of recall, memory, or even praxis for normal voice production. We do not think that the articulatory mechanism is susceptible in a similar way to the effects of nonuse, illustrating again the special nature of the larynx and phonation.

* * *

D.S., a five-year-old boy, was found to have small bilateral vocal nodules. His speech clinician placed him on complete voice rest, which unfortunately was enforced for five continuous months. At the end of five months, the nodules had disappeared, and the child was instructed by both the physician and speech pathologist to renew normal phonation. Despite all efforts by the child, he could only whisper. He became completely aphonic, but conversed easily with all people with much animation and relative comfort. This functional aphonia remained for two months after he was instructed, "Go back and talk the normal way, Davey." The child gestured that he wanted to use his voice but that he could not "find it." Therapy efforts to restore the phonation were begun some seven months after the child's natural phonation had ceased (Boone, 1977).

SUMMARY

1. Voice may provide clues to underlying personality in normal individuals; however, research to prove this assumption is fraught with problems of defining personality, vocal parameters, and acceptable research methodology.

2. Specific changes in voice quality, pitch, and loudness have been associated with discrete emotional states, environmental stress, depression, and schizophrenia.

3. Psychogenic voice disorders are muteness, aphonia, and dysphonia in the absence of organic laryngeal disease, or with disease that is insufficient to explain the voice disorder. These voice disorders can be traced to the anxiety or depression produced by life stress, to psychoneuroses, or to personality disorders.

4. Musculoskeletal tension due to environmental stress can produce a variety of dysphonias, sometimes even aphonia, that are the effects of hypercontraction of the extrinsic and intrinsic laryngeal musculature.

5. If hypercontraction of the musculature caused by musculoskeletal tension is combined with vocal abuse, the tissue reactions of inflammation, a vocal nodule, or contact ulcer can develop, causing further dysphonia.

6. A vocal nodule is a small white or grayish protuberance on the free margin of the vocal fold at the junction of the anterior and middle third, unilaterally or bilaterally. It is a protective tissue reaction to trauma.

Vocal nodules occur in children of both sexes, and most commonly in adult females who use their voices excessively by screaming, yelling, excess talking, or singing.

More often than not, children and adults with vocal nodules give a history of interpersonal conflict, often tied in with family problems, and have an aggressive and controlling personality.

7. A contact ulcer is a superficial ulceration of the mucosa overlying the medial surface of the arytenoid cartilage at the junction of the posterior third of the vocal fold. It develops at the tip of the vocal process of the arytenoid cartilage, unilaterally or bilaterally.

The ulcer is caused by forceful and damaging contact between the opposing arytenoid cartilages during forceful phonation under conditions of heightened muscular tension and reduced pitch.

Contact ulcer has a predilection for males in their 40s who come from occupational backgrounds involving greater-than-average voice use and who show personality characteristics of aggressiveness and competitiveness.

Smoking, alcohol consumption, and air pollution are often associated findings in the histories of patients who have contact ulcer.

8. A conversion voice disorder is muteness, aphonia, or dysphonia in which there is an involuntary loss of control over the muscles of phonation as an unconscious attempt to avoid unpleasant confrontations.

9. Voice disorders can occur in patients who have problems of emotional maturity and sex identification. Mutational falsetto (puberphonia) is the failure of adolescent voice change, most often in males, despite normal laryngeal growth.

10. Whether organic or psychogenic, all voice disorders produce adverse secondary psychologic effects on the speaker, increasing the severity of the primary voice disorder.

11. Iatrogenic voice disorders are those caused inadvertently in the course of treatment of other medical or surgical problems and as a result of injudicious advice, the most notable of which is voice rest.

SUGGESTIONS FOR ADDITIONAL READING

Aronson, A.E., Peterson, H.W., Jr., and Litin, E.M.: Psychiatric symptomatology in functional dysphonia and aphonia. J. Speech Hear. Disord., 31:115–127, 1966.
This article illustrates the strong influence of interpersonal problems on the development and maintenance of dysphonia and aphonia.

Bady, S.L.: The voice as curative factor in psychotherapy. Psychoanal. Rev., 72:479–490, 1985.
This article on the importance and meaning of voice for patient and psychotherapist alike makes extremely interesting reading. The author goes into considerable detail about how the therapist's voice can facilitate therapy and how the patient's voice indicates that person's emotional status. The act of verbalizing one's thoughts is analyzed as a physical as well as psychologic one, having almost tactile effects.

Elias, A., Raven, R., Butcher, P., and Littlejohns, D.W.: Speech therapy for psychogenic voice disorder: A survey of current practice and training. Br. J. Disord. Commun., 24:61–76, 1989.
This article is worth reading for information on the attitudes and practices of speech clinicians in the United Kingdom toward patients with psychogenic dysphonia and aphonia. This survey revealed some interesting opinions and practices concerning the inadequacy of their undergraduate education in psychology and psychiatry and the extent to which such education served them later in practice. From the study, the authors were led to conclude that much more background in psychology and psychiatry was necessary in the practical treatment of patients with psychogenic voice disorders. (See Chapter 11 for more details about this study.)

Hartman, D.E., and Aronson, A.E.: Psychogenic aphonia masking mutational falsetto. Arch. Otolaryngol., 109:415–416, 1983.
An interesting case illustrating the coexistence of two psychogenic voice disorders, the second caused by the first.

Kramer, E.: Judgment of personal characteristics and emotions from nonverbal properties of speech. Psychol. Bull., 60:408–420, 1963.
An excellent, unbiased critical review of the literature on the relationship between voice, personality, emotions, and psychopathology.

Peacher, G.: Contact ulcer of the larynx: Part IV. A clinical study of vocal re-education. J. Speech Disord., 12:179–190, 1947.
One of a series of four landmark studies on the etiology, symptomatology, and therapy of contact ulcer. Check its bibliography for the remaining three. They're well worth reading.

Ziegler, F.S., and Imboden, J.B.: Contemporary conversion reactions: II. Conceptual model, Arch. Gen. Psychiatry, 6:279–287, 1962.
An absolute must for anyone who works with psychogenic voice disorders because it explains so well the modern interpretation of conversion and hysteria.

REFERENCES

Andrews, M., and Shank, K.: Some observations concerning the cheerleading behavior of school-girl cheerleaders. Lang. Speech. Hear. Serv. Sch., 14:150–156, 1983.

Arnold, G.E.: Vocal nodules and polyps; laryngeal tissue reactions to habitual dysphonia. J. Speech Hear. Disord., 27:205–217, 1962.

Aronson, A.E., Peterson, H.W., Jr., and Litin, E.M.: Psychiatric symptomatology in functional dysphonia and aphonia. J. Speech Hear. Disord.: 31:115–127, 1966.

Bady, S.L.: The voice as curative factor in psychotherapy. Psychoanal. Rev., 72:479–490, 1985.

Barker, K.D., and Wilson, F.B.: Comparative study of vocal utilization of children with hoarseness and normal voice. Paper presented at the convention of the American Speech and Hearing Association, Chicago, 1967.

Boone, D.R.: The Voice and Voice Therapy. Englewood Cliffs, Prentice-Hall, 1977.

Bralley, R.C., Bull, J.L., Gore, C.H., and Edgerton, M.T.: Evaluation of vocal pitch in male transsexuals. J. Commun. Disord., 11:443–449, 1978.

Brown, B.L., Strong, W.J., and Rencher, A.C.: Fifty-four voices from two: The effects of simultaneous manipulations of rate, mean fundamental frequency, and variance of fundamental frequency on ratings of personality from speech. J. Acoust. Soc. Am., 55:313–318, 1974.

Chevrie-Muller, C., Dodart, F., Sequier-Dermer, N., and Salmon, D.: Étude des parameters acoustiques de la parole au cours de la schizophrenic de l'adolescent. Folia Phoniatr., 23:401–428, 1971.

Costanzo, F.S., Markel, N.N., and Costanzo, P.R.: Voice quality profile and perceived emotion. J. Counsel. Psychol., 16:267–270, 1969.

Davitz, J.R.: The Communication of Emotional Meaning. New York, McGraw-Hill, 1964.

Duncan, S., Rice, L., and Butler, J.M.: The therapists' paralanguage in peak and poor psychotherapy hours. J. Abnorm. Psychol., 73:566–570, 1968.

Eldred, S.H., and Price, D.B.: The linguistic evaluation of feeling states in psychotherapy. Psychiatry, 21:115–121, 1958.

Fairbanks, G., and Hoaglin, L.W.: An experimental study of the durational characteristics of the voice during the expression of emotion. Speech Monographs, 8:85–90, 1941.

Fairbanks, G., and Pronovost, W.: An experimental study of the pitch characteristics of the voice during the expression of emotion. Speech Monographs, 6:87–104, 1939.

Fiedler, I.: Vocal rest. ASHA, 19:4, 307–308, 1977.

Friedman, M., and Rosenman, R.H.: Association of specific overt behavior pattern with blood and cardiovascular findings: Blood cholesterol level, blood clotting time, incidence of arcus senilis, and clinical coronary artery disease. J.A.M.A., 169:1286–1696, 1959.

Friedman, M., Brown, A.E., and Rosenman, R.H.: Voice analysis for detection of behavior patterns. J.A.M.A., 208:828–836, 1969.

Glassel, W.L.: A study of personality problems and vocal nodules in children. Paper presented at the American Speech and Hearing Association Convention, San Francisco, 1972.

Goldfarb, W., Brownstein, P., and Lorge, I.: A study of speech patterns in a group of schizophrenic children. Am. J. Orthopsychiatry, 26:544–555, 1956.

Goldfarb, W., Goldfarb, N., Brownstein, P., and Scholl, H.: Speech and language faults of schizophrenic children. J. Austism Child. Schizophr., 2:219–233, 1972.

Green, G.: Psycho-behavioral characteristics of children with vocal nodules: WPBIC ratings. J. Speech Hear. Disord., 54:306–312, 1989.

Greene, M.C.L.: The Voice and Its Disorders. Philadelphia, J.B. Lippincott Co., 1972.

Hargreaves, W.A., and Starkweather, J.A.: Voice quality changes in depression. Lang. Speech, 7:84–88, 1964.

Huttar, G.L.: Relations between prosodic variables and emotions in normal American English utterances. J. Speech Hear. Res., 11:481–487, 1968.

Jensen, P.: Hoarseness in cheerleaders. ASHA, 6:406, 1964.

Kalra, M.A.: Voice therapy with a transsexual. Paper presented at the American Speech and Hearing Association Convention, Chicago, 1977.

Kazan, E.: A Life. Doubleday, New York, 1988.

Khachatur'yants, L., and Grimak, L.: Cosmonaut's emotional stress in space flight. N.A.S.A. Space TT, F-14, p. 654, 1972.

Levin, H., and Lord, W.: Speech pitch frequency as an emotional state indicator. IEEE Trans. Sys. Man Cybernet., 2:259–272, 1975.

Luchsinger, R., and Arnold, G.E.: Voice—Speech—Language. Belmont, California, Wadsworth Publishing Co., 1965.

Mallory, E., and Miller, V.: A possible basis for the association of voice characteristics and personality traits. Speech Monographs, 25:255–260, 1958.

Markel, N.N., Bern, M.F., and Phillis, J.A.: The relationship between words and tone-of-voice. Lang. Speech, 16:15–21, 1973.

Moore, W.E.: Personality traits and voice quality deficiencies. J. Speech Hear. Disord., 4:33–36, 1939.

Mosby, D.: Predominant personality characteristics of 25 children with voice disorders. Paper presented at the American Speech and Hearing Association Convention, Chicago, 1967.

Moses, P.J.: The Voice of Neurosis. New York, Grune & Stratton, 1954.

Moskowitz, E.: Voice quality in schizophrenic reaction type. Doctoral Thesis. New York, New York University, 1951.

Nemec, J.: The motivation background of hyperkinetic dysphonia in children: A contribution to psychologic research in phoniatry. Logos, 4:28–31, 1961.

Newman, S.S., and Mather, V.G.: Analysis of spoken language of patients with affective disorders. Am. J. Psychiatry, 94:912–942, 1938.

Ostwald, P.F., and Skolnikoff, A.: Speech disturbances in a schizophrenic adolescent. Postgrad. Med., 40:49, July, 1966.

Peacher, G.: Contact ulcer of the larynx: Part IV: A clinical study of vocal re-education. J. Speech Disord., 12:179–190, 1947.

Peacher, G., and Hollinger, O.: Contact ulcer of the larynx: The role of re-education. Arch. Otolaryngol., 46:617–621, 1947.

Perellò, J.: Dysphonies fonctionnelles: Phonoponose et phonoevrose. Folia Phoniatr., 14:150–205, 1962.

Popov, V.A., Simonov, P.V., Frolov, M.V., and Khachatur'yants, L.S.: The articulatory frequency spectrum as an indicator of the degree and nature of emotional stress in man. N.A.S.A. TT, F-13, p. 772, 1971.

Reich, A., McHenry, M., and Keaton, A.: A survey of dysphonic episodes in high school cheerleaders. Lang. Speech Hear. Serv. Sch., 17:63–71, 1986.

Rosenman, R.H., Friedman, M., Straus, R., Wurm, M., Kositchek, R., Hahn, W., and Werthessen N.J.: A predictive study of coronary heart disease: The Western Collaborative Group Study. J.A.M.A., 189:15–22, 1964.

Saxman, J.M., and Burk, K.W.: Speaking fundamental frequency and rate characteristics of adult female schizophrenics. J. Speech Hear. Res., 11:194–203, 1968.

Scherer, K.R., London, H., and Wolf, J.: The voice of confidence: Paralinguistic cues and audience evaluation. J. Res. Personal., 7:31–44, 1973.

Sedlácek, K., and Sychra, A.: Die melodie als faktor des emotionellen ausdruchs. Folia Phoniatr., 15:89–98, 1973.

Senturia, D.H., and Wilson, F.B.: Otorhinolaryngolic findings in children with voice deviations. Ann. Otol. Rhinol. Laryngol., 77:1–15, 1968.

Simonov, F.V., and Frolov, M.V.: Utilization of human voice for estimation of man's emotional stress and state of attention. Aerospace Med., 44:256–258, 1973.

Skinner, E.R.: A calibrated recording and analysis of the pitch, force and quality of vocal tones expressing happiness and sadness, and a determination of the pitch and force of the subjective concepts of ordinary, soft, and loud tones. Speech Monographs, 2:81–137, 1935.

Takahashi, R., Hinohara, T., Ohmori, K., and Saruya, S.: Psychosomatic aspects of the complaint of foreign feelings of the pharyngolaryngeal region. In Ear, Nose and Throat Studies, Dept. of Otorhinolaryngology, Jikei University School of Medicine, Tokyo, 1971, pp. 723–729.

Tarrasch, H.: Muscle spasticity in functional aphonia and dysphonia. Med. Wom. J., 53:25–33, 1946.

Toohill, R.J.: The psychosomatic aspects of children with vocal nodules. Arch. Otolaryngol., 101:591–595, 1975.

Van den Berg, J.: Modern research in experimental phoniatrics. Folia Phoniatr., 14:81–149, 1962.

Vaughn, C.W.: Current concepts in otolaryngology: Diagnosis and treatment of organic voice disorders. N. Engl. J. Med., 307:333–336, 1982.

Williams, C.E., and Stevens, K.N.: Emotions and speech: Some acoustical correlates. J. Acous. Soc. Am., 52:1238–1250, 1969.

Williamson, A.B.: Diagnosis and treatment of 72 cases of hoarse voice. Q. J. Speech, 31:189–202, 1945.

Whitman, E.N., and Flicker, D.J.: A potential new measurement of emotional state: A preliminary report. Newark Beth Israel Hosp., 17:167–172, 1966.

Wilson, F.B., and Lamb, M.M.: Comparison of personality characteristics of children with and without vocal nodules on Rorschach protocol interpretation. Paper presented at the American Speech and Hearing Association Convention, Atlanta, 1973.

Zaliouk, A., and Izkovitch, I.: Some tomographic aspects in functional voice disorders. Folia Phoniatr., 10:34–39, 1958.

Ziegler, F.S., and Imboden, J.B.: Contemporary conversion reactions: II. Conceptual model. Arch. Gen. Psychiatry, 6:279–287, 1962.

Zuberbier, E.: Zur Schreib-und Sprechmotorik der Depression. Psychother. Med. Psychol., 7:239–249, 1957.

SUPPLEMENTARY STUDIES IN PSYCHOGENIC VOICE DISORDERS

VOCAL NODULE AND PERSONALITY AGGRESSIVENESS

The following case study was selected to illustrate the inseparability between the development of vocal nodules and vocal acting out, basic personality, and family conflict in children who develop this disorder.

* * *

Speech Pathology
   History: This is a 9½-year-old boy who was brought to the clinic for evaluation of a voice disorder of four years' duration. Otolaryngologic examination revealed small, bilateral vocal nodules. He has had four years of voice therapy without benefit.
   Examination: This child has a moderately breathy voice consistent with vocal nodules.
   The psychosocial history obtained from the mother is positive. She describes her child's personality as a "type A." She says that he is "aggressive, hard on himself, perfectionistic, always the first in line, and very competitive." She emphasizes that the two of them get into daily, escalating yelling matches if he can't have his way or when she restricts his activities. "His first tendency is to yell when he gets emotional. He needs a lot of discipline and control." The mother, interestingly, describes herself as having had a similar relationship with her parents. She describes herself and her husband as high achievers with a high degree of self-expectation.
   Impression: Vocal nodules secondary to vocal abuse from yelling, inseparable from personality aggressiveness and argumentative disputes with parents over daily activities.
   Recommendation: Because the vocal nodules are not simply caused by vocal abuse but are actually the end products of the verbal acting out of conflicts with his parents over discipline, both parent and child need to be seen by Child Psychiatry for further diagnosis and recommendations. The mother was most appreciative of this suggestion, and an appointment has been made in Child Psychiatry.
   Voice therapy has not helped this child because he cannot suppress his anger and the manipulative use of his voice. His nodules and complaints of chronic sore throat might improve with a change in the family interrelationships.

Child Psychiatry: This child entering the fourth grade was referred because of hoarseness associated with vocal nodule suspected as being related to family conflict.
   He is the oldest of two children. His parents feel that he has always been a highly stressed child, needing to be first and reluctant to fail. He will cry after a soccer match if he loses. In the second grade he had a teacher who was excessively critical, and he frequently refused to do his homework or clenched his fists at home. He will put himself down at home when he is punished or disciplined, saying, "I'm no good, I'm a failure." There is no history of depression, obsessive or compulsive thinking, phobias, or sleep disturbances. His younger brother, age 6, is more easy-going.
   The child's mother identifies the child with her father, who has always been hard-driving and achievement-oriented. She felt that, in her childhood, her parents gave her very little attention. Consequently she has had a low concept of herself growing up and was determined that this would not happen to her son. She is highly invested in his success.
   In my interview with the child, he presented himself in a measured and guarded way. He talked freely about his interest in soccer, sports, airplanes, and collecting things. He did not describe any chronic dysphoria, fears, or anxieties. His chief unhappiness was when he did not have something that he wanted. He thinks of himself as a good student. He makes friends well in school but has no close friends in his neighborhood. He seemed somewhat immature in his

way of conversing and had a mild suggestion of a serious frown to his demeanor. He described a happy relationship with both of his parents and a happy life together for both of them, but he thought of his father as being more absent from the family circle.

Impression: Although this is an essentially normal child, he has perfectionistic behavioral characteristics. Although no specific therapy recommendations were given, we discussed means of helping him to increase his self-esteem. His father could spend more time with him and increase the father–son identification and diminish somewhat the strong identification and dependency relationship that he has with his mother.

* * *

HOARSENESS, CONTACT ULCER, AND PSYCHOLOGICAL STRESS

The common association between contact ulcer, vocal misuse, and life stress is demonstrated in the following case study.

* * *

History: A 26-year-old college student was referred by Otolaryngology, having been diagnosed as having bilateral contact ulcer granulomas attributed to vocal misuse or abuse.

The patient began having throat and voice difficulties six to eight months ago when he began noticing a sensation of "swelling, tightness or lump" in his throat.

Examination: This patient has a rough hoarseness consistent with contact ulcer. He also has musculoskeletal pain in response to pressure in the laryngeal-hyoid region.

The psychosocial history is strongly positive. Although he does not admit to continuous voice misuse, he does say that he has to raise his voice daily in order to discipline children who ride in the school bus which he drives approximately 15 hours a week in order to help support himself through college. He is also carrying a full academic load. He also admits speaking loudly against background noise in "dance bars."

At approximately the time the patient began having trouble with his voice he was beginning to have difficulties in his relationship with his fiancé, who terminated their relationship because of extreme differences in outlook. From that time to the present the patient has been depressed, unable to sleep or to concentrate, and has increased his use of alcohol and marijuana to counteract his feelings of depression and rejection.

Impression: This patient's contact ulcer would appear to have resulted from the combined effects of vocal abuse, chemical abuse, and chronic depression.

Recommendation: (1) The patient was advised to reduce the quantity and intensity of voice use until healing of the contact ulcer. (2) Psychological counseling was strongly recommended, which the patient accepted with almost immediate insight.

* * *

HOARSENESS, CONTACT ULCER, AND PSYCHOLOGICAL STRESS

Anger and yelling go hand-in-hand with the development of contact ulcer as in the following case study.

* * *

History: A 50-year-old executive began complaining of throat and voice trouble seven months ago. He describes its beginning as a feeling of something like a "fish hook" in his throat. He was not aware of any voice change at the time but was concerned about the discomfort and its implications. He consulted an otolaryngologist who diagnosed contact ulcer granuloma of the left vocal fold. After having been placed on modified voice use he was reexamined five months later when it was found that the granuloma had remained.

Examination: This patient has a rough hoarseness and excessively low-pitched voice consistent with contact ulcer.

The psychosocial history during the time of onset and development of his contact ulcer is highly positive. In addition to being the vice president of a large corporation, the patient is a community leader, using his voice to a much greater than average extent in carrying out his responsibilities as a public speaker and as a member of several boards.

The major stress that has affected his life has been occurring at home. For the past five years his wife, who is 15 years younger than the patient and whom he describes as "beautiful, well educated, and well liked," has been having increasing problems with alcohol. During the past year her alcohol consumption has increased alarmingly to the point that she now has a daily habit pattern of drinking that begins late in the afternoon and lasts throughout the evening. The patient often returns home after work to find his wife intoxicated. Her disinhibited behavior when under the influence of alcohol has become increasingly disturbing to the patient, whose anxiety about the possibility that his wife's behavior might become known to the small community in which they live has intensified, fearing that her behavior will negatively influence their status as a family and affect his business.

Particularly during the past year, the patient has had violent arguments with his wife consisting of angry vocal exchanges of long duration occurring two to three times a week. He exclaims, "If we could get her out of that habit everything would be great." Unfortunately, during the time of his vocal abuse from arguments with his wife, the patient himself has increased his own alcohol consumption.

Impression: Voice disorder due to vocal and alcohol abuse resulting in contact ulcer, inseparably related to a major upheaval in the patient's domestic life.

Recommendation: This highly intelligent executive has known for a long time that he and his wife need psychological counseling but has avoided obtaining it because of the fear that to do so will become known in the small community in which they live. Unfortunately, their local physicians have played into this failure to obtain help for the patient and his wife because, in their small town, they are personal friends of the patient.

A long discussion ensued pertaining to two major problems: (1) The need to reduce vocal abuse and to allow the ulcer to heal; (2) The immediate need to confront this deteriorating family situation caused by the wife's alcohol abuse. From the standpoint of vocal abuse, the patient was advised to avoid the volatile arguments taking place at home and to reduce his public speaking schedule to a minimum until his contact ulcer has healed. He must also avoid the use of alcohol during this period. He was instructed to cough and clear his throat as gently as possible. And, finally, the patient was strongly advised to consider psychiatric consultation for both him and his wife. The patient appeared gratified at the opportunity to bring out the problem into the open and said he will strongly consider the recommendations given to him. He will return for laryngology and speech pathology re-examination in two months.

* * *

PSYCHOGENIC MUTENESS IN A PATIENT WITH MULTIPLE SCLEROSIS

This case history illustrates the differential diagnostic problem that can arise in patients who have underlying neurologic disease who develop communicative disorders that may or may not be of neurologic origin.

* * *

Neurology: This 39-year-old nurse's aide was seen last year with symptoms of dysarthria and clumsiness of her right arm. Her MRI showed an increase in T2 signals in her white matter. Her CSF and IgG index were elevated. Her previous neurologic examination led to the diagnosis of multiple sclerosis.

Her neurologic complaints seemed to improve until three weeks ago when she developed acute head shaking and inability to produce any speech whatsoever. These symptoms lasted several hours during which the patient had no trouble with language comprehension. She communicated by writing, which she noted was much slower.

On examination the patient is mute; she cannot speak or whisper. She has a mild gait ataxia, but there is a "functional overlay," the patient taking slow, deliberate steps and balancing precariously from side to side. She is able to stand on one foot with little difficulty.

Impression: This patient has underlying multiple sclerosis, but her speech problem seems psychogenic as does her gait. It is difficult to be certain about how much of what we see is organic and how much is "functional." Will get a Speech Pathology consultation and a repeat MRI.

Speech Pathology: This 39-year-old nurse's aide who works for a nursing home was referred by Neurology with a diagnosis of multiple sclerosis. Her speech was diagnosed as ataxic dysarthria during her previous visit to the Clinic. She was referred this time because of a complete loss of her speech approximately 1½ weeks ago. Writing her answers to the examiner's questions, she states that her speech loss began with "slurring" which rapidly deteriorated to complete inability to talk. She says that there have been brief periods of normal speech from the time of onset of her mutism.

Examination: This patient entered the examination without any ability to speak whatsoever, laboriously writing notes as a means of communication and complaining that it is more difficult to write since the onset of her multiple sclerosis.

The oral-physical examination shows normal symmetry and strength of her speech musculature. Although she is unable to phonate, she can produce a sharp coup de glotte and cough. Despite normal lip, tongue, and velopharyngeal non-speech movements, she cannot voluntarily produce lateral, alternating tongue movements, her tongue remaining in the midline and quivering in that position. When she tries to produce alternate motion rate for p-t-k, she has tonic blocking of her labial and lingual musculature. She is able to sustain a vowel with very breathy quality.

Within 15 minutes of symptomatic speech therapy the patient could speak normally, having been led from isolated sound production to simple, familiar words. Beginning with counting she progressed from a few single digits to several, her phonation and articulation becoming stronger as she did. She was then able to transition to contextual speech. However, when she did, her speaking was "telegraphic," i.e., devoid of articles of speech, which rapidly began to fill in until her syntax and grammar were normal. As her speech emerged she produced sounds with *tonic stutteringlike blocking* on the initial phonemes of words.

We entered into a psychosocial history once the patient was able to speak with relative ease. However, inquiry into interpersonal problems or other life stresses was met with denial that anything might have been bothering her on or about the time of her speech loss. Despite having been asked four times in different ways as to whether or not she was having personal problems, she steadfastly denied their existence. But, when her daughter was asked to come into the room, she revealed that her mother has, in fact, been upset recently by the following situations:

1. Her 21-year-old son, who had been having serious behavior problems from the age of 17, suddenly left home at that time and had not been heard from in four years until the family managed to find him. Contacting him a few weeks before the patient lost her speech, he had agreed to come home but then cancelled this agreement, promising to come later in the month.

2. A second disappointment is that the patient's parents decided against coming up north to witness their granddaughter's graduation, a decision which deeply hurt the patient.

Impression: Conversion muteness. It is important to note that these events have occurred in a patient who admits to having been "raised not to show anger." Her daughter says that when her mother becomes angry she goes into her bedroom and shuts the door. Outwardly, the patient denies that these events have angered her.

Recommendation: (1) Normal speech with symptomatic voice therapy. (2) Consider psychiatric consultation. Will discuss with Neurology.

* * *

PSYCHOGENIC BREATHINESS

This case study was selected to demonstrate that continuous breathiness is yet another voice sign of interpersonal problems, reminding us of the wide spectrum of abnormal voices that stem from unresolved emotional conflict.

* * *

History: This 35-year-old, married mother of two children began having episodes of dysphonia and aphonia six years ago. She says that most of these bouts of abnormal voice were preceded by "viral infections." The first time she had trouble with her voice followed what she thought was a viral infection. Her voice returned to normal, but several weeks later she inhaled smoke from burning leaves which produced coughing immediately followed by voice loss. Since then, whenever she has a respiratory infection she loses her voice.

Her throat feels tight when she is in a dusty atmosphere, and her voice becomes breathy, hoarse, or whispered.

She was placed on voice rest and tried to comply with this recommendation, even to the point of developing hand signals with her children, but she says that reducing her speaking activities is driving her "stir-crazy," cutting her off from her friends.

Examination: This patient has a continuously breathy voice quality of moderate severity during both contextual speech and vowel prolongation. Her most recent episode of abnormal voice began one month ago. Her coup de glotte and cough are normal. She has severe musculoskeletal tension pain in the laryngeal-hyoid region in response to palpation.

The psychosocial interview uncovers a major interpersonal problem that the patient has had with her mother, whom she describes as a "martyr-dictator," a woman who has tried to control her life, who is prone to emotional outbursts, and who is unreasonable and unpredictable in her demands upon the patient. The patient and her mother have been treated by two psychologists in the past with modest improvement in their relationship.

While describing her defective relationship with her mother, the patient cries frequently. She insists that she has finally come to understand that her mother cannot help herself and that she must look to other sources of satisfaction, namely her husband and her children. She sees her mother approximately once a month and talks to her once or twice a week on the telephone. Her husband has been supportive throughout.

Despite her frank and open disclosure of her relationship with her mother, the patient's voice did not change. However, musculoskeletal tension reduction improved her voice to 70 percent of normal.

Impression: It is not certain that all of this patient's dysphonia is psychogenic, although her concurrent frustration in her relationship with her mother is highly suggestive.

Recommendation: This patient was ill-advised to reduce the amount of her voice use. She does not have a vocal abuse or misuse disorder. During the interview she gave the strong impression that these suggestions had created inhibitions to full voice use and may have increased the musculoskeletal tension of her phonatory musculature. The patient was strongly advised to return to full voice use. In spite of the unfortunate relationship that this patient has with her mother, the patient did not ask for, nor did she seem to be in need of, immediate psychological help. It was decided to defer recommendation of psychological help until after determining the effect of returning to full voice use.

* * *

PSYCHOGENIC HOARSENESS

This case reinforces the principle that the overwhelming majority of patients with psychogenic voice disorders are unable to express their emotions when confronted with a disturbing life situation that demands a verbal response in order to balance the scales.

* * *

History: Here is a 28-year-old, married woman who was referred by Otolaryngology because of a voice disorder and throat pain. Her voice troubles go back three years when she lost her voice for five days and then a month later for three weeks, during all of which time she "whispered." Her latest episode of voice disorder began four months ago, beginning with a cold and hoarseness. Rapidly she became aphonic (whispered speech), her voice improved and then worsened. Laryngologic examination was normal.

Examination: During the examination the patient's voice is mildly and continuously hoarse. She has mild-to-moderate musculoskeletal tension pain in the left laryngeal-hyoid region in response to palpation, a pain which she says spontaneously migrates to her left ear at times.

The psychosocial history is positive. Throughout the examination it becomes apparent that this sensitive, moderately religious woman has been in conflict with herself about the perplexing and anger-producing behavior of her sister over the past few years. The patient loves her sister very much and became extremely upset when her sister began having marital problems and indulging in extramarital affairs which violated the patient's and family's moral convictions. Recently, her sister's marital situation ended in divorce.

What disturbs the patient most of all is that her sister is angry at her for not supporting her decision to divorce, accusing the patient of being self-righteous and lacking in understanding. Taking these accusations to heart, the patient has felt "sad, angry, and guilty." The patient is now in a dilemma, because she perceives that her sister, who is barely on speaking terms with the rest of the family, wants her support for what she has done, but the patient cannot find it within herself to give that approval.

It is important to note that on the night before her recent voice loss she had had a depressing conversation with her mother about her sister during which the patient reiterated her sister's accusations. The patient said, "Kiddingly, after I lost my voice I compared myself to a biblical character who loses his voice after some kind of conflict." The patient became aphonic on the same night she had this conversation with her mother.

Contributing to her dysphonia is the injudicious advice given to her by another clinician that she raise the pitch of her voice as a means of therapy which has most assuredly contributed to her elevated musculoskeletal tension and pain.

Impression: Psychogenic hoarseness with associated musculoskeletal tension and pain in the laryngeal-hyoid region.

Recommendation: A long discussion ensued about how the patient has taken her sister's accusations and blamed herself rather than recognizing her rights to her own opinions. She seemed to understand the relationship between her being emotionally upset with her sister and her voice disorder and throat pain. It was decided that she would talk over the entire situation with her husband, to try and understand that it is not she who is to blame for her sister's problems, and that it might be beneficial were she to express her disapproval of her sister's behavior more openly without feeling guilty. She was advised that, should the situation remain unresolved, that she should call and an appointment for psychological counseling will be arranged.

Finally, the patient was told to disregard any advice to change the pitch or loudness of her voice. The patient appeared to appreciate the results of this consultation, and there is a good chance that it may result in an overall improvement in her voice, throat discomfort, and her manner of dealing with her sister's demands.

*   *   *

PSYCHOGENIC BREATHY HOARSENESS AND DIPLOPHONIA

The following case study reinforces the fact that an acoustically wide variety of abnormal voices can be signs of the same underlying life conflicts, and that each patient acquires his or her own unique type and severity of abnormal voice.

*   *   *

History: This is a 41-year-old, married woman who was referred by Otolaryngology after laryngologic examination failed to show any significant laryngeal pathology other than irritation of the vocal folds, which was incongruous with the severity of the patient's dysphonia.

Her voice complaints began eight months ago, from which time she has been continuously dysphonic.

Examination: The patient's voice during contextual speech can be described as continuously harsh, breathy, and diplophonic. She has moderately elevated laryngeal-hyoid musculoskeletal tension and pain in response to palpation of this area. Her larynx is elevated at rest. *Brief kneading in the thyrohyoid region, although painful, produced immediate and significant voice improvement indicating a musculoskeletal tension-related voice disorder.*

This patient has a highly positive psychosocial history. Almost immediately after being asked about her personal life, she breaks down and cries, citing the following conflicts that have existed during the past three to four years.

Her husband strongly disapproves of her twin sister, believing that she is manipulative and dishonest in her relationships with the family. At the same time, the patient wants to have a closer relationship with her sister now that they are getting older and particularly during the past three to four years, following her nephew's suicide at age 18. The patient's husband, who regards himself, and whom she regards, as the patriarch in the family, will have nothing to do with the patient's sister and objects to the patient seeing her. He will not discuss the situation and becomes angry when the patient attempts any social contact with her sister or tries to discuss the subject with him.

While all of this has been going on, she has been chronically upset about her obesity and about always being tired. But she cannot grapple with these issues, because her husband prevents her from asserting herself in ways that might make her life better. He always has the last word on matters of discipline, money, and other family matters. More than once she has considered getting psychiatric help, but her husband controls the purse strings and will not allow her to see anyone because "he doesn't believe in it. He's always right and others are always wrong." She cries, "I'm confused and mixed up. I don't know what to do."

Impression: This patient has a *psychogenic dysphonia secondary to suppressed anger and depression* in response to chronic conflict between her need for a reconciliation with her sister and her fear of her husband's disapproval. Other issues in this patient's life are also unresolved because of her inability to negotiate with her husband on a reasonably even plane.

It is important to note that *this patient's voice becomes completely normal during periods of emotional disclosure of her feelings during this interview.*

Recommendation: Despite this patient's capability for normal voice, voice therapy is not the solution to her problem. Whatever gains would be made from symptomatic voice therapy would be short-lived owing to the potency of the conflict that she is experiencing. We talked at considerable length about her need to consult a psychiatrist, psychologist, or psychiatric social worker to discuss her situation in much greater depth. Even if her husband is intransigent, she might be able to become more assertive in order to achieve what is best for her future happiness.

Movement in this direction is hampered by the patient's not knowing where to turn. She says she can't confront her husband with what she has learned here because "there is no way he would understand." Her sole conduit to getting psychological help and persuading her husband of its importance is through her local physician, "the only person my husband will listen to." She was strongly encouraged to contact this family doctor on her return home and who would be provided with information necessary to persuade him that this patient's voice problems are directly and seriously related to her defective communicative relationship with her husband.

* * *

PSYCHOGENIC HIGH PITCH AND INITIAL DENIAL OF PSYCHOLOGICAL PROBLEMS

This case study of a patient who developed an excessively high-pitched voice of psychologic origin illustrates the *common tendency on the part of patients who have psychogenic voice disorders to deny or fail to recognize emotional problems in their lives early in the examination but who divulge them later on.*

* * *

History: Last Christmas this 47-year-old, married woman began having episodes of excessively high-pitched voice which began with a cold or cough. There are times when she whispers as well. However, she says that she whispers voluntarily because it is "easier to talk that way." She also complains of chest pains. She has also been fatigued and worn out since Christmas, complaining of shortness of breath. She has an "ache" in her throat and "chest pains" in the upper part of her sternum and substernal region. She has just come from a general medical and otolaryngologic examination where she has been cleared of any laryngeal pathology or general medical illness as explanation for her chest complaints.

Examination: The patient has an excessively high-pitched, strained, mildly breathy voice. She has moderate musculoskeletal tension and pain in her left thyrohyoid region in response to palpation.

At first the psychosocial history was negative, the patient *repeatedly denying* that she had any problems in her life whatsoever. Finally, she admitted that she has been upset for many years over her sister's and brother-in-law's alcoholism and the effect that it has been having on their teenage children. She considers her 14-year-old and 16-year-old nephews as being neglected. Both parents begin drinking at the local tavern at about 4:00 in the afternoon and can be found there frequently intoxicated. Both teenage boys, particularly the 14-year-old, are depressed and prefer to spend time in the patient's home rather than their own. The patient admits that she is chronically anxious that the teenage children will abuse alcohol as well and that they will be killed in an automobile accident.

The patient relates this information without apparent emotion. Reluctantly, she admits that she is ashamed over her sister's alcoholism and crudeness and that, recently, she has decided that she must talk to her sister about their alcoholism and what it is doing to their children. She anticipates that this will be at least a delicate, and possibly disastrous, encounter because her sister is "quite touchy and has a very mean streak."

It is important to note that the moment the patient began speaking about her sister, brother-in-law, and their children, *her voice returned to normal.*

Impression: Psychogenic high pitch based on a normal laryngologic examination, positive musculoskeletal tension and pain, a positive psychosocial history, very possibly signifying ambivalence and fear in communicating with her sister and brother-in-law about her concerns over their alcoholism, and the patient's voice returned to normal as she was discussing these deep concerns.

Recommendation: It is not certain how much insight this patient is able to develop concerning the relationship between her feelings and her voice. She was guarded and protective about disclosing personal information, even though she was quite pleasant and cooperative in doing so. She said she would think seriously about what we had discussed, and a return appointment was made to review the situation after she has talked with her sister and brother-in-law.

* * *

EXCESSIVE LOUDNESS OF PSYCHOGENIC ORIGIN

Excessive loudness is not a particularly common psychogenic voice disorder. However, in certain patients, speaking too loudly may indicate a psychological adjustment disorder.

* * *

History: This 35-year-old, single female called directly for an appointment in order to discuss what she describes as a problem of excessively loud voice. As a secretary, she was recently reprimanded for speaking too loudly and says that she has had a lifelong inability to keep the intensity of her voice down to an appropriate level. She decided that the time has come for her to do something about this tendency before it has any more serious vocational or social repercussions.

Examination: The patient is a pleasant, attractive, but obese, woman who converses in a low-pitched, clear voice. Although she conversed more loudly than the average person, she demonstrated ample ability to maintain a normal vocal loudness level. The voice and allied motor speech examination failed to reveal any evidence of motor speech disorder.

The psychosocial history is that the patient, one of eight children, had to use her voice and speech as a means of defense while growing up. While still in high school she was repeatedly reminded that she was too loud. She admits that all of her life she has been verbally aggressive and defensive and offers the opinion that, as far as she is concerned, loudness is equated with anger.

The patient has a past history of psychological problems surrounding her poor self-image and lack of self-acceptance, having been in psychotherapy to learn to accept herself to a greater extent than she has, not to become angry with herself, or "to take the blame for all relationships that go bad." During much of this discussion the patient cries quietly. Her attitude is that "the world is not fair," but she recognizes that she is the one who will have to change. She is now acutely aware that she is considerably overweight, having recently become concerned about her personal appearance. One of her immediate objectives is to diet and learn to dress in a more sophisticated manner.

Impression: This patient's excessive loudness appears to be secondary to her lifelong manner of adapting to her environment when she was growing up, the surface of a deeper problem of hostile reactions to others. Fortunately she is intelligent, has considerable insight into her problem and is motivated for change. She believes that the psychotherapy that she is now receiving is benefiting her self-concept.

Recommendation: Because her excessive loudness is psychogenic and related to her aggressiveness, poor self-image, and hostile relationships with others, improvement psychologically ought to benefit her loudness problem. But, she also needs symptomatic voice therapy to teach her to reduce her vocal loudness on a voluntary basis as well, as it is important that her voice disorder not worsen her employment situation in the immediate future.

Summary of Subsequent Reports: By the end of three speech therapy sessions, the patient reports that she is doing much better in her ability to control her loudness during conversations with others at work and socially. People have remarked to her that she is less in evidence. "I don't know where you are anymore," one said. She proudly reported that she was successful in controlling her loudness during a recent argument with a friend, although some days it is an effort to remain aware of the need for such control, she says.

She continues with her program of self-improvement—has gone for a "color analysis," learning how to wear different make-up, and she intends to modify her wardrobe and to work on her diet. She is still seeing her psychiatrist and reports fewer and less intense bouts with depression. During a discussion about insights that she has achieved in her psychotherapy, she offers the opinion that her loudness has been the main reason for her previous job and interpersonal failures that would result in "punishment" for her; that it became a "self-fulfilling prophesy," that perhaps she felt a "need to fail," and her speech was "a direct route to the alienation of others." She feels she does not need to do this any longer.

Subsequent meetings with the patient disclosed ups and downs in her ability to control her loudness level. It is at its worst when she is at home where their poor family rapport and destructive communication habits irritate her; "it's like a zoo when we're together." She volunteers that she is having continuing problems with her self-esteem, is tearful throughout the interview, and complains that she is not seeing her psychiatrist often enough to work more deeply into her feelings about her relationships with others. The psychiatrist is now seeing her "only during an emotional crisis."

A follow-up visit by the patient indicates that she is now seeing her psychiatrist more often at our request. She has seen him for four sessions since our last meeting and says that they are already getting down more deeply into her emotions, and she is learning to trust herself and others more than she has.

In the meantime, her loudness control is very good, and both patient and clinician have been impressed with the extremely close relationship between her voice and her adjustment problems.

Her last visit resulted in the following information. She has been able to control her loudness quite well. During the session her speech was well modulated with no signs of loss of loudness control.

This was the last contact with the patient until three years later when she called to say that she had completed her psychotherapy, that she has learned to regard herself in a much better light, that she doesn't need to be angry, and that she has almost no difficulty controlling the loudness of her voice. She expressed gratitude for the voice therapy and psychological support given to her during more difficult times.

*   *   *

EFFECTS OF EMOTIONAL STRESS ON THE SINGING VOICE

The voices of singers and actors are particularly vulnerable to psychological stress. Although personal problems causing mild to moderate depression and anxiety may not affect the speaking voice, these dysphoric affective changes can interfere with subtle control over the voice for professional purposes.

* * *

History: A 20-year-old music major has had difficulty controlling the pitch of her voice and has been experiencing sore throat while singing. She was suspected of vocal abuse or allergy; however, consultations with an otolaryngologist and an allergist failed to disclose any evidence of structural lesions of the vocal folds or allergies to any substances within the patient's environment.

Examination: All speaking voice parameters on examination were normal. However, the patient had mild musculoskeletal tension pain in the region of the thyroid notch in response to palpation.

During the psychosocial interview, the patient at first denied any depression or anxiety. However, on repeat questioning later in the examination she tearfully reported that she has been upset since learning that her singing teacher, with whom she had a close relationship, was diagnosed as having cancer and had to discontinue teaching. Since then the patient has been shifted from one teacher to another. She admits that she has been extremely upset about her teacher's illness, and was on the verge of crying as she described her feelings. Both she and her mother agree that the patient has a lifelong tendency to keep her feelings to herself.

Impression: Although it is not certain that this patient's singing problems are related to her current unhappiness about her teacher's illness and the unsettled teaching situation that she describes, the concurrence between her singing problem and these personal problems indicate that they may be closely related to each other. The patient admitted that she is still harboring sadness, even grief, concerning her teacher's illness, and it was recommended that she talk with a professional person about her feelings concerning this illness and her dissatisfactions and disappointments surrounding the unsatisfactory teaching situation that she is currently experiencing.

* * *

PSYCHOGENIC ADDUCTOR SPASTIC DYSPHONIA WITH INHALATORY STRIDOR

The following case study is of a patient who presented with adductor strained voice arrests but with the uncommon accompaniment of inhalatory stridor which, because of its unusualness, led others to suspect a neurologic inability to abduct the vocal folds during inhalation. As the case study will demonstrate, the stridor was integral with the spastic dysphonia and both of psychogenic origin.

* * *

History: Otolaryngology referred this 57-year-old businessman primarily because of adductor laryngospasms during inhalation producing laborious and audible stridor. However, otolaryngologic examination failed to show evidence of abductor paralysis of the vocal folds during quiet inhalation. Only during speech did studies indicate that the vocal folds were not abducting. The patient notes that his stridor worsens toward the end of the day. He occasionally chokes on liquids and solids.

Examination: The patient is pleasant and straightforward in describing his complaints. He has inhalatory stridor at rest and during inhalation for speech. On exhalation for speech he has adductor laryngospasms producing the acoustic features of *adductor spastic dysphonia.*

Oral-physical examination does not disclose any evidence of weakness or asymmetry of his speech musculature, and the remainder of the motor speech examination was normal.

The psychosocial history has been positive during the approximately one-year duration of his respiratory and voice complaints. He describes serious emotional setbacks that go back for more than three years which have become more intense during the past year.

His first marriage ended after his wife asked for a divorce. Five children were involved. Three years ago he divorced his second wife and at the same time encountered serious financial reverses resulting in bankruptcy.

Following that divorce he met the widow of a wealthy businessman and with this woman entered into both a romantic and a business relationship. Approximately one year ago, when his respiratory and voice symptoms began, she decided to terminate this relationship. Her decision caused the patient great pain on both a personal and financial basis. Because he had, in effect, given up his own business plans and had become dependent upon her for his financial well-being, he now found himself without financial resources and unable to find a decent job.

The patient describes himself as a very sensitive person and broke down and cried during the examination. He admits to having been severely depressed over the past year and hinted vaguely at suicide.

It is important to note that both his dysphonia and inhalatory stridor virtually disappeared during his description of the emotionally traumatic events of the past year.

Impression: Prior to taking the psychosocial history, because of the adductor laryngospasms during speech and on inhalation particularly, a neurologic laryngeal dyskinesia was strongly suspected. However, because the psychosocial history revealed concurrent depressing life events and, particularly the disappearance of his dysphonia and stridor during disclosure of these events, we are unavoidably led to the conclusion that both the dysphonia and the stridor are psychogenic.

Recommendation: To assure us that no neurologic components are contributory, a neurologic examination is being scheduled. Irrespective of the neurologic findings, we frankly discussed the need for psychiatric consultation to which the patient responded affirmatively.

★   ★   ★

PSYCHOGENIC ABDUCTOR SPASTIC DYSPHONIA

The following case study was selected to illustrate that abductor spastic dysphonia can be psychogenic.

★   ★   ★

History: This patient is a 26-year-old minister referred by Otolaryngology for evaluation of a voice disorder. The laryngologic examination showed normal structure and function of the vocal folds.

The patient began having an intermittently breathy voice approximately two years ago that has remained the same or has gotten slightly worse.

Examination: The oral-physical examination is normal. The motor speech examination does not give any evidence of dysarthric phonatory, resonatory, or articulatory disturbances. Vowel prolongation is carried out with a steady vocal tone and without evidence of the breathy air releases heard during contextual speech. His coup de glotte is normal.

The psychosocial history is positive and appears to be related to his voice disorder. When his voice problems began two years ago, the patient was under considerable stress while attending a religious college, a very strict and authoritarian school that expelled him when they learned he had become engaged to the woman who is now his wife, because they did not approve of her social behavior.

Upon discussing his relationship with his wife, he reveals his need for obedience from her, as a religious principle. He says that he "lives in constant fear when she will disobey me next." *It is important to note that during this discussion the patient's voice becomes completely normal.* His wife, also raised in the same religious tradition, supports the idea of the dominant husband in the family ("God made the man head of the family"), but she says that even she has her limits and resists being ordered around and expected to obey his every command. If he should ask her to perform certain household chores or social obligations and she fails to do so, he becomes "depressed," although he does not openly lose his temper, trying to retain control of himself and to change her behavior through reasoning. Even he admits that at times he goes overboard in his authoritarianism and wishes he were more tolerant of her needs for independence, but he keeps reverting back to certain absolutes based on his religious teachings.

Impression: Abductor spastic dysphonia, the psychosocial history strongly indicating psychogenic etiology.

Recommendation: This personable young man is willing to recognize the possibility that his abnormal voice may be related to his inability to express his anger and disappointment toward his wife. The desirability of a psychiatric examination and exploration of the relationship between the voice disorder and the patient's intolerance of his wife's noncompliance with his demands was recommended. He considers this recommendation potentially valuable, and so does his wife, saying, "Anything that will help him with his voice is desirable."

Both the patient and his wife do not believe they have a fundamental marital problem, although both concede that they have a conflict over the subject of obedience, that this is a contaminant in their marriage, and that they are concerned about setting the "proper example" for their daughter. Toward the end of the interview, the patient became adamant that whoever they saw in Psychiatry or Psychology must agree with his religious views and should not be a female.

* * *

PSYCHOGENIC ADDUCTOR-ABDUCTOR SPASTIC DYSPHONIA

Adductor and abductor spastic dysphonia of psychogenic origin can exist simultaneously in a patient in which the adductor strained hoarseness and voice arrests are intermingled with abductor breathy air releases.

* * *

History: This 38-year-old waitress and bartender has had three episodes of abnormal voice within the past five months, each coming on suddenly and lasting about one week followed by spontaneous voice return. The second dysphonic episode occurred two months after the first, and the third about two weeks ago, which has persisted. She complains that at times she is "unable to get any voice out," and that her throat "feels swollen inside."

One week after her first episode she consulted an otolaryngologist who found that her vocal folds were clear and fully mobile, although he found a very small web in the region of the posterior commissure. But, the laryngologist emphasized that the laryngologic examination was, for the most part, normal and could not account for the patient's severely abnormal voice. She has been in good health otherwise.

Examination: This pleasant, smiling woman has intermittent adductor voice arrests inter-spersed by intermittent breathy air escapages during conversational speech. Vowel prolonga-tion is produced in a normal voice, however. She had moderate musculoskeletal tension of her laryngeal-hyoid sling and pain over the left side of her neck over the hyoid bone and in the thyrohyoid space. She also has pain just lateral to the thyroid notch and over the superior border of the thyroid cartilage. The thyrohyoid space is significantly reduced by excess approximation of the thyroid cartilage and the hyoid bone.

This patient has a highly positive psychosocial history. Tearfully throughout the remainder of the examination she disclosed three aspects of her life that have upset her, although she has consciously tried not to think about them.

1. Her impending divorce following 20 years of marriage.
2. Her children's rejection of her current boyfriend.
3. An automobile accident within the recent past which killed three of her girlfriends with whom she had been very close.
4. A situation in her job in which the patient is not being paid for extra work that she has had to do while another employee has been on maternity leave.

During a more detailed explanation of these concerns, the patient gives further insight into her marriage of 20 years to a man who was alcoholic, who gambled, and who indulged in marital infidelities. A year-and-a-half ago she walked out. She says she would have done so sooner, but what finally precipitated her action was that she fell in love with another man, which gave her the courage to leave. This decision was very difficult for her because of her children, ages 2, 18, and 19, who now live with their father. Since moving out her children have been angry with her, blaming her boyfriend for the marital break-up, and they will have nothing to do with him. This attitude upsets the patient, who would like her children to have an amicable relationship with her boyfriend, whom she intends to marry. Their rejection of him prevents her from seeing her children at the same time she sees her boyfriend.

The patient expresses guilt feelings about the death of her girlfriends in the automobile accident. She wishes she had spent more time with them, and now they are gone. At first she said they were killed a few months before the onset of her voice disorder, but later she thinks that she may have been mistaken about the date and that the accident actually might have occurred very shortly before her voice disorder began.

By personality, the patient admits a lifelong tendency to suppress her feelings rather than to admit them openly. For example, she allowed herself to be taken advantage of by not being paid for work that she had to take over while her fellow employee went on maternity leave. She feels she should have complained about this situation to her supervisor but admits that she is unable to muster the courage. In the same way, she has never stood up to her husband, fearing physical abuse. Instead of arguing with him when his drinking and womanizing would surface, the patient would "just cry." All in all, she says smiling through her tears, "It's been a crazy year."

Impression: Psychogenic, probably conversion, adductor-abductor spastic dysphonia.

Recommendations: During the course of her disclosures concerning her personal problems, *her voice improved approximately 50 percent, and became completely normal during laryngeal-hyoid musculoskeletal tension reduction therapy.*

We discussed at some length the interrelationship between suppressed grief and anger and the development of voice disorders and throat discomfort as a sign of contraction of the throat muscles. Although the patient was frankly surprised that her dysphonia turned out to be caused by her being emotionally upset, she appeared to understand the connection.

Finally, we discussed future avenues of remediation of the conflict between her older children and her boyfriend, namely to obtain conjoint counseling at home during which all parties would have a chance to rationally come to some understanding of one another. It was also suggested that the patient obtain individual counseling in order to help her to learn to express her feelings more openly, to bring out into the open her incompletely expressed grief over the death of her friends and over the impending dissolution of her marriage. The patient appeared to accept these recommendations as reasonable and volunteered that she would pursue counseling upon return home.

* * *

"GLOBUS," THROAT DISCOMFORT, AND EPISODIC DYSPHONIA

Abnormal voice is not the only laryngeal manifestation of psychologic stress. Patients with and without abnormal voice can develop feelings of tightness, sometimes described as a ball or other obstruction in the throat, historically known as "globus," as a sign of psychologic stress.

* * *

History: This 24-year-old economics major was referred by Otolaryngology because of episodes of "hoarseness" and "sore throat" that have gone on for the past six or seven years. However, her complaints have worsened over the past few months. Laryngologic examination, except for mild erythema around the vocal processes of the vocal folds, was normal.

Examination: The patient's voice is normal on examination. She complains of throat discomfort, describing a feeling of a "baseball in my throat."

She has a highly positive psychosocial history. Over the past 15 years the patient has accumulated a tremendous amount of unexpressed anger toward her father and, especially, her stepmother and stepsisters for the way in which they have treated her. "I have been made to feel unwanted, and my stepmother has created a 'her kids-our kids' conflict." After spending a year away from home, she returned only to discover that her angry feelings have mushroomed almost beyond her control. And, although her lifelong tendency has been to keep her feelings under wraps, she has found herself unable to keep from communicating her anger and resentment toward members of her family. Saying that she has been always taught to suppress her anger, she considers her current feelings and inabilities to keep them to herself as "scary," and equates the expression of anger with "violence and revenge." In the final analysis she admits, "I don't know what to do with anger."

From the moment she is asked about her personal life she begins crying and continues to do so on and off during the remainder of the examination. As she tells of her relationships with other members of her family, she emphasizes that her stepmother is "kind of ridiculous" as a mother, an alcoholic. "I am tired of being treated like dirt. I have a lot of anger but you can't do that. I have been stomped on for years and years. I think I must be upset at myself for taking this for so many years. Now, I feel like I should say stuff, but it's pretty scary. No one has ever seen me angry or raise my voice." The other day when she was crying and expressing anger and hurt toward her stepmother, she felt much better, but that happens very infrequently because of her strong censorship of her feelings.

Contributory to her laryngeal musculoskeletal tension producing her throat discomfort and feelings of tightness, and her episodes of dysphonia, is that she leads a stressful life, working hard as a student, holding down a job as a secretary, and pushing herself extremely hard. Last year she had mononucleosis and thinks she did not recover completely from it, frequently feeling tired and not getting enough sleep.

Impression: There is a strong likelihood that this patient's episodes of dysphonia and throat discomfort are primarily due to elevated musculoskeletal tension associated with the building up of unexpressed anger toward members of her family, particularly her stepmother, occurring in a young woman who has always regarded the expression of anger as repellant.

Recommendation: The patient was seeing a psychological counselor about once a month until recently. One receives the impression that they never got down to the heart of this patient's problems. We spent a considerable amount of time devoted to explaining to the patient the relationship between abnormal voice, laryngeal muscle tension, and suppressed anger. Not unexpectedly, the patient finds it difficult to accept this explanation because it signifies to her that she is "weak." Nevertheless, by the time the session had ended she could hardly avoid recognizing the connection between her throat problems and her emotions. She was strongly advised to consult another psychologist, or a psychiatrist, in order to get into the long history of suppressed emotions, to enable her to express her feelings more openly and to view them more rationally.

*   *   *

Chapter Seven

ADDUCTOR SPASTIC DYSPHONIA

"When we approach the problem of spastic dysphonia we see so many different opinions about any of its many aspects that we come to the conclusion that one of the following two things has happened: either we are not speaking about the same thing or we look at the same thing with different eyes. And these "eyes" depend upon our culture and on the understanding that even scientific "truths" are, frequently, provisional."

—Bloch

PROLOGUE AND DEFINITION

Spastic dysphonia is an example of the way in which the meanings of words change with time and the expansion of knowledge, and the confusion that accompanies such change. Early in the history of this disorder, those few clinicians who wrote about it seemed to be in reasonable agreement that spastic dysphonia was intended to mean a single entity, distinct from other voice disorders, which conformed to fairly narrow criteria. The original definition of adductor spastic dysphonia, reviewed by Arnold (1959), is paraphrased as follows:

1. A voice that is variably squeezed, strained, choked, staccato, stuttering-like, jerky, grunting, groaning, effortful, pinched, grating, and has periodic breaks in phonation. It has a tendency to be monopitched and reduced in loudness, and vowels are initiated with hard glottal attacks.

2. The abnormal voice occurs only during voluntary phonation for communication purposes and not during singing, vowel prolongation, laughing, or crying.

3. The abnormal voice is the effect of hyperadduction of the true and false vocal folds.

4. The disorder is caused by psychoneurosis from either occupational stress or emotional trauma, such as family conflicts, accidents, terrifying events, or accumulated frustrations.

What needs to be remembered is that this definition originated with a few otolaryngologists and psychiatrists, whose experience with patients who had this kind of strained voice was limited and whose knowledge of both the psychiatric and neurologic characteristics of their patients paralleled the relatively undeveloped state of both specialties. The first article written on the subject by Traube in 1871, setting into motion and directing subsequent thought on this disorder, described it as "a spastic form of nervous hoarseness." At least a half dozen other writers before 1900 also linked the disorder to psychoneurosis (Kiml, 1963). Their early impressions about psychogenic etiology, given at the dawn of modern psychiatry and psychology, have ultimately proved to be correct. However, subsequent experience has shown—particularly during the past 20 years—that what these clinicians had failed to notice, understand, and document during the early years was that there were people whose voices sounded very much like the spastic dysphonia as defined originally but were caused by neurologic, not psychogenic disorders. This, too, is understandable because the specialty of neurology at the turn of the century was in a similar state of primitive evolution, as were psychiatry and psychology.

With the passage of time, more clinicians began to witness cases of strained hoarseness of different types, many of which were eventually found to be of neurologic etiology, and still others for whom neither psychoneurosis nor neurologic substrates could be demonstrated. Although these

161

patients failed to conform to the early criteria for spastic dysphonia, their disorders were called *spastic dysphonia* nevertheless, mainly because that was the way they *sounded*.

Terminology being vitally important to clarity, we are faced today with the following dilemma: Either there is only one *true* spastic dysphonia, the specific criteria for which was set down by the early writers on the subject and just listed in this chapter, and all other strained voices are not true spastic dysphonia and should be called something else, or all strained voices should be called "spastic dysphonia," but the term should be modified to specify etiology.

The viewpoint taken in this book is that the latter course is preferable to the former because it recognizes the ever-widening recognition of the multiple origins of adductor laryngospasm. Therefore, the following definition and criteria pertaining to the voice disorder concept of spastic dysphonia is recommended, based on evidence to be presented later in this chapter:

1. The term "spastic dysphonia" should be preserved for reasons of historical precedent and common usage.*

2. The term "adductor" should be used as a prefix to designate a class of voice characteristics produced by hyperaddduction of the vocal folds.

3. Continuing along this line of thinking, then, "adductor spastic dysphonia" is a *perceptual* term that refers to a strained, groaning, staccato, effortful voice, no different from the original definition.

4. It varies within and among patients according to severity and detailed voice characteristics.

5. It may be of psychogenic, neurologic, or of unknown etiology.

6. If data lead the clinician to conclude that the laryngospasms are psychogenic beyond a reasonable doubt, then the term used should be *"psychogenic adductor spastic dysphonia."*

7. If data lead the clinician to conclude that the laryngospasms are neurologic beyond a reasonable doubt, then the term used should be *"neurologic adductor spastic dysphonia."*

8. If data fail to prove either psychogenic or neurologic etiology, then the term *"idiopathic adductor spastic dysphonia"* should be used.

In summary, a modern interpretation of the term "adductor spastic dysphonia" is that it applies to a family of strained voices produced by adductor laryngospasm that arise from different etiologies. To distinguish among them is not a trivial academic exercise. It has considerable importance to clinicians responsible for establishing a differential diagnosis of laryngospasms in patients who need to know the truth about their abnormal voices and whose treatment may depend on the type of adductor spastic dysphonia that they have.

PATHOPHYSIOLOGY

The common denominator underlying all types of adductor spastic dysphonia is *adductor laryngospasm*. While keeping in mind that within and among patients the degree and frequency of adductor laryngospasms vary considerably, the following kinds of laryngeal adductor, and sometimes even sphincter, actions have been observed during videofluoroscopy and videofiberoptic laryngoscopy (McCall et al., 1971; Parnes et al., 1978).

1. *Adductor spasms of the true vocal folds only.* Hyperaddduction of the true vocal folds alone occurs in mild cases of these disorders. Although the degree of adductor force cannot be seen readily during such spasms, the midline separation between the ligamentous portions of the vocal cords may be obscured owing to compression of one vocal fold against the other. The vocal folds can be seen to snap shut synchronous with each voice arrest.

2. *Adductor spasms of both the true and false vocal folds.* During moderate to severe strained voice or voice arrest, the false or ventricular vocal folds close over and obscure the true folds.

---

*Throughout its history, the disorder has had many synonyms that have only served to confuse an already complex subject. An incomplete list includes spasmodic dysphonia; lalophobia, phonatory glottic spasm; mogiphonia, aphthongia, psychophonasthenia, stammering of the vocal cords (Kiml, 1963).

3. *Supraglottic constriction.* Severe strained voice or voice arrests are accompanied by constriction of the hypopharynx, i.e., the inferior pharyngeal constrictor just above the level of the false vocal folds. The shape of the lumen during such closure is not an anteroposterior, elongated one, as in true and false vocal fold hyperadduction alone, but is sphincteric or circular. Moreover, the true and false cords hyperadduct along with the pharyngeal constrictors. What appears to be true, then, is that the more severe the adductor laryngospasms, the greater the vertical extent of intrinsic laryngeal muscle participation. As tightness of spasms increase, constriction progresses superiorly from the true folds to involve the ventricular folds, and, ultimately, the pharyngeal constrictors (Fig. 7-1, 7-2, and 7-3).

Although hypercontraction of the intrinsic laryngeal and pharyngeal muscles is fundamental to the adductor spastic dysphonias, moderate to severe laryngospasms are accompanied by synchronous movements of the *entire* larynx, most often in a superior direction, as shown in the succeeding figures. Associated laryngeal movements implicate the extrinsic laryngeal muscles as well. Such movement can also be seen through the skin of the neck. Downward and forward displacement of the larynx occurs less often. As expected, increased amplitude of electromyographic potentials in the general neck region have been recorded during such spasms (Tarrasch, 1946). It is important to realize, then, that the adductor spastic dysphonias are disorders not just of the true and false vocal folds, but the supraglottic pharyngeal constrictors also participate, and so do the strap muscles, responsible for moving the body of the larynx. The neuroanatomic implications of these facts is that

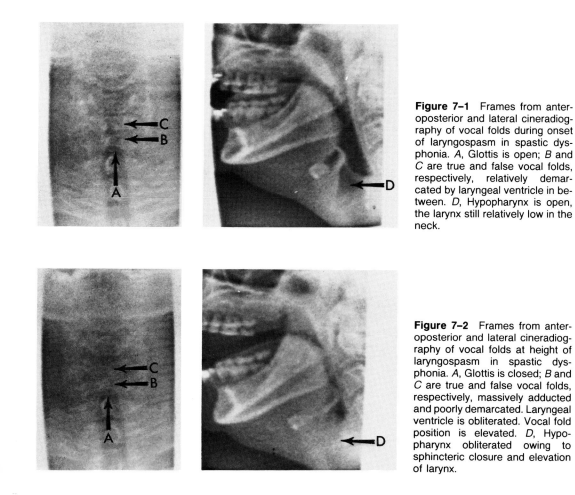

Figure 7–1 Frames from anteroposterior and lateral cineradiography of vocal folds during onset of laryngospasm in spastic dysphonia. *A*, Glottis is open; *B* and *C* are true and false vocal folds, respectively, relatively demarcated by laryngeal ventricle in between. *D*, Hypopharynx is open, the larynx still relatively low in the neck.

Figure 7–2 Frames from anteroposterior and lateral cineradiography of vocal folds at height of laryngospasm in spastic dysphonia. *A*, Glottis is closed; *B* and *C* are true and false vocal folds, respectively, massively adducted and poorly demarcated. Laryngeal ventricle is obliterated. Vocal fold position is elevated. *D*, Hypopharynx obliterated owing to sphincteric closure and elevation of larynx.

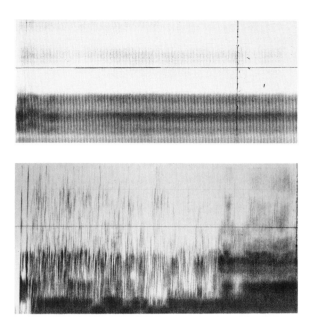

Figure 7–3 Sonogram of normal voice and spastic dysphonia. *A,* Normal regularity of fundamental frequency and higher harmonics on /a/ vowel prolongation. *B,* Spastic dysphonia. Irregular breaks in the fundamental frequency and noise in the harmonic range on /a/ vowel prolongation.

not only the Xth nerve, innervating the intrinsic laryngeal muscles, but also the IXth nerve to the pharynx and the cervical spinal nerves to the extrinsic laryngeal muscles, transmit nerve impulses responsible for the spasms.

Aberrant respiratory movements often accompany the laryngospasms. The clinician can see sudden, jerky arrests and other dysrhythmic movements of the thorax and abdomen synchronous with strained voice or voice arrests. Respiratory dysfunction in spastic dysphonia, most probably, is the secondary *effect* of the uncontrolled glottic closures, i.e., during adductor spasm, more exhalatory effort is required to force air through the glottis. If an adductor spasm is particularly abrupt, the exhalatory muscles react to the sudden laryngeal arrest of exhaled air by contracting more quickly and forcefully, actions that can be seen with the naked eye. The speaker, in effect, is caught in the throes of a series of involuntary effort closures or Valsalva maneuvers. The normal speaker can simulate adductor spastic dysphonia realistically by trying to phonate while straining or bearing down. Notice how exhalatory arrests are accompanied by sudden, visible abdominal and thoracic movements. Severe laryngospasm produces other visible features, such as flushing of the face. Silent lip movements may occur during moments of voice arrest. Even stuttering-like articulatory repetitions during inaudible voice are common as the patient struggles, by repetition, to compensate for moments of unintelligibility. Other signs of struggle are excessive contractions of the neck muscles, shoulder girdle, and upper arm. Typically, patients with severe, long-standing adductor spastic dysphonia will present with a strained facial expression consisting of frowning, squinting, and downward turning of the angles of the mouth. What is unseen by the observer is the intense physical effort and fatigue felt by the patient. So tiring is speaking that many patients elect to whisper because of the freer airflow that it provides. It should come as no surprise then that therapeutic alleviation of laryngospasm is as much a physical relief as it is a contribution to voice improvement.

INCIDENCE

The incidence and prevalence of adductor spastic dysphonia in the general population is unknown. However, limited data on frequency of occurrence, age, and sex in individual practices are available. The reader must bear in mind two kinds of errors in reporting: (1) Most past and even current reports do not identify the spastic dysphonics studied according to etiologic type. Patients are chosen almost exclusively on the basis of the sound of their voices. Quite likely, then, these are not homogeneous populations. More probably, they represent mixtures of psychogenic, neurologic, and idiopathic types. (2) In collecting statistical data on spastic dysphonia in clinical practice, some clinicians fail to recognize the disorder when confronted by it, and others identify it falsely when it does not exist. These sources of error must be considered, particularly the first, when critically reading studies reported here and elsewhere. The following data and those later in this chapter are given with awareness of these limitations.

The consensus is that adductor spastic dysphonia is rare. Most clinicians witness only a few cases over a lifetime, and some have never had any direct experience with such patients. Table 7-1 shows the number of cases reported in several studies.

AGE OF ONSET

Most research publications cite middle age as the time of onset. Aronson (1968) reported distribution of age of onset in spastic dysphonia in 34 patients. The average age was 44 years (range, 28 to 69 years): 20 to 29 years, 9 percent; 30 to 39 years, 24 percent; 40 to 49 years, 29 percent; 50 to 59 years, 20 percent; and 60 to 69 years, 18 percent. Brodnitz (1976) reported a mean age of 50.2 years in 130 patients with the following distribution: 20 to 30 years, 10 percent; 31 to 40 years, 16 percent; 41 to 50 years, 27 percent; 50 to 60 years, 29 percent; older than 60 years, 18 percent. His youngest patient was 27, his oldest, 76. In another study of 100 patients, Aronson (1979) found a median age of onset of 50. The incidence by age in this study can be found in Table 7-2.

SEX RATIO

The male to female ratios reported in different studies range from approximately 1:1 to 1:4. Because patients usually present themselves for examination they introduce a self-selection factor that may not be a true indication of incidence in the general population. Table 7-1 summarizes several studies reported by Kiml (1963) modified to include later ones.

ONSET AND COURSE

With rare exception, adductor spastic dysphonia begins insideously as a nonspecific hoarseness, at first fluctuating in severity, with intervening periods of normal voice. Then, gradually, the strained adductor laryngospasms intrude, breaking up the hoarseness. The disorder may plateau or continue to worsen until phonation during speech is all but impossible. From a follow-up study of 100

Table 7–1 Sex Ratio of Patients with Adductor Spastic Dysphonia

SOURCE	NO. CASES	RATIO M:F	REFERENCE
Bauer (Heidelberg)	19	1:1.7	Kiml (1963)
Brodnitz (United States)	34	1:1.4	Kiml (1963)
Fritzell (Göteborg)	3	1:0.5	Kiml (1963)
Kiml (Praha)	8	1:1	Kiml (1963)
Perellò (Barcelona)	8	1:1	Kiml (1963)
Van Thall (London)	6	1:2	Kiml (1963)
Robe et al. (United States)	10	1:4	Robe et al. (1960)
Aronson et al. (United States)	34	1:1.4	Aronson et al. (1968a)
Brodnitz (United States)	130	1:1.3	Brodnitz (1976)
Aronson (United States)	100	1:1.04	Aronson (1979)
Izdebski et al. (United States)	200	1:2.3	Izdebski et al. (1984)

Table 7-2 Age of Onset of Spastic Dysphonia*

AGE RANGE (YR)	MALES		FEMALES		ALL PATIENTS	
	NUMBER	PERCENT	NUMBER	PERCENT	NUMBER	PERCENT
21–29	3	8	6	9	9	9
30–39	4	11	7	11	11	11
40–49	12	33	17	27	29	29
50–59	15	42	22	34	37	37
60–69	1	3	7	11	8	8
70–79	1	3	5	8	6	6
Total	36	100	64	100	100	100

*Unpublished data.
+Median age of onset for males, 48 years; females, 50 years. Range for males, 21–72; for females 22–77.

patients, Aronson (1979) found that the median time necessary for spastic dysphonia to develop into its full-blown state from onset was approximately one year in both males and females. Although some patients consulted a specialist almost immediately after onset, others waited as long as eight years. The median period from onset until consultation was two months. These patients consulted an average of four specialists, although some had gone to as many as 25 in search of help. Izdebski et al. (1984), in a survey of 200 patients, found gradual onset in 84 percent of patients; the remainder reported sudden onset. They found that in patients whose disorder had begun gradually, the voice declined and reached a plateau within six to nine months. Patients whose voices intermittently fluctuated between abnormal and normal from onset deteriorated and reached a plateau after about 23 months. Once the disorder takes hold, remissions are rare unless the spastic dysphonia is of the conversion reaction type. In an 18-year follow-up study of 10 spastic dysphonic patients, Borenstein et al. (1978) found that in all 10 the disorder had remained; four reported no change during the intervening years, two reported that their voices had worsened slightly, three had mildly improved, and one improved substantially.

Factors Affecting Severity

During the life of the disorder, patients report unexpectedly wide fluctuations in severity. Periods of emotional stress make the disorder worse. Talking on the telephone and to authority figures is especially difficult, and the voice is vulnerable to moods of anxiety and depression. Physical labor also can cause the voice to worsen. One patient reported that if he knew he needed an especially good voice for some occasion, he would refrain from lifting, pushing, or digging. The temptation is to conclude from such testimony that voluntary effort closure increases susceptibility to spasm. Yet, at other times, the spasms can be mild, prompting many patients to claim periods of nearly normal voice. These moments of relief are usually accompanied by feelings of relaxation and freedom from anxiety. For that reason, the voice is often much better while the patient is on vacation. One patient reported that while on a trip to Hawaii, her voice began to improve incrementally in proportion to the distance from the California coast, so that by the time she had reached the islands her voice was the best it had ever been. On her trip home, the closer her plane got to the mainland, the worse her voice became. By the time the plane had landed, her spastic dysphonia was as bad as when she had left. These patients have a baffling ability to produce normal voice when surprised or taken off guard, such as when they are greeted by a passer-by or spoken to from behind. The common factor seems to be a high level of situational spontaneity in which the patient does not have time to think before speaking. The more patients concentrate on what they wish to say, the worse their voices become. Many patients report that even the affective content of their thoughts and mood fluctuations can alter severity; that when thinking pleasant thoughts their voices are better, the reverse being true for unpleasant ones. Normal voice during singing was one of the earliest criteria for spastic dysphonia described. For this type of spastic dysphonia, therefore, it is logical to conclude that spasms are linked to volitional, intellectual, or executive speech functions and disappear during uninhibited, emotional, automatic, nonintellectual speech.

Factors Associated with Onset

The clinician's ability to uncover factors associated with onset of any disorder is contingent upon the patient's ability to remember or willingness to disclose such information. Even when patients report events antecedent to or concurrent with onset of spastic dysphonia, there is a danger that the examiner will conclude they are necessarily cause and effect.

Upper respiratory infections, as discussed elsewhere in this book, are commonly reported as associated with the onset of adductor spastic dysphonia. Asked if their disorder had occurred after a cold, sore throat, or laryngitis, 35 percent of patients answered in the affirmative, and 17 percent said it occurred after a "flu-like" illness (Aronson, 1979). Izdebski et al. (1984) found that 15 percent of their patients reported nonspecific vocal tract illness as well as colds and viruses as being associated with onset. What remains unknown is whether these laryngeal and respiratory illnesses were true infections that had some physical bearing on the disorder, or whether they were unconscious simulations of respiratory infections that provided the psychologic rationale for announcing the disorder, as is known to occur in psychogenic voice disorders as a group.

An unavoidable fact, again not necessarily indicative of cause and effect but in many cases highly suspicious and even compelling, is the co-occurrence of spastic dysphonia and acute or chronic psychologic stress. In their survey of stress and emotional trauma, Izdebski et al. (1984) found that approximately 16 percent of patients thought that stress had caused their spastic dysphonia. Brodnitz (1976) found that 40 percent of his patients had described what he called trigger incidents: death of a relative, severe automobile accident in which the patient was not physically harmed, witness to murder of a relative, divorce of a relative, unremitting work stress, marital conflict, and perpetually demanding responsibility. The term "trigger incident" is an apt one in any discussion of cause and effect, for later in this chapter the distinction will be made between stress as a *primary* psychogenic cause and stress as a trigger or *precipitant* of a latent neurologic disorder. Meanwhile, one should resist the temptation to conclude that all of these cases of spastic dysphonia are *primarily* psychogenic merely on the grounds that the disorder coincided with upsetting life circumstances.

In a study of 100 spastic dysphonia patients, Aronson (1979) found an extraordinarily high percentage of patients who had reported a close temporal relationship between stress and the onset of their voice disorder. Did spastic dysphonia occur after a sudden emotional event? Forty-five percent said it had. Had spastic dysphonia been accompanied by a continuous, ongoing stressful situation? Fifty-five percent answered affirmatively.

The following are samples of patient reports of *acute* emotionally traumatic events shortly after which spastic dysphonia surfaced: "Auto accident; family death; son got divorced; angered at work over a situation I could not handle; death in family followed by marital, family and business stress; dispute over property; daughter's marriage; unmarried daughter became pregnant; brother killed in auto accident and husband died of heart attack in close succession." On a frequency of occurrence basis, family illness and death rank high as precipitants of adductor spastic dysphonia.

Typical *chronic* stress situations reported were: "Hectic worried life; unemployment; hospitalizations; pushing self too hard; continuous job pressure; under tension because of husband's business; having marital difficulties; passed over for promotion; responsibility for caring for alcoholic brother; responsibility for caring for aged mother; taking care of invalid husband and his eventual death; own cancer surgery; homosexual son living at home and his objectionable friends who come to visit."

Many patients have no recollection of physical illness or emotional stress at the time of onset of their dysphonias. Whereas in some cases they have forgotten, in others, they are guarding or repressing sensitive information. In still others, no event occurred at the time of onset. An attempt will be made to clarify the implications of these variations in the section on etiology.

PSYCHOSOCIAL EFFECTS

It does not matter if the etiology of adductor spastic dysphonia is psychogenic, neurologic, or of unknown cause; the voice disorder in its own right is a threat to the patient's psychologic equilibrium. Self-consciousness, feelings of inadequacy, paranoid ideation, diminished interpersonal communication, social withdrawal, alcoholism, depression, and even suicidal tendencies are found in a majority of these patients to some degree. The intensity of these emotions is roughly proportional to the severity and duration of the voice disorder and to the importance of communication in the patient's daily life. Some patients are prime candidates for psychiatric and psychologic help strictly on the basis of the *voice effects* alone. These patients prove how considerably important normal voice is to the maintenance of a secure self-image and how alienated we become with ourselves and society when our self-image, epitomized by our voices, is threatened by our own and others' adverse reactions to it.

Spastic dysphonia affects the emotional, social, and occupational life of each person differently, depending upon each patient's premorbid personality and life circumstances. The extent of incapacitation depends upon the patient's reliance upon speech occupationally and socially. Occupational effects can be devastating in those whose livelihood is heavily dependent upon oral communication, e.g., teachers, attorneys, physicians, clergy, entertainers—any human endeavor in which the personality, ethos, or persuasiveness of the speaker is integral to that person's need to communicate. In a survey of the effects of spastic dysphonia on job performance, Izdebski et al. (1984) found that spastic dysphonia seriously interfered with job performance in 93 percent of men and 77 percent of women, and, as a result, 26 percent of men and 37 percent of women were forced to change jobs or to be reclassified, usually with adverse financial and emotional consequences. Aronson (1979) found that 64 percent of spastic dysphonic patients surveyed reported having become socially withdrawn and depressed after developing the condition. Forty-one percent said it interfered with their earning a living. The following are excerpts from that survey.

Occupational Effects

1. "It caused me to retire. I could no longer work like I used to."
2. "I had to be placed on disability pension."
3. "In my work, the ability to communicate is essential. My voice has resulted in my passing up or not doing some things I might have done otherwise for added income, like negotiating teacher contracts."
4. "By the time I reached retirement age I was ineffective on the telephone, inadequate in communicating with employees or in participating in management sessions. I had to quit."
5. "I live in a secluded world and don't apply the potential I know I have. I don't work toward a better life."
6. "I have missed several promotions due to my voice situation."
7. "I have kept my job as a college professor by using "self-paced" nonlecture methods of teaching. But, this requires more time, and my productivity has dropped."
8. "Mine is a small business and I cannot find help. I have to wait on customers and communicate with them. I become very worn out and tired, angry at myself and depressed."
9. "My job as a consultant consists of sales pitches directly, and due to my voice problem, I haven't been able to communicate properly with customers. I work on a commission basis, and sales have dropped."
10. "How can clients have confidence in me as their attorney with a voice like this? Some of them look at me strangely, and when there is any office noise they can't hear me. Trial work is impossible, now. I let my partner do that."

Social Effects

1. "I no longer want to go to social events or meet with people."
2. "I try to avoid talking to people. I avoid meetings of any kind; going to people's houses or having guests at home. It's embarrassing."

3. "I cannot speak comfortably in crowded rooms, automobiles, buses, or airplanes."

4. "I have been hesitant and have withdrawn from taking office in several clubs and fraternal activities where use of the voice is involved."

5. "People shy away because they cannot hear, and I, in turn, do likewise, because I am aware of their discomfort."

6. "I am unable to carry on a conversation without straining my throat and am silent most of the time, even at home. When I am with other people I listen and seldom enter the conversation."

7. "It's embarrassing to talk, because people stop and stare. Children and teenage boys ridicule me."

8. "I can't visit as I would like. Sometimes my experiences have been knowledgeable, and I would like to express them, but I cannot, and it appears to others that I am stupid."

9. "I used to sing in the church choir. Now my singing is horrid."

10. "I'm not completely withdrawn but am more selective. I try to avoid one-on-one social events and tend more to group events. Also, I try to socialize with those who have heard me and understand my problem."

Emotional Effects

1. "I try to talk and words won't come out. I get frustrated and feel like crying or just getting away from people. I get frustrated, then angry, but it's hard to get angry when you can't raise your voice."

2. "I really freaked out and was put in the hospital for two weeks under sedation. After I came home it was several months before I had any interest in living. I even contemplated suicide, but I felt I couldn't do that to my family."

3. "Lack of vocal confidence is a very emotional experience when you have talked normal all of your life and then your voice becomes less proficient; you tend to become depressed. The question Why? is always present."

4. "Certainly, any person who enjoys life and people would be depressed. It's hell not being able to communicate."

5. "I have been depressed much of my life; always had suicidal tendencies; couldn't communicate with the world, and children especially."

6. "Black moods. Hopelessness. Helplessness. Haplessness."

7. "I feel like my life is being wasted and that I'm being a burden to my husband."

8. "It's hard to put into words, but I feel shut away from the world."

9. "My self-concept has become much more negative. I withdraw socially and become depressed when I think of how well I used to do things, like meet people and make friends. It also had an effect on my marriage. I feel it was the cause of our separation."

10. "I began to feel very sorry for myself. I felt I was being punished for something I had done wrong in life. My marriage problems grew worse as I focused more on myself. I was very unsure of everything."

The preceding testimony on the destructive life effects of adductor spastic dysphonia does not mean every patient who acquires this disorder is destined to suffer in this way. Many patients after a time learn to live with the disorder. They adopt a philosophic point of view, but usually these are not the more severe cases. These patients are the more stable and self-sufficient ones, who do not rely heavily on speech as a means of emotional expression or social satisfaction, and who do not use speech as a primary means of earning a living.

ETIOLOGY

Adductor spastic dysphonia should not be regarded as a single disorder or disease entity but as a voice sign of any one of several different causes. These causes should be specified whenever possible. In order to specify cause, thorough clinical studies of each patient are necessary.

Psychogenic Adductor Spastic Dysphonia

Whether or not a sign or symptom is psychogenic is usually based on indirect, circumstantial, and impressionistic evidence. The credibility of evidence for psychogenicity as a primary cause of any disorder is proportional to the time devoted to the interview; skill, wisdom, and judgment of the clinician; and the honesty, insight, and verbal ability of the patient. It is not difficult to find lives ridden with conflict, strife, disappointment, tragedy, insecurity, rage, hostility, suspiciousness, and other signs of emotional turmoil. It would be too simple, and erroneous, to assign a speech complaint to any change of job or an argument with a spouse. However, when the following relationships can be demonstrated, a strong likelihood that a voice disorder is psychogenic must be considered:

1. The onset of the voice disorder and the stressful life event occur in reasonable proximity to one another.
2. Verbal communication is important to the patient in the conflict, however trivial it might appear to others.
3. During disclosure of delicate or confidential information to the clinician, the voice becomes appreciably improved or normal.
4. During trial symptomatic voice therapy, the voice improves appreciably or becomes normal.
5. When the conflict is moderated, or the patient takes a vacation, the voice improves considerably or becomes normal.

Diagnosis of psychogenicity might not be possible until the clinician has begun trial therapy. Few people would argue against the diagnosis of psychogenic adductor spastic dysphonia if, during the course of the psychosocial interview or reduction of musculoskeletal tension, the voice returned to normal and remained that way for a reasonable duration. Organic, neurologic voice disorders do not fluctuate to such extremes or disappear completely.

ADDUCTOR SPASTIC DYSPHONIA OF CONVERSION REACTION

A review of the early literature on spastic dysphonia indicates that the majority of clinicians perceived their patients to be psychoneurotic and thought their strained, groaning, effortful voices were directly caused by and were manifestations of such psychoneurosis. Specifically, the spastic voice was regarded as a *conversion reaction* (Bloch, 1965; Kiml, 1963). Contemporary experience sustains the validity of this initial etiologic conceptualization. The evidence, then and now, is based upon the logical relationship between the dysphonia and certain life events surrounding its development, and the ease and manner in which the dysphonia is alleviated during the verbalization of emotional conflict and by symptomatic voice therapy. A review of the theory of conversion reaction in Chapter 6 and references given there will remind the student of the strong and symbolic relationship between unresolved conflict and abnormal voice.

Spastic dysphonia can be a sign of conversion reaction no different from conversion aphonia or dysphonias of other voice descriptions. The spastic dysphonia serves to erect a barricade against the dangers of self-revelation. The squeezed, groaning, effortful voice communicates suppression of intense aggression and fear of verbal expression. Psychoanalytically oriented psychiatrists view the disorder as a regressive phenomenon parallel to primitive laryngeal reflexes, such as coughing, gagging, wretching, vomiting, and swallowing. Heaver (1959), one of a handful of psychiatrists, convincingly established the conversion reaction type of spastic dysphonia. The following study by Heaver, and other cases, can be found in Bloch (1965), and these should be read for their psychologic correlative evidence. The student should always ask in contemplating single case and group research studies here and elsewhere, "What is the likelihood that these stories are reasonably, symbolically, and temporally related to the voice disorder? Or, to what extent are these life storms and the dysphonia merely coincidence?" The following is a synopsis of Heaver's classic case of conversion adductor spastic dysphonia.

* * *

This is the case of a 56-year-old woman, married to a pharmacist. She manifested envy for her husband's several academic degrees and was driven to engage in outside activities. Four years before admission, the patient gradually became completely aphonic. It was necessary for her daughter to learn lipreading. Her aphonia, the patient said, followed a series of "severe emotional shocks." The son was in battle in the South Pacific, the husband for a time was thought to have throat cancer, she had a painful thrombophlebitis, and was concerned over her son's impending divorce. . . . This last was connected very closely to her voice symptoms. When the divorce question arose she was no longer permitted to see her grandchildren. The son was doing poorly economically. Her daughter broke off two successive engagements.

The ear, nose, and throat examination showed a larynx of normal size with injected mucosa. The mobility of the congested cords appeared spastic and sphincterlike. During phonation, there was congestion of the external jugular veins. Vocal analysis revealed spastic respiration, low pitch, choked timbre, rigid inflection, hoarse quality, weak volume, a limited range, and spastic vocal attacks. It was noted that the singing voice was not affected. Diagnosis: typical spastic dysphonia with marked laryngeal sphincter action.

The initial Rorschach study revealed a personality structure characterized by much energy and strong self-will, a need to maintain control of others and to exert her influence on all about her. Marked childish narcissism was coupled with general negativism, aggression, and hostility. Strong self-doubts and concern over self-image of failing sexual attraction. In group therapy she sat apart, interrupted others with comments, and seemed to enjoy herself.

Minor degree of improvement occurred with voice therapy. She was not cooperative regarding the advice received during psychotherapy. Her voice ran into total spastic aphonia and even intermittent mutism. It was recommended that voice therapy be combined with dramatic and suggestive but nonprobing psychotherapy. Gradually, her mutism returned to the previous spastic dysphonia. She expressed her underlying aggressive and hostile feelings toward her family, friends, and medical staff covertly disguised by facetious and joking attitudes. She maintained evasiveness and resistance to any effort, no matter how superficially leveled, to analyze her attitudes and voice problem. Her behavior is erratic and histrionic; her urge to dramatize her feelings is strong, as it is to attract attention. Whenever she neared discussion of emotionally charged personal material, she conjured some rationalization to discontinue her visits temporarily. Her most extended period of absence of spastic voice symptoms occurred during the second year of therapy with the second therapist. For almost three weeks, she spoke in her previous normal fashion. With her mother's death, her spastic syndrome rapidly returned. Since then, she is sometimes a little improved, sometimes notably worse, and on a few transitory occasions she was free of dysphonia.

* * *

Hostility, verging on rage, inability to verbalize aggression, and entrapment in life circumstances with no apparent means of escape, so common in the conversion reaction type of adductor spastic dysphonia, is further exemplified in the following case study of a 45-year-old woman who had been diagnosed as having adductor spastic dysphonia several years before this interview:

* * *

C: When did you first start having trouble with your voice?
P: Well, seven and a half years ago when I was pregnant with my little girl.
C: Had you ever had any such trouble before?
P: Yes. Nine years ago I had a little boy, he was seven months old, he is nine now, and I would just have flashes of something and . . .
C: Similar to what you have now?
P: Yes, it was frightening whatever it was; I couldn't seem to control it. It only happened a few times and I went on a vacation and it came back.
C: Same kind of voice that you had seven and a half years ago?
P: Well, I can't really remember it.
C: But the present problem began in earnest seven and a half years ago.
P: Yes.
C: What did you notice first? Was it the same kind of voice that you have now, or was it something different?

P: Oh . . . well, I can't really remember it. It is just hard to speak. Sometimes shakiness. I had left my husband. I was living with my daughter who was going to college, and I've had a lot of trauma the last nine years.

C: Do you remember exactly or approximately when the voice trouble began? Was it while you were pregnant or after the birth of your child?

P: While I was pregnant, and then that summer all of a sudden I had gone back on the ranch and I couldn't speak at all, it didn't really happen suddenly but probably over a period of a week.

C: And has the voice trouble been present ever since?

P: More or less. Sometimes it does get better.

C: Has it ever disappeared completely?

P: No. Only three times when I drank way more than I should have. Usually drinking makes it worse.

C: Under what conditions will it be better?

P: Well, I can't really say.

C: Under what conditions will it be worse?

P: Well, when I'm under extreme stress, and talking about it makes it worse.

C: And what previous help have you sought for the problem?

P: First, seven and a half years ago, I went to a throat specialist twice. The first time he gave me cortisone and I went home and took it faithfully, and then after two days I couldn't talk at all. My husband had to call him back, so I went back and he gave me Valium, and that is the last time I ever saw him.

C: So, except for a brief episode or two about nine years ago, the voice trouble really started about seven years ago.

P: Yes.

C: Now, was that period in your life a significant change over the way it was before that time?

P: Well, I guess, because I have a troubled marriage, that got worse. It has never gotten better. Well, I had left, and after my baby was born I had gone back. It was just a real bad time.

C: At the present time what would you consider the major problem in your life?

P: My marriage.

C: Would you describe that in as much detail as you can?

P: Well, it's bad. I don't see any way out, because I have these two perfectly delightful children who are happy and secure and they have a wonderful home in a small town. There life is just ideal, and I just can't ruin it for them.

C: Why do you say that there is no way out?

P: Well, I've been married for 30 years, and now I was thinking about it last night, for the last year I think I've just had a few emotions. My love for my children and then all the rest of them are just completely negative. All hate, which I know is the worst thing that you can . . . it is very devastating.

C: What do you mean hate?

P: Well, I just don't like my husband.

C: Why not?

P: Oh, it has gone on for so long. When I was 18 I thought he was great; he is seven years older than I am, and I just kind of married him out of, just for security. I was kind of the first hippie, or I feel like I was, and I thought he was nice, but now I've grown up and I know what he is like, and I'm sure, well, we just both tried to destroy each other. I feel as though he has tried to destroy me, and I feel like I've given him way, way more, but he is very, very unyielding and completely unable to . . . I work very, very hard and have tried to suppress all kinds of emotions or feelings. The only time I really let go is in a screaming fight.

C: How is your voice during those fights?

P: Well, it comes out pretty good. That's why he says "there is nothing wrong with your voice now." Of course, it is still very forced, but sometimes I feel like my voice is a substitute for crying, because I have quit crying. I decided a long time ago that that is really useless to do. Sometimes I think it was good for me to cry, and now I can't. I had breast cancer a year ago last February and had a mastectomy, and my husband knew that I had a lump for four to six weeks. When I discovered it I knew immediately that it was bad, and I called him into the bathroom and he said, "Oh I knew you had that four to six weeks ago, and I said 'why didn't you tell me.' " And he had come up behind me and grabbed me which makes me want to kill, and I guess I elbowed him or he said, "Oh, you're so mean" or something, and now I'm really very bitter about that. I keep telling him that I can't forgive him for it, but he is the kind of person that he can't even yield enough to say, well I did make a mistake, or I don't know why I did that. He can't even do that. He just says, "Well, if you're so stupid that you can't find your own lump" more or less to that effect. Oh this is so painful.

C: It was four weeks before . . .

P: He said four to six weeks.

C: So when was that?

P: Well, I had my mastectomy a year ago, last February.

C: So that certainly didn't improve the situation.

P: No. Not my marital situation. I don't think it affected my voice any.

C: But it reinforced your feelings toward your husband.

P: I don't understand. I do understand him in a way, because I know the rest of his family.

C: But the marriage was in trouble before your voice trouble started wasn't it?

P: Yes.

C: And yet you had no trouble with your voice seven years ago.

P: No. I love to talk. I used to, but, of course, now I don't.

C: Well, what do you see for yourself in the future?

P: Well, about the only solution, he says that he will go to a marriage counselor. He is such a contradictor. He has gotten totally dependent on me. He annoys me because he thinks he has to talk about everything. It's like someone thinking aloud. He just talks me to death telling me what he is going to do. If he is going to go up the hill and feed the horse he has to tell me. He feels threatened, I know, about all kinds of things.

C: Like what?

P: Well, I know that he thinks that I am independent and strong, and I'm sure that he feels threatened by that, and when I do things on my own I know that he feels threatened by that. He is terribly jealous. Terribly, and we don't like the same people, or he doesn't fit in with the people that I like. Of course, in the town I live in I don't have . . . I like where I live. I love my home, and it would be very hard to leave, but I don't really have any close friends that I relate to. I have the kind of friends that I have to use poor grammar around every once in a while, or they would think that I'm, you know, trying to be something else. I hate to say it without sounding snobbish, because I really am fond of the people that are good to me, but sometimes I'd like to go to the university and take a course in creative writing and an art course. I do a lot of painting, I do some rosemaling, and I feel deprived in that way. I really don't feel like a martyr for my children, because they are the most important thing that I have.

C: So you have said, then, that your husband has felt jealous and threatened and at the same time you'd like to go back to school and take some courses.

P: You asked me what I saw ahead. I told you what I'd like to see. This is what I do see ahead. He did say that he would see a marriage counselor. I don't know what they are like, but I know we have to work something out; we have to. We just can't go on like we have this summer. But last summer he changed. I think possibly he could have been having affairs, but that doesn't bother me all that much really, but it has been bothering me that he seems to be regressing. I feel as though he is growing old without ever growing up. He doesn't have any interests; he is not doing anything in particular. He just likes to hang around the house.

C: Is that threatening to you?

P: Well, it annoys me, because he doesn't have any, you know, I think he should have interests. The people in his family have an idea that the older you get the easier you should take it. You know, you should just sort of roll into a steady decline. And my life isn't going to be long enough for me to do all the things I want to do, and I just can't stand people like that. And he doesn't like it; he hates my reading; he doesn't like books. He is very scornful of people . . . and he never reads. He does better than he did when I first married him, because he only read comic books then. I should have realized then that a 25-year-old man that read comic books was a little bit . . . But he is intelligent.

C: Why do you say that you are not going to live long enough?

P: Well, I mean I have so many things I want to do. I don't have any idea that I'm not going to last very long, because I promised my kids that I'll live forever. No, I don't want you to think I'm making a death wish or anything. No.

C: So you and he think something needs to be done?

P: It has to be. We can't go on this way, because finally I've given up keeping a pretense by trying to move out of his bedroom. Up until a month ago I still tried to be pleasant by talking to him as much as I could, but finally he wanted to drag me to an alumni thing at his old high school, and I just couldn't face it, especially not with my voice being bad. People I don't care for and I just couldn't face it. And we had just had a disastrous trip.

C: Disastrous?

P: Well, it was just disastrous. We hated it. I hated him. We went to see my daughter, and she was having difficulties with her husband. Her husband is quite a bit older than she is, and he is the very same kind of person. They both have the very same ideas about what a woman or a wife should be and do, and what a man should be and do, and how it should be, and the two of them were buddy-buddy. So when he wanted me to go on this trip, I knew everything was going to hit the fan, and I knew it wasn't very smart of me, but I'm so tired of pretending. I just said I made up my mind when I got back that I'm not even going to ride in town with him let alone go on a weekend trip. And of course, you can guess what all that led to.

C: What?

P: Well, just terrible, terrible things that I said to him and he said to me. But we don't fight in front of the kids. No one but my closest friends know that I'm anything but Miss Mary Sunshine. My voice. This is the worst it has been, just talking about these things. It is very difficult, but usually when I go into town and buy groceries and take the kids to the swimming pool I can get by, but my whole life is a pretense except when I'm with my kids.

C: Again, your whole life is a pretense.

P: Well, I mean because I am keeping up a front, you know, you don't go around telling everybody you're not happy.

C: Have you been getting unhappier as the years have gone by?

P: Yes, well, we've hit a new low.

C: Why?

P: Because we're fighting.

C: You are fighting more this summer than ever before you think?

P: Yes.

C: Why do you think that is so?

P: Well, because I finally just told him I, well, something has happened to me, because I was always able to try and come around and say, Oh he's not such a bad guy, and I guess I'll be able to stick it out till, you know . . .

C: Could you summarize for me what it is about him that you find so objectionable?

P: I feel that he is unyielding and he is a chauvinist. He just can't accept letting me just be.

C: What is the nature of this relationship that makes you feel as antagonistic toward him as you do? What is there about him?

C: He has a cruel streak. Very cruel.

P: What do you mean?

C: Oh, things that he says to me. Of course, I say cruel things to him, too. But I think he hits deeper than I do, I don't know. I hated my father. I just completely disassociated myself from my mother and sisters. Oh I didn't want to get into that. I don't know . . . Oh, I said I hated my father. Well he reminds me of my father.

C: Your husband has many of your father's traits?

P: Yes, in fact most of them I think. But he certainly would have been a complete opposite as far as I can see when I married him.

C: You didn't see that other side to him?

P: No. I didn't deliberately choose someone who was like my father.

C: What has the sexual part of the marriage been like for the past seven years?

P: Oh, pretty fair. Of course, there hasn't been any sex for the past probably four months. And for me I don't want him to touch me, ever.

C: Up until that time you were having a normal sexual relationship?

P: I would say that it has never been enough for him, which turns me off.

C: But, for the past four months there has been no sexual activity at all.

P: No.

C: What caused that?

P: Well, I don't know. I just plain moved out of the bedroom.

C: Why did you do that?

P: Because . . . he just repells me.

C: Why now . . . ?

P: Well, I don't like him. If you don't respect . . . you certainly have to like someone you have sex with and I don't like him.

C: Have you told him that?

P: Well, I think it is obvious to him that I don't like him.

C: What was his reaction to this move on your part?

P: Well, his idea of a confession is to, after we've had a big fight, never to admit anything but to come up and say "Can I mix you one?" "Can I get you a cup of coffee?" And that is supposed to be his wanting to make up. Everything is just supposed to be forgotten. He has made these overtures to me wanting to just forget the whole thing, and he hasn't said a word about my moving out of the bedroom. We don't even talk about sex any more. It used to be a big hassle but there, it's just, I can't give you any answers without talking for an hour on each thing. I can hardly do it. (Pause)

C: We are not completely sure that this voice disorder is caused by marital problems, but I think in this case there is a good chance that it is.

P: Except that there have been times when I've been extremely happy, at least thought I was, and relaxed and it has still been bad.

C: At any rate, before saying it is or it isn't, I think we are going to need a psychiatric opinion about this. I have a colleague in Psychiatry who has been seeing patients of mine who have voice disorders for several years. And I would like him to see you if that is all right with you.

P: Yes.

C: Even if you had no voice problem, it would still be definitely indicated for you to see somebody, as I'm sure you have already concluded that yourself.

P: I know.

C: "Something has got to be done" those are your words and there is no time like the present, in my opinion. What is yours?

P: The same. That's why I'm here. Oh, something else. Did I mention the fact that I'm sure that he has never wanted me to have, to do anything about my voice? I'm sure of that.

C: What makes you say that?

P: Well, because he has never encouraged me to, or never said, "Why don't we. . .," he says he loves me but he has never said "Why don't we take you somewhere and see what we can do?". I had a few sessions with a speech pathologist last summer, and it kind of helped because just, temporarily, I was enjoying the idea that I was doing something about it, but he never asked me a question about it. Or he didn't say "You're better," or "How are you doing?" or "What are they doing with you?" or anything. Not one word. And when I wanted to come here my husband informed me that he wasn't going to pay for any trip. So I borrowed the money to come here.

*   *   *

In a study of the possible psychiatric background in patients with adductor spastic dysphonia, Aronson et al. (1968) submitted 29 of 34 patients to psychiatric interviews averaging two hours in duration. In 18, or 62 percent, the psychiatrists judged the histories and personality characteristics to be indicative of psychoneurosis. Five had significant psychiatric problems; 13 presented with equivocal psychiatric findings, and 11 were psychiatrically normal.

As a group, the 62 percent who had emotional problems of varying degrees—regardless of whether or not these problems can be considered causally related to spastic dysphonia—possessed the following traits: (1) They were compulsive and perfectionistic, not very tolerant of error in others or themselves, and had to do things "right." (2) They had a tendency to suppress their anger resulting from their relationships with other people. (3) They had lifelong tendencies toward verbal repression rather than free expression of ideas. (Not all patients had all three traits.) The psychiatrists agreed that:

> Generally, these patients were rigid, conscientious people who took their responsibilities very seriously. They tended to be worriers and perfectionistic. In addition, and common to many psychiatric conditions, their means of dealing with their feelings of anger, resentment, and irritation were faulty and inefficient; instead of expressing their angry feelings in a socially acceptable way, they usually would choose to keep their anger to themselves . . . With disconcerting frequency, these patients described themselves as "the quiet ones" in their families, from childhood on. One or both parents or a sibling was often the dominant one as far as verbal expression was concerned and these patients had little opportunity or need to participate verbally (Aronson et al., 1968, p. 215).

A review of the Aronson et al. (1968) study shows reasonable psychogenic certainty in five of the 29 patients who had undergone psychiatric examination. However, 13 produced equivocal information and 11 were thought to be free of any evidence of psychiatric disorder. Only in retrospect do these discrepancies become explainable. The study had been done when its authors were just beginning to become aware of neurologic etiology. To be noted is that 71 percent of the patients in the study had *voice tremor*. Probably the authors had reported on the psychologic results of a heterogeneous group of adductor spastic dysphonic patients whom they had regarded as homogeneous. The neurologic patients, in other words, were mixed in with the psychogenic types.

Brodnitz (1976) describes 53 of his spastic dysphonia patients who volunteered, under *careful* probing during the initial interview, what they considered to be the events that triggered the development of their disorders. Examples are death of a near relative, 13 cases (five from laryngeal cancer); severe automobile accident without personal injury, eight cases; climactic marital crisis, eight cases (one starting suddenly in a divorce court after verbal abuse by the opposing attorney); laryngeal surgery for removal of benign lesions, five cases. One woman became dysphonic after her husband threatened to kill her, another after her husband was murdered, a third after her brother was shot to death in a holdup, a fourth after observing her child's first seizure.

> A young psychiatrist was told that his training in analysis was complete. A few weeks after his cutting of the analytical umbilical cord he developed spastic dysphonia. He discussed it with his analyst who agreed to take him back for three more months. Immediately his voice became normal only to revert to the dysphonia when the analyst told him at the end of these three months, that he should now be able to stand on his own two feet (Brodnitz, 1976, pp. 212–213).

> Aside from these 53 patients who could pinpoint the onset of the disorder, there were 28 who exhibited many of the characteristics of severe neuroses. Eight of them had already had long periods of psychiatric treatment before they developed spastic dysphonia. This leaves only about one third of the cases reported in this paper where no obvious psychogenic background could be found. This is not an unusual situation in psychosomatic disorders, particularly in manifestations of conversion hysteria. Of course, everybody who has had frequent contact with cases of spastic dysphonia has entertained the suspicion that an organic neurologic factor may be the etiological basis of the more severe forms of the disorder. Possibly, future research with more refined methods may demonstrate such a connection in some cases (Brodnitz, 1976, p. 213).

ADDUCTOR SPASTIC DYSPHONIA OF MUSCULOSKELETAL
TENSION REACTION

Some patients develop the voice of adductor spastic dysphonia on the basis of a relatively simple muscle tension reaction also called vocal hyperfunction. Although these dysphonias are technically psychogenic, caused by heightened anxiety, tension, or depression, they are not the more serious conversion reaction types.

Increased musculoskeletal tension as a cause of the voice symptoms of adductor spastic dysphonia has been called the tension-fatigue syndrome, the components of which are hoarseness, often of the strained variety, vocal fatigue, poor respiratory support, and pain on phonation. The dysphonia of musculoskeletal tension or the tension-fatigue syndrome can have all of the earmarks of adductor spastic dysphonia. This category of voice disorder is highly amenable to symptomatic voice therapy (Koufman and Blalock, 1988).

Neurologic Adductor Spastic Dysphonia

This section endeavors to demonstrate that strained, staccato, effortful voices within the perceptual definition of adductor spastic dysphonia can be caused by, and are often signs of, two major categories of neurologic disease or syndromes and their subsidiaries:

1. Organic (essential) tremor
2. Dystonia
    a. Meige's syndrome
    b. Spasmodic torticollis
    c. Mixed dystonia-tremor

The following preliminary points about these syndromes should be noted:

1. The adductor spastic dysphonia perceived during contextual speech is superficially indistinguishable from the psychogenic forms. Unless neurologic signs in addition to the dysphonia are present—and often either they are not, or they are so subtle as to go unnoticed—it is almost impossible to tell the neurologic from the psychogenic spastic dysphonias.

2. The above syndromes are established organic disorders recognized by academic and clinical neurologists.

3. They are caused by a lesion or lesions within the extrapyramidal system.

4. The motor signs of these syndromes do not express themselves identically in all patients, who differ from one another according to: how much of the body is involved, the range extending from a single muscle group to the entire body; the onset of the disease, which may begin in one organ or structure and spread to others, or, the disease may remain confined to a single organ; severity, which may range from threshold to severe levels; if the disease affects the respiratory, phonatory, resonatory, and articulatory musculature, in which case the result is a hyperkinetic dysarthria of which strained, effortful, or staccato voice is but one component; and the site of the disease. When the disease expresses itself solely or predominantly in the larynx, the shift of perceptual attention to the voice induces the clinician also to shift the terminology to spastic dysphonia. Technically, then, the adductor spastic dysphonia of these neurologic syndromes are dysarthrias or components thereof.

5. The unusualness and often bizarreness of the movements in these syndromes routinely lead less experienced clinicians of all specialties to diagnose them incorrectly as psychogenic and to explain the unusual movements—e.g., ticlike contractions, facial grimaces, and blepharospasm (squinting and frequent eye blinking)—as secondary psychogenic struggle reactions when, in fact, they are the main signs of the disease.

6. Confusing and misleading to clinicians unless they have been forewarned is that *neurologic movement disorders are often forced into the open for the first time by acute emotional trauma or chronic stress* and, once in evidence, usually worsen with the pressures of daily life or fatigue and improve when the patient is relaxed. Emotional stress as the trigger of organic disease, well known in general illness, is common throughout the histories of patients who develop many different kinds of neurologic diseases. The idea that sudden shock or protracted aggravation can produce irreversible structural or neurochemical changes in the nervous system may tax credibility, but experienced neurologists who have witnessed this correlation unreservedly support this concept.

ADDUCTOR SPASTIC DYSPHONIA OF ORGANIC (ESSENTIAL)
VOICE TREMOR

Noted previously in Chapter 5 are several important points. (1) The quavering voice called organic or essential voice tremor is often a component of the essential tremor syndrome. (2) The voice tremor can involve the larynx only. (3) The rate of the voice tremor ranges from 5 to 12 c/sec. (4) Onset can be sudden or gradual. (5) The voice tremor can be best demonstrated during vowel prolongation. (6) The perceived tremor is produced by alternating adduction and abduction of the true and, often, false vocal folds, which may be synchronous with vertical oscillations of the larynx. (7) The voice tremor can be smooth, (Fig. 7–4a), or it can be interrupted by hoarse voice stoppages or voice arrests. (8) *When organic voice tremor becomes sufficiently severe, the range or amplitude of the adductor phases of most or all of the vocal fold tremor cycles is so extensive that the folds momentarily meet in the midline and seal the glottis, producing a strained or staccato voice arrest. Repeated voice arrests cause the voice to lose its qualities of tremor and take on those of adductor spastic dysphonia* (Fig. 7–4b). (9) Clinically, adductor spastic dysphonia of organic tremor can be confirmed by rhythmic, semirhythmic, or irregular voice arrests during vowel /a/ prolongations that may or may not be separated by several cycles of voice tremor;* or by associated tremor of the head, lips, mandible, tongue, velum, pharynx, and thorax during phonation and of the upper extremities

---

*In very severe cases, the spasms may be sufficiently intense to produce a continuously strained voice rather than tremor on vowel prolongation. Raising the pitch level may enable voice tremor to break through.

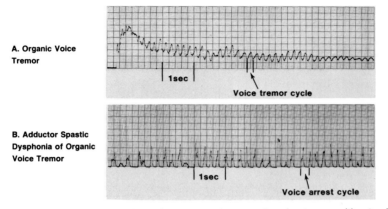

A. Organic Voice Tremor

1sec

Voice tremor cycle

B. Adductor Spastic Dysphonia of Organic Voice Tremor

1sec

Voice arrest cycle

Figure 7–4   Oscillographic tracings comparing organic voice tremor without voice arrest and with voice arrests during vowel prolongation. *A,* Organic voice tremor without voice arrests. *B,* Adductor spastic dysphonia of organic voice tremor. Note the rhythmic voice arrests. *From* Aronson, A.E., and Hartman, D.E.: Adductor spastic dysphonia as a sign of essential (voice) tremor. J. Speech Hear. Disord., 46: 52–58, 1981.

when extended. However, these corroborative signs may be absent or so mild as to go unnoticed by all except those trained to recognize them.

The evidence linking adductor spastic dysphonia to essential tremor follows.

1. Spastic dysphonia in two patients with heredofamilial tremor was reported by Critchley (1939, 1949).

2. In a neurologic study of 10 spastic dysphonia patients, all 10 had scattered neurologic signs. One of the patients had heredofamilial tremor involving the head and both upper extremities (Robe et al., 1960).

3. A neurologic and psychiatric study of 31 patients with adductor spastic dysphonia disclosed regular voice tremor during vowel prolongation in 71 percent of patients. Six patients had accompanying head or hand tremor (Aronson et al., 1968).

4. A videofluoroscopic study of three spastic dysphonia patients showed intermittent voice stoppages associated with complete glottic and supraglottic closure and tremor of the larynx, hypopharynx, and tongue during quiet respiration and contextual speech and were consistent with the patients' tremulous voice quality. Tremor amplitude increased markedly during intermittent voice stoppages (McCall et al., 1971).

5. In a study of 21 patients with voice tremor, 10 were described as having spastic dysphonia. In three there was a family history of tremor. Vowel prolongations showed irregular intervals of complete voice arrest at around 6 c/sec. (Dordain and Dordain, 1972).

6. In 12 patients diagnosed as spastic dysphonic, tremulous, quavering phonation was found in at least three patients, and postural tremor in three patients. In one case tremor elsewhere in the body appeared five years after onset of spastic dysphonia; in another, one year after onset. In one patient, tremor had appeared 20 years before onset of the voice disorder (Aminoff et al., 1978).

7. A study compared three groups of patients, one consisting of 14 essential tremor patients without voice arrest, a second of 16 essential tremor patients with occasional voice arrests, and a third of 22 patients suspected as having the tremor type of adductor spastic dysphonia. On vowel prolongation median voice tremor frequencies of 5.7, 5.0, and 5.5 c/sec. were found in the three groups, respectively. The differences were statistically insignificant. Tremors in other parts of the body were found in 93 percent of the first group, 81 percent of the second group, and 50 percent of the third group (Aronson and Hartman, 1981).

Emotional Stress as a Precipitant of Adductor Spastic Dysphonia or Organic (Essential) Voice Tremor. One would hope for the sake of simplicity that all psychogenic adductor spastic dysphonias showed a history of acute or chronic emotional stress, and that absence of such a history would characterize the neurologic types. Regrettably, and remarkably, such is not the case, for convincing evidence from several different sources shows that both essential voice tremor and the adductor spastic dysphonia of essential tremor frequently follow emotional stress. That stress can produce permanent neurologic change is based upon indirect data correlating life history with onset of the neurologic disorder. However, the time and circumstantial relationship is so close in single case and group studies as to be highly convincing. As noted elsewhere, the concept that stress can precipitate incipient neurologic disease, or be a primary cause of it, is accepted doctrine in medicine and is not considered to be particularly unusual.

1. A 72-year-old woman with a 20-year history of face and hand tremor developed voice tremor shortly after the death of her husband (Ardran et al., 1966).

2. In three patients who had the tremor types of spastic dysphonia, the voice and associated tremors occurred after emotional shock several days after the traumatic event (Dordain and Dordain, 1972).

3. Emotional stress was associated with onset in two groups of essential voice tremor patients, 29 and 25 percent, and in 41 percent of adductor spastic dysphonias of essential tremor (Aronson and Hartman, 1981).

The kinds of stress that precipitate adductor spastic dysphonia of organic voice tremor are not qualitatively different from those responsible for the psychogenic type. Death of a relative and violation of mores within the family are common themes responsible for both the psychogenic and neurologic types. However, many more neurologic than psychogenic patients give histories free of such stresses and appear to have well-adjusted personalities.

ADDUCTOR SPASTIC DYSPHONIA OF DYSTONIA

Evidence strongly supports the concept that adductor spastic dysphonia can also be a laryngeal sign of dystonia. As already noted in Chapter 5, the larynx can be involved in the hyperkinetic dysarthrias of which dystonia is one type. Dystonia is a general term referring to a group of isolated neurologic signs or complete syndromes. Potentially confusing are several synonyms used to describe these signs: Meige's syndrome, Brueghel's syndrome, orofacial dyskinesia, and focal dystonia. Spasmodic torticollis, athetosis, and writer's cramp also fall within the purview of the dystonias. Spasmodic torticollis as a specific type of dystonia can coexist with dyskinetic facial and lingual movements and even tremor.

Dystonia refers to patients who have relatively slow, adventitious, uncontrolled, nonrhythmic contractions of the lips, mandibular muscles, tongue, velopharyngeal muscles, larynx, thorax, or extremities. Dystonias are caused by lesions of the extrapyramidal system. The contraction of different muscle groups can occur in any combination. Often they are confined to one region of the body, such as to the head and neck musculature. They can even involve a single muscle group, especially in the early stages of the disorder if it is progressive; in many patients it is static.

The evidence will show that adductor spastic dysphonia can be an example of a dystonia isolated to the larynx, i.e., a focal laryngeal dystonia, or it can be one component of a more generalized dystonia. As mentioned in the previous section on spastic dysphonia of organic voice tremor, when dystonia is focal to the larynx, the tendency is to describe the effect as spastic dysphonia. When additional speech muscles are affected, the tendency is to call the entire speech disorder hyperkinetic dysarthria.

Meige's Syndrome. Meige's syndrome, originally called medial facial spasm, is a type of dystonia that consists of symmetric dystonic spasms of the facial muscles, which may first involve the eyes, producing blepharospasm, and later the remainder of the facial muscles, producing lip retraction and uncontrolled jaw opening and closing. Day-to-day fluctuations are typical, aggravated by stress, improved by sedation, and disappearing during sleep. A similar syndrome is called

Brueghel's syndrome or blepharospasm-oromandibular dystonia syndrome (Tolosa and Klawans, 1979).

Jacome and Yanez (1980) described a 49-year-old man who had typical spastic dysphonia for three years that began with blepharospasm, symmetric facial spasms, and mild jaw retraction. Symptoms improved with rest and were worse under stress. He could talk and sing normally at times. "We believe this patient has a combination of Meige's disease and spastic dysphonia,* with blepharospasm and medial facial spasms as described by Meige, as well as typical spastic dysphonia." Marsden and Sheehy (1982) found that the most common speech difficulty of patients with the dystonic spasms of Meige's syndrome was "having to force air through a tight throat and mouth resulting in a strained, monotonous, slurring speech, which resembled closely the classical description of spastic dysphonia. . . . Since spastic dysphonia may occur in the same syndrome, *it is quite likely that isolated spastic dysphonia itself may be a sole focal manifestation of dystonia* [emphasis mine]. Indeed, we have encountered a small number of patients with speech disturbance indistinguishable from that seen in Meige Syndrome, patients who would be classified as cases of spastic dysphonia but which we believe to be examples of isolated focal laryngeal dystonia."

Jankovic and Ford (1983) studied 100 patients with signs of dystonia. Twenty-one were found to have spastic dysphonia. In 15 the dysphonia was accompanied by blepharospasm, orofacial movements, and tremor. *In six patients spastic dysphonia was the only sign.* In view of the previous discussion of emotional stress as a *precipitating,* not a causal, factor in essential tremor and the spastic dysphonia of essential tremor, it is important to note that the dystonic patients in this study yielded similar psychiatric signs: "Although we found no evidence to support hysterical origin of the facial movements, many patients had psychiatric problems which were preceded, followed by, or associated with the movement disorder. These include marked depressions (one-quarter of the patients), anxiety, obsessive-compulsive personality, 'schizoid' personality, space phobia, and a variety of other psychological abnormalities."

In a study of 10 patients with Meige's syndrome during neurologic examination, Golper et al. (1983) documented laryngospasm in five of the patients studied. One was described as having an alternating strained/strangled voice quality and voice stoppages; a second voice stoppage on vowel prolongations; a third voice stoppages and phonation on inhalation; a fourth strained/strangled voice, and a fifth, a question of voice tremor.

In 1875 Schnitzler (Kiml, 1963) described two patients with spastic dysphonia who had dystonic movements of the arms and legs.

In three of 12 spastic dysphonic patients studied by Aminoff et al. (1978), one had torsion dystonia, a second had buccolingual dyskinesia, and a third had blepharospasm. The authors stated:

> Our own findings would certainly suggest that spasmodic dysphonia should be regarded as a focal dystonia of the laryngeal musculature. . . . The high incidence of tremor among our patients with spasmodic dysphonia accords with the high incidence reported in patients with torsion dystonia . . . or related movement disorders such as spasmodic torticollis.

Spasmodic Torticollis. Spasmodic torticollis, also once thought to be a psychiatric disorder, is now regarded by most neurologists as a dystonia caused by a lesion within the extrapyramidal system. People who acquire this disease experience an uncontrollable pulling, twisting, or tilting of the head to one side. Variations may be a retrocollis in which there is an extension of the head backward, or a procollis, in which there is flexion of the head forward. The disease often shows signs of dystonic facial movements, blepharospasm, and dysarthria, including voice tremor. But, in addition to these classic signs, adductor spastic dysphonia may precede, follow, or parallel the development of spasmodic torticollis. Since Critchley's (1939) early report of a patient with spastic dysphonia who had spasmodic torticollis, the association between the dysphonia and this disease has been observed by many clinicians, particularly when the illness is in its full-blown stage. The

---

*They might have rephrased their statement to say Meige's disease, of which spastic dysphonia was a *sign* or *component,* for that is probably what they had intended.

association between torticollis, dystonia of other types, and tremor indicates the more than casual interrelationship among these various extrapyramidal syndromes. Schaefer (1983) also recognized the close connection between adductor spastic dysphonia and spasmodic torticollis because of the frequent existence of both diseases in the same patient, the association of tremor in both diseases, and the similarities in the historical controversy as to whether spasmodic torticollis was psychogenic or neurologic. Once considered to be psychogenic, few would argue against the fact that spasmodic torticollis is now well accepted as neurologic.

Looking back, what has been emerging is a picture of one form of adductor spastic dysphonia as a solitary, or coexisting sign of any one of several extrapyramidal movement disorders. These, it should be emphasized, are syndromes of the central nervous system. During a brief period in the search for neurologic etiology, the notion was advanced that the voice disorder could arise from a peripheral nervous system lesion, specifically of the Xth nerve, and was of viral origin (Dedo et al., 1977; Bocchino and Tucker, 1978). These clinicians based their hypotheses on the finding of what they thought were demyelinated nerve fibers in specimens taken from adductor spastic dysphonic patients during nerve resection. However, Ravits et al. (1979) were unable to find any evidence of differences between the nerve fibers in spastic dysphonic and normal subjects. On other grounds, it is unlikely that such a peripheral nerve lesion could produce massive spasticity; flaccidity is usually the result of such lesions. The hypothesis also could not account for periods of normal voice in many spastic dysphonic patients.

Idiopathic Adductor Spastic Dysphonia

The term "idiopathic adductor spastic dysphonia" is reserved for patients in whom no convincing evidence of psychogenic or neurologic etiology can be found. Some clinicians have a tendency to infer etiology without adequate proof, interpreting the patient's spastic dysphonia according to their own biases. To do so is not in the best interest of the patient or conducive to scientific thought. Loose diagnostic formulations given to the patient are usually taken to heart and can adversely influence the patient's self-concept.

The category of idiopathic adductor spastic dysphonia is not diagnostic, but a means of placing the diagnosis in suspense until further data have been acquired to show a definite etiology. If the patient is suitably followed over a long period of time, a psychogenic or neurologic etiology often will reveal itself, permitting a change of classification. One example is that of a 34-year-old attorney who was referred by an otolaryngologist who cited adductor spastic dysphonia as the only complaint. The psychiatric history and neurologic examinations failed to disclose any evidence of cause from either discipline. Three years later on the patient's return to the clinic, dystonic leg movements and procollis were found on neurologic examination, in addition to a worsening of his adductor spastic dysphonia.

SUMMARY

1. Adductor spastic dysphonia is characterized by a strained, groaning, effortful, staccato voice varying in qualities of these components among different patients and also in severity.

2. The strained, effortful voice is the product of hyperadduction of the true, and often false, vocal folds and accompanied by excessive extrinsic laryngeal muscle action that usually elevates the body of the larynx in synchrony with the spasms.

3. The psychogenic causes of adductor spastic dysphonia are conversion reaction or muscu-loskeletal tension.

4. The neurologic causes are organic (essential) tremor, orofacial dyskinesia or dystonia (Meige's syndrome), and spasmodic torticollis. These extrapyramidal diseases can occur singly or in combination. Their spastic dysphonias can occur in isolation in the beginning, and as the disease progresses, other signs will appear. Often the dysphonia may be the only sign or the predominant one.

5. It is advocated, therefore, that the type of adductor spastic dysphonia be designated in any ultimate diagnostic categorization, e.g., adductor spastic dysphonia of essential tremor, adductor spastic dysphonia of dystonia. If no specific cause can be found, the term "idiopathic adductor spastic dysphonia" should be employed.

6. In most cases, adductor spastic dysphonia, regardless of etiologic type, begins gradually in the middle years, somewhere between the ages of 40 and 50 years, although studies have shown onset in childhood. The ratios of males to females ranges from 1:1 to 1:4, depending upon studies consulted.

7. For both psychogenic and neurologic types, a high percentage of patients experience onset as associated with emotional stress, causal in the former type and as a triggering of the neurologic disease in the latter.

8. Regardless of cause, adductor spastic dysphonia usually *produces* serious occupational, social, and emotional disturbances.

SUGGESTIONS FOR ADDITIONAL READING

Aronson, A.E., Brown, J.R., Litin, E.M., and Pearson, J.S.: Spastic dysphonia. I. Voice, neurologic and psychiatric aspects. J. Speech Hear. Disord., 33:203–218, 1968a.

Aronson, A.E., Brown, J.R. Litin, E.M., and Pearson, J.S.: Spastic dysphonia, II. Comparison with essential (voice) tremor and other neurologic and psychogenic dysphonias. J. Speech Hear. Disord., 33:220–231, 1968b.

Aronson, A.E., and Hartman, D.E.: Adductor spastic dysphonia as a sign of essential (voice) tremor. J. Speech Hear. Disord., 46:52–58, 1981.

Blitzer, A., Brin, M.F., Fahn, S., and Lovelace, R.E.: Clinical and laboratory characteristics of focal laryngeal dystonia: Study of 110 cases. *Laryngoscope,* 98:636–640, 1988.

This article contains statistical data on the incidence of spastic dysphonia in a large group of patients who had dystonic movement disorders, illustrating that *one type* of spastic dysphonia, in all probability, is a manifestation of an extrapyramidal movement disorder of the dystonic variety.

Block, P.: Neuro-psychiatric aspects of spastic dysphonia. Folia Phoniatr, 17:301–364, 1965.

The most voluminous and comprehensive article on spastic dysphonia extant. Has considerable historical significance. Psychoanalytically oriented. Hundreds of references.

Marsden, C.D., and Sheehy, M.P.: Spastic dysphonia and Meige disease. *Neurology* (NY), 30:349, 1980.

These four articles should be read for a background to both the psychogenic and neurologic forms of adductor spastic dysphonia.

Robe, E., Brumlik, J., and Moore, P.: A study of spastic dysphonia. Laryngoscope, 70:219–245, 1960.

A landmark study, probably the first comprehensive one that advocated that at least one form of spastic dysphonia was neurologic. It served to shift research and clinical thinking about the causes of adductor laryngospasms during speech in new directions.

REFERENCES

Aminoff, M.J., Dedo, H.H., and Izdebski, K.: Clinical aspects of spasmodic dysphonia. J. Neurol. Neurosurg. Psychiatry, 41:361–365, 1978.

Ardran, G., Kinsbourne, M., and Rushworth, G.: Dysphonia due to tremor. J. Neurol. Neurosurg. Psychiatry, 29:219–223, 1966.

Arnold, G.E.: Spastic dysphonia: I. Changing interpretations of a persistent affliction. Logos, 2:3–14, 1959.

Aronson, A.E.: Spastic dysphonia: Retrospective study of one hundred patients. (Unpublished manuscript), 1979.

Aronson, A.E., Brown, J.R., Litin, E.M., and Pearson, J.S.: Spastic dysphonia. I. Voice, neurologic, and psychiatric aspects. J. Speech Hear. Disord., 33:203–218, 1968a.

Aronson, A.E., Brown, J.R., Litin, E.M., and Pearson, J.S.: Spastic dysphonia, II. Comparison with essential (voice) tremor and other neurologic and psychogenic dysphonias. J. Speech Hear. Disord., 33:220–231, 1968b.

Aronson, A.E., and Hartman, D.E.: Adductor spastic dysphonia as a sign of essential (voice) tremor. J. Speech Hear. Disord., 46:52–58, 1981.

Block, P.: Neuro-psychiatric aspects of spastic dysphonia. Folia Phoniatr., 17:301–364, 1965.

Bocchino, J., and Tucker, H.: Recurrent laryngeal nerve pathology in spasmodic dysphonia. Laryngoscope, 88:1274–1278, 1978.

Borenstein, J.A., Lipton, H.L., and Rupick, C.: Spastic dysphonia: An 18-year follow-up. Paper presented at the American Speech and Hearing Association, San Francisco, 1978.

Brodnitz, F.S.: Spastic dysphonia. Ann. Otol. Rhinol. Laryngol., 85:210–214, 1976.

Critchley, M.: Observations on essential (heredofamilial) tremor. Brain, 72:113–139, 1949.

Critchley, M.: Spastic dysphonia ('inspiratory speech'). Brain, 62:96–103, 1939.

Dedo, H.H., Izdebski, K., and Townsend, J.: Recurrent laryngeal nerve histopathology in spastic dysphonia. A preliminary study. Ann. Otol. Rhinol. Laryngol., 86:806–812, 1977.

Dordain, M., and Dordain, G.: L'epreuve du "a" tenu au cours des tremblements de lu voix (tremblement idiopathique et dyskinesie volitionnelle, leurs rapports avec la dysphonie spasmodique). Revue, Laryngol. Otol. Rhinol., 93:167–182, 1972.

Golper, L.C., Nutt, J.G., Rau, M.T., and Collman, R.O.: Focal cranial dystonia. J. Speech Hear. Disord., 48:128–134, 1983.

Heaver, L.: Spastic dysphonia: II. Psychiatric considerations. Logos, 2:15–24, 1959.

Izdebski, K., Dedo, H.H., and Boles, L.: Spastic dysphonia: A patient profile of 200 cases. Am. J. Otolaryngol., 5:7–14, 1984.

Jacome, D.E., and Yanez, G.F.: Spastic dysphonia and Meige disease. Neurology (NY), 30:349, 1980.

Jankovic, J., and Ford, J.: Blepharospasm and orofacial-cervical dystonia: Clinical and pharmacological findings in 100 patients. Ann. Neurol., 13:402–411, 1983.

Kiml, J.: Le classement des aphonies spastiques. Folia Phoniatr. 15:269–277, 1963.

Koufman, J.A., and Blalock, D.P.: Vocal fatigue and dysphonia in the professional voice user. *Laryngoscope,* 98:493–498, 1988.

Marsden, C.D., and Sheehy, M.P.: Spastic Dysphonia, Meige disease, and Torsion Dystonia, Neurology (NY), 32:1202, 1982.

McCall, G.N., Skolnick, M.L., and Brewer, D.W.: A preliminary report of some atypical movement patterns in the tongue, palate, hypopharynx, and larynx of patients with spasmodic dysphonia. J. Speech Hear. Disord., 37:466–470, 1971.

Parnes, S.M., Lavarato, A.B., and Myers, E.N.: Study of spastic dysphonia using videofiberoptic laryngoscopy. Ann Otol. Rhinol. Laryngol., 87:322–326, 1978.

Ravits, J.M., Aronson, A.E., Desanto, L.W., and Dyck, P.J.: No morphometric abnormality of recurrent laryngeal nerve in spastic dysphonia. Neurology (NY), 29:1376–1382, 1979.

Robe, E., Brumlik, J., and Moore, P.: A study of spastic dysphonia. Laryngoscope, 70:219–245, 1960.

Schaefer, S.D.: Neuropathology of spasmodic dysphonia. Laryngoscope, 93:1183–1202, 1983.

Tarrasch, H.: Muscle spasticity in functional aphonia and dysphonia. Med. Wom. J., 53:25–33, 1946.

Tolosa, E.S., and Klawans, H.L.: Meige's disease. Arch. Neurol., 36:635–637, 1979.

Traube, L.: Spastische form der nervosen heiserkeit. Pathol. Psysiol., 2:677, 1871.

Chapter Eight

ABDUCTOR SPASTIC DYSPHONIA

DEFINITION

"Abductor spastic dysphonia" is a term used in reference to a perceptually distinctive voice in which normal or hoarse voice is suddenly interrupted by brief moments of breathy or whispered (unphonated) segments (Aronson, 1973). The term "abductor spastic dysphonia" was chosen because it appeared as if the vocal fold physiology responsible for the voice disorder was the opposite of that which occurs in adductor spastic dysphonia, i.e., instead of spastic or spasmodic hyperadduction of the vocal folds producing moments of strained voice or voice arrest, the vocal folds *spasmodically hyperabduct,* releasing bursts of unphonated air. Although the disorder has not been long recognized, evidence is beginning to show that, as with the adductor forms, abductor spastic dysphonia may not be due to a single cause, but may have either psychogenic or neurologic substrates.

PATHOPHYSIOLOGY

Fiberscopic viewing of the vocal folds during connected speech discloses that, with each breathy air release, a synchronous and untimely abduction of the true vocal folds occurs exposing an extremely wide glottic chink. Frequently, bowed vocal folds may be found on laryngoscopic examination. These abductor spasms are triggered by consonant sounds, particularly the unvoiced ones, especially when they are in the initial positions of words. For example, in some patients it is possible to inhibit the breathy release of air entirely by having the patient read material containing only voiced consonants. Conversely, it is possible to precipitate rampant bursts of breathiness by asking the patient to read passages saturated with unvoiced consonants. The duration of breathy segments evoked by initial stop consonants has been measured at two to three times normal, but the total duration of words can remain normal nevertheless; the period of aspiration intrudes into the vowel segment, depleting its energy (Zwitman, 1979).

Figure 8–1 shows spectrographs of a normal speaker and an abductor spastic dysphonic speaker producing the sentence: "Berries are good to eat." The abductor breathy segments can be detected by the diminished or absent voice fundamental frequency energy at the following points: (1) a prolonged interval between the /z/ ending the word "berries" and the /a/ vowel beginning the word "are"; (2) between initiation of the sound /g/ and the vowel /ʊ/ in "good" with some loss of sound energy during the vowel; (3) a prolonged interval between the final /d/ of "good" and the initial /a/ of "on"; and (4) during production of the /b/ and /r/ phonemes of the word "bread." Aspiration time occupied 96 of 260 msec. or 36.5 percent of the word, whereas no aspiration occurs during normal production of the word. However, sentences spoken with abductor breathiness can take longer than normally phonated ones as noted in a study of Merson and Ginsberg (1979) in which one patient required 2150 msec. compared with a normal control who spoke the same sentence in 1775 msec., and whose mean airflow rate was 77 ml/sec. compared with the dysphonic person's airflow of 400 ml/sec.

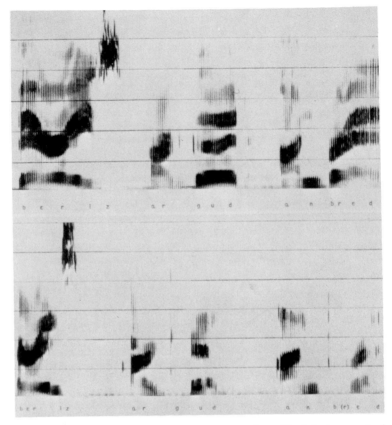

Figure 8–1. Spectrographs of a normal speaker (A) and a patient with abductor spastic dysphonia (B) producing the sentence: "Berries are good on bread." (*From* Zwitman, D.H.; Bilateral cord dysfunctions: Abductor type spastic dysphonia. J. Speech. Hear. Disord., 44: 373–378, 1979.

ONSET, COURSE, AND FACTORS AFFECTING SEVERITY

Abductor spastic dysphonia usually begins insidiously, not essentially differently from onset in patients who develop adductor spastic dysphonia. The voice may begin as a nonspecific hoarseness or breathiness and over a period of days or weeks begin to show signs of intermittent breathy air release.

Severity of the dysphonia fluctuates under conditions similar to the adductor type. When the patient is relaxed and free of tension, pressure, or worry, the voice can be nearly normal. It can be better or nearly normal during conditions of anger or laughter. It is much worse when the patient is emotionally upset, when required to speak with figures of authority, or when the communicative content of speech is more than usually critical. Severity can be temporarily reduced by avoiding voiceless consonants and by phonating at higher pitch levels.

Factors Associated with Onset

Factors associated with onset are not essentially different in these patients as in those who have adductor spastic dysphonia. The disorder can occur in the absence of any known associated event, or it can follow laryngitis with sore throat or domestic or work-related emotional stress.

The history of previous dysphonias and factors associated with onset in five patients who today would be designated as having abductor spastic dysphonia were reported by Aronson et al. (1964), who found that three had had previous episodes of pure whispered (aphonic) speech, all five had had previous hoarseness, in two the onset had been associated with cold or influenza, in all five the onset had been associated with fatigue or exhaustion, and in two the onset had been associated with feelings of tightness in the throat.

ETIOLOGY

With the continual gathering of data, a pattern appears to be emerging in which abductor spastic dysphonic patients, like their adductor counterparts, may be divisible into psychogenic, neurologic, and even idiopathic types, and that psychologic stress may precipitate the neurologic ones. In a study by Hartman and Aronson (1981), 10 of 13 patients (77 percent), had a scattering of neurologic signs: deterioration in writing, synkinetic facial movements, hyper-reflexia, ataxic gait, nasal regurgitation, and dysphagia. However, more importantly, this study also uncovered a neurologic parallel to one form of adductor spastic dysphonia—essential tremor. In five (30 percent) of the 17 patients, voice tremor on vowel prolongation was documented within the range of 4.5 to 6.0 Hz, which is well within the limits of the essential tremor syndrome. On laryngoscopic examination, in some patients the abductor spasms are rhythmic, and a breathy release of air occurs on the abductor phase of each tremor cycle. In other patients voice tremor without breathy air releases are audible on vowel prolongation (Fig. 8–2a). Four (31 percent) of the 13 patients in the study who had been given

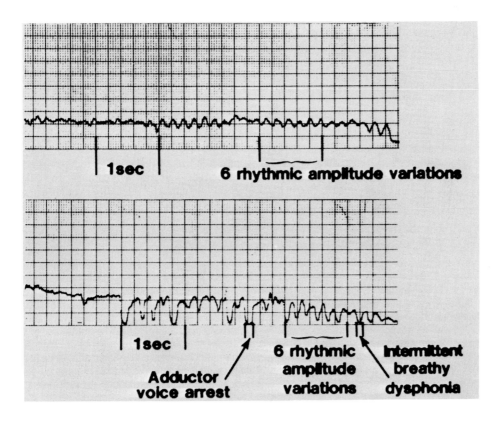

Figure 8–2.   Oscillographic tracings of (A) an abductor spastic dysphonic patient of the essential tremor type during vowel prolongation. The patient has almost continuous tremor. Patient (B) has mixed abductor-adductor spastic dysphonia of the essential tremor type. Note moments of both adductor and abductor (intermittent breathy dysphonia) spasms. (From Hartman, D.E., and Aronson, A.E.: Clinical investigations of intermittent breathy disphonia. J. Speech Hear. Disord., 46: 428–432, 1981.

neurologic examinations had tremor of the head, face, and extremities. There may be, then, at least one definable neurologic type of abductor spastic dysphonia that parallels the adductor form—*abductor spastic dysphonia of essential tremor*.

Some patients have a mixed abductor-adductor spastic dysphonia; moments of breathiness occur alternately with moments of strained-harshness or voice arrest (Fig. 8–2*b*). Noting the co-occurrence of abductor and adductor laryngospasms, Connito and Johnson (1981) made the interesting proposition that, rather than adductor and abductor spastic dysphonia being separate disorders, they are on a continuum, a view that is not only plausible but one that would help to explain their similarities pertaining to nature of onset, factors influencing severity, and multiple etiologies.

Convincing evidence is also accumulating to show that there is a psychogenic form of abductor spastic dysphonia. In a psychiatric study, seven patients, who had what was then called "intermittently whispered-phonated speech," before the coining of the term "abductor spastic dysphonia," had various combinations of the following: histories of chronic stress, clinical signs of hysterical personality, histories of other conversion reactions, marital discord, repressed anger, immaturity and dependency, neurotic life adjustments, mild to moderate depression, and "conversion V" on the Minnesota Multiphasic Personality Inventory test (Aronson et al., 1966). Voice signs of abductor spastic dysphonia of conversion reaction were found in the following patients.

* * *

A 46-year-old housewife and beauty salon operator had been under chronic stress from several sources. Her 25-year-old son had a behavior problem. She harbored unspoken hostile feelings toward her husband, who had never adequately supported the family and who was unemployed. She was perpetually irritated with her employees for their inability to measure up to her standards, but she was unable to express her feelings to them. She had chronic and overwhelming fatigue by early afternoon and would have to retire to her bed. Her marginal insight into her problem was evident from her statement that "I am afraid my employees think I am angry with them when I lose my voice and can't talk" (Aronson et al., 1966, p. 117).

* * *

A religious, perfectionistic woman had a long-standing disappointment in her married daughter who drank and read "unacceptable" literature. She disapproved of the way her daughter was raising her children. The patient asked if "being frustrated and never letting anyone know" could cause her to "lose" her voice. Later in the interview, she came closer to the central issue. "My only daughter annoys me constantly, but I never let her know. . . . Where did we fail with this daughter? . . . I can't reprimand her. I can't get on her back, because it may be something I have done that's wrong. . . . I don't admire people who show anger. I think you should control it. I have been so angry that I have felt actually warm inside, but no one has known that I was angry. . . . Joy and love are emotions to be expressed, but not anger" (Aronson et al., 1966, p. 120).

* * *

A 45-year-old married woman has had intermittent moments of breathiness for the past two years. Laryngologic examination shows normal vocal cord structure and function.

The patient's voice disorder began during an intensely troubled period of her life. Active in a women's service organization and in line for the presidency, she was defeated for this office by a false rumor that she had misused the organization's finances. When the patient learned of this plot, she was furious and resentful and was strongly tempted to express her contempt toward the membership, but decided against this course of action because she could not bring herself to express the unladylike feelings she felt toward them.

During this time of anger, frustration, defeat, and violent arguments at meetings of the organization, she began to detect feelings of tension in her throat followed shortly thereafter by a gradual change in her voice. As the arguments grew in ferocity, her voice symptoms became increasingly disabling.

One month after the first signs of the voice change, she became involved in an extramarital affair. She recalls, "I was a sitting duck to get involved." After one year it was discovered by the man's wife. "She came over and called me every name in the book. I was ashamed, humiliated, furious."

Her voice disorder, by now well entrenched, became progressively worse following this confrontation. At present, she feels tremendously guilty toward her husband, whom she describes as "so good and unsuspecting." She would like to tell her husband of the affair but is so "deeply in love" with the other man that she cannot give him up. As a result she is caught in a perpetual conflict (Aronson, 1973, p. 51).

*   *   *

This chapter closes with an interview with a patient who came to the Clinic with moderate to severe abductor spastic dysphonia. The etiology remains unclear from the interview and examination, and the disorder has to be considered idiopathic until the accumulation of further evidence. The interview was selected because of the patient's exceptional ability to describe the onset and course of his voice disorder, its symptoms, efforts toward therapy, and his reactions to the disorder. It is also illustrative, rather typically in many ways, of the pilgrimage many patients enter into to find a cure for their voice disorders.

*   *   *

C: Could you tell me now, first of all, your age.
P: I'm 38.
C: And what is your occupation?
P: A corporate representative.
C: Are you married?
P: Yes.
C: Do you have any children?
P: I have three children.
C: Had you ever had any voice trouble like this before as a child or as an adolescent?
P: No.
C: Tell me when this first started.
P: It first started about 6 years ago. I had a very bad cold one weekend and when the cold got a little better, I was left with laryngitis, and that was the outset of the thing. The laryngitis got a little better within about a week, but after that it was difficult to say certain words. To begin with it was just every so often and just one particular sound, which was a hard "c" like "Carol" or "cam," or a "k" sound like in "keep". It was barely noticeable, but then it seemed like each year it got a little bit worse and there would be new sounds that would prove more difficult.
C: What came next?
P: It seems like it was anything like a "p" or "t" going into vowels, and I remember most specifically "Porsche" because I was selling foreign cars then. Then it seems like maybe "s" and "h" came next.
C: How long after the laryngitis did the breathy trouble start?
P: Oh, it was the next week.
C: The laryngitis disappeared.
P: The laryngitis disappeared but the other didn't. And then it has just gotten progressively worse through the years, and it can be a great deal better one day and a great deal worse the next.
C: What kinds of things make it better or worse?
P: I think the things that make it better are almost complete relaxation. If I can get into a super relaxed position and get my voice into a real low level, then it tends to operate fairly well. Many people who might meet me in this circumstance might think that I don't really have any voice problem. Unfortunately, the world that we live in doesn't permit us necessarily to operate at this voice level.
C: Are you saying that the louder you talk . . .
P: The louder I talk the worse it gets.
C: Let's hear you count to five softly and then do it loudly. (Patient follows instructions.)
C: It does make a difference, doesn't it?
P: You were asking what makes it a little better, and I think anybody who runs into something like this makes compensatory adjustments. I know which words I'm going to have difficulty with to a large degree, so I can avoid those words. For instance, I know that I can't say the

word "hard" so I don't say it. I say "difficult." I started to say "words that I can say" and it was like a trigger; you can't say that, so I didn't say "say" I said pronounce.

C: Does time of day make it better or worse?

P: Yes. Usually it is easier early in the morning and it gets, depending on what I do during the day, progressively worse.

C: If you should go on vacation or be involved in some other release from work, will it be better?

P: To a degree. Very early on the degree might have been greater when, say, I went to the lake or something and just did nothing but lay on a beach or go fishing. The degree that it gets any better is less now than it was very early.

C: Let's go back to the beginning of this voice disorder. I wish you would think about the answer to this question very carefully. Before or during the time that you had this laryngitis and developed the voice disorder, were you under any unusual stress different from what might have been under usual life circumstances?

P: I'm not giving you a quick answer, because I have thought about this a lot, because the question has been asked a lot. The only thing that I can remember as being unusual is, I knew for six months in advance of the voice trouble that I was being considered for a promotion. I know that I was pushing, because I wanted it, and the weekend that the voice disorder came on was when I got the promotion.

C: Were you looking forward to the promotion?

P: Yes, I wanted the promotion. I was not looking forward, and I have to say this in all honesty, to the prospects of having to work very closely with the owner of the company that I would be working directly with. He was a very abrasive, intimidating individual, and I knew I was going to have to work with him if I got the promotion. I'll be as honest as I can be; I am sure that gave me some apprehension, because he was a very intimidating individual.

C: Well, you've left that company since.

P: Yes, that company went out of business.

C: How long were you working for this individual before that happened?

P: Three years.

C: And during that time your voice disorder got gradually worse.

P: Yes.

C: Did the relationship between you and this man work out to be as threatening as you thought it would be?

P: No.

C: Was it as traumatic as you had anticipated?

P: No, it wasn't.

C: And so here you are another three years after parting company with this individual still with the voice disorder.

P: Right.

C: We want to be careful not to assign effects to erroneous causes.

P: Oh, I understand.

C: Two things that happened in close proximity don't necessarily mean that they are cause and effect. Did any of the psychologists or psychiatrists you had consulted attach any importance to the anticipation that you had about the promotion as it might relate to the voice disorder?

P: Not any major importance. They didn't really think there was any direct relation there.

C: And as far as you know there were no other emotionally upsetting family or business problems.

P: Not at that point. There have been since then, but not at the outset.

C: And stresses that have happened since. Have they worsened your voice?

P: Well, I don't know whether they worsened my voice or whether it would have gotten worse anyhow. There has been a fairly progressive deterioration through the years. There probably has not been any deterioration this year. Maybe the last two years it has been fairly stable.

C: How would you honestly assess the effects of the voice on your professional, domestic, and social life?

P: I don't want to use the word devastating, because that seems to be a little too much, but it has had a very dramatic effect.

C: In what way.

P: For instance, I'll talk about just little things. When I was coming over here today on the bus there was a gentleman sitting in the seat beside me. I would normally be very eager to strike up a conversation with him, but I am very reticent to do that because it is going to be embarrassing, so as a result I don't seek out people. I avoid saying anything just in day to day conversation; when you go to a restaurant and something is amusing and you want to tell somebody about it, I don't. I don't participate.

C: Why is that?

P: Because the words don't happen. The words don't come out, and it's embarrassing.

C: Have you had abnormal reactions from other people?

P: Not generally. People normally don't have anything to say about it. That is on a very basic level. On a professional level, it does affect me, particularly with new customers. I will avoid going to see people whom I should go see, customers or potential customers. Even if there were no voice problem there would be a certain amount of stress involved in going to see these people anyhow due to the nature of their business, the size of their business, the nature of the individual, or whatever. Just recently I was being considered for a promotion in my company, and my boss, quite candidly, said that I would not get it as a result of the speech disorder. He told me that as a friend as much as anything else, because the particular position would involve a great deal of sales training, which is getting in front of a group and teaching them about machinery, which I am good at. I'm as good as anybody I have ever seen at sales training, at taking a group of people and keeping them interested in what they are learning as they sit there an hour or two hours. I can do that, and I can do it well, but I can't do it under the circumstances that I am working with now. So, instead of looking for opportunities to do that, I look for ways to avoid it. In social situations if I'm at a party or something, rather than seeking out people to talk to I try to get into a corner or get where I can talk with just somebody that I know rather than getting into a threatening situation.

C: Has the total effect of the voice made you periodically or chronically depressed?

P: Periodically, yes. I would be the first to admit that.

C: How bad is it?

P: Here again, sometimes it is worse than others. The last two and a half years have added to my voice problem. I went into business, which failed. My wife became seriously ill. So, in answer to your question, do I ever get depressed, yes I do but I really make an effort not to. As a matter of fact the people in my office, the people that I talk with daily over the telephone, they say, "Golly, I've never known anyone who stays up like you do. How do you do that? You just always seem to have something nice to say." I really work at doing that because I don't want to be the other way.

C: What therapies have been tried from the very beginning to help the voice.

P: At the very beginning I went to the regular doctor, and he said I had an inflammation and then gave me penicillin, or something, which did nothing. Then I went to an ENT specialist, and he tried a couple of medicines on me, I don't remember what they were, and then he said maybe you need to try speech therapy. So I went to the Speech and Hearing Center for nine months.

C: Any benefit?

P: None. Then several months after that I went back to the ENT doctor, and he didn't really know what to do. Then I went to a regular GP, and immediately, he said "I think this is something that has an emotional base," so he set up an appointment for me to see a psychiatrist. I said, "that's great. I'll go see a psychiatrist." So I went to see a psychiatrist for about six months, and he said one day, "Mr.——, we can keep doing this, but I don't think I'm doing you any good, and I don't think there is any evidence of a hysterical reaction, or hysterical conversion. There is just nothing that leads me to believe that so I really don't think we ought to continue." So I didn't do anything there again for a bit. I went to another throat specialist, did that for several months. I ended up at another GP, and he said, "I think you ought to try hypnosis." I said, "O.K. I'm open. I'll do it." So he said, "all right let's do that." He was trained in hypnosis. I did that for about three months. He said, "it just doesn't seem to be doing any good and I don't understand it. I thought that it would." Another doctor referred me to a second speech pathologist. She is the one that first used the word "spastic dysphonia." She said, "there is really nothing that you can do for spastic dysphonia other than speech therapy, and there is a psychologist here who specializes in this with hypnotherapy, and I want you to go see him." I said "all right, I've been through it once, but maybe I wasn't at the right place." I went to the hypnotherapist there and was there once a week for about a month, and it just didn't do anything even though my speech was a little better under hypnosis. I can do that to myself just by relaxing, so they weren't really doing anything. I went back to the ENT doctor and he said the only thing he could do was refer me for speech therapy. I had already been through it once but thought maybe I just didn't have the right person, so I went back into speech therapy for little over a year, and at the end of about a year she helped to a degree. I think she would help anybody with speech to a degree, and she did work with me on breath control and relaxation techniques and some of the compensatory techniques. For instance, like, if you can avoid attacking a word, just to roll through a word. If I were to say "trouble" then it is difficult if I just attack that word "trouble," but if I'm talking to you about "somebody-in-trouble" then it rolls right on in there. So she helped me to that degree.

C: So the learning how to attack the words helped somewhat, but it didn't really make. . .

P: No. Then another doctor said "there is a psychologist who has treated spastic dysphonia patients. I spoke with her and she thinks she can help you with therapy." I'm off again. That was last year. I had begun to get a little bit of information that this thing may have something to do with neurology or neurologic condition.

C: Before you get onto that, you had some more psychotherapy with the psychologist. Did it benefit?

P: No. It didn't help at all.

C: How long did that go on?

P: That went on for almost a year.

C: Then you started. . .

P: Then I went to a neurologist just about when I started going to that psychologist. He was very honest. He gave me a neurologic exam. He said, "I just did not see any evidence of a neurologic condition, but I will if you are interested in doing this, be happy to prescribe some medicines that are used to treat certain movement disorders, which might be of some benefit. If they do any good that is great. If they don't do any good, then we will stop and try something else."

C: There were several different kinds?

P: There were about six.

C: And after that. . .

P: And after that I haven't really been doing anything, because I really didn't know what to do. Then, about six months ago I went back to therapy a little bit, we used a voice masker, the Edinburgh Voice Masker, and that had a little positive effect when I first put it on and then after I used it for just a few minutes the effect diminished but I felt like maybe if I wear that enough that will help, so I ordered the Edinburgh Voice Masker. When I did that I got on somebody's mailing list for stuttering. I got a newsletter from —— University, the stuttering center. So, I wrote, and they wrote back and said there is really nothing we can suggest other than speech therapy and I am sure there is a very good speech pathologist in your area if you'll get in touch with somebody." Then, you wrote me and here I am.

C: Did the university people talk to you on the telephone?

P: No.

C: I wonder if they didn't think you had the other kind of spastic dysphonia.

P: I would imagine that they did.

C: You understand there are two kinds and the kind that is most familiar to people is the kind in which the vocal cords come together excessively.

P: The adductor.

C: They probably thought what you meant by "spastic dysphonia" in your letter was the adductor type, but you really meant abductor.

P: Well, I didn't know that until I talked to you.

* * *

SUMMARY

   1. "Abductor spastic dysphonia" is a term that describes abrupt breathy releases of air owing to sudden hyperabduction of the true vocal folds.

   2. Evidence indicates that these spasms can be due either to psychogenic (conversion reaction) or neurologic (essential tremor) causes, or it can be idiopathic.

   3. There is a propensity for the abductor spasms to occur most strongly during the production of unvoiced consonants, to a lesser extent during voiced consonants, and least of all during vowels.

   4. Like the adductor spastic dysphonias, onset of the disorder is gradual and often associated with psychologic stress.

REFERENCES

(All of the following references are suggested for additional reading on this disorder, about which the literature is limited.)

Aronson, A.E., Peterson, H.W., and Litin, E.M.: Psychiatric symptomatology in functional dysphonia and aphonia. J. Speech Hear. Disord., 31:115–127, 1966.

Aronson, A.E., Peterson, H.W., and Litin, E.M.: Voice symptomatology in functional dysphonia and aphonia. J. Speech Hear. Disord., 29:367–380, 1964.

Cannito, M.P., and Johnson, P.: Spastic dysphonia: A continuum disorder. J. Commun. Disord., 14:215–223, 1981.

Hartman, D.E., and Aronson, A.E.: Clinical investigations of intermittent breathy dysphonia. J. Speech Hear. Disord., 46:428–432, 1981.

Merson, R.M., and Ginsberg, A.P.: Spasmodic dysphonia: Abductor type. A clinical report of acoustic, aerodynamic and perceptual characteristics. Laryngoscope, 89:129–139, 1979.

Zwitman, D.H.: Bilateral cord dysfunction: Abductor type spastic dysphonia. J. Speech Hear. Disord., 44:373–378, 1979.

Chapter Nine

INTRODUCTION

ANATOMY AND PHYSIOLOGY OF THE
VELOPHARYNGEAL MECHANISM

ORGANIC AND PSYCHOGENIC HYPERNASALITY AND
NASAL AIR EMISSION

ORGANIC HYPONASALITY

MIXED NASALITY

CLINICAL EXAMINATION

Nasal Resonatory Disorders

For when we wish to emit voice or breath through the mouth only, which may happen in the pronunciation of the letters which I shall name explosives, we shut the passage of the nostrils, as with a valve.

—Amman, 1700

INTRODUCTION

The Velopharynx in Life

The isthmus between the oral and nasal cavities must be closed during swallowing and speech, or else food will be regurgitated out the nares, vowels will be excessively resonated in the nasal chambers, pressure consonants will lose their characteristic explosive and friction noises, and air will be audibly emitted through the nares. In Chapter 1 we noted that phonation was a phylogenetically recent acquisition among vertebrates and that the vital functions of the larynx were respiratory and protective of the airway. Much the same can be said about velopharyngeal function. The velopharyngeal port was not designed primarily as a means of coupling or uncoupling the oral and nasal cavities for speech. Rather, velopharyngeal closure exists primarily to:

1. Seal off the nasal from the oral cavities in order to isolate the oropharyngolaryngeal tract from atmospheric pressure during deglutition, producing a partial vacuum to facilitate compression of the food bolus by the tongue, cheeks, and pharynx, and thereby forcing it into the esophagus.
2. Open the eustachian tube during swallowing in order to ventilate the middle ear.

In only three phonemes of English, the nasal semivowels, is it permissible for the velopharyngeal valve to remain open, coupling the oral with the nasal cavities: /m/, /n/, and /ŋ/ (as in sing). The remainder of English phonemes are correctly produced with the velopharyngeal port closed, meaning all vowels and consonants. If the port is left open, voiced consonants will be excessively resonated in the nasal cavities, and intraoral air pressure for plosives, fricatives, and affricates will be reduced or absent. In an attempt to produce them, air escapes through the nose and results in a weak, nasally distorted production of the target sound. It should also be mentioned that a certain amount of nasal resonation of vowels is normal. The borderline between normal and pathologic hypernasality often is a matter of perceptual preference.

What must be remembered is that the nasal resonatory defect of hypernasality is not the only one produced by velopharyngeal insufficiency. Hypernasality is the primary one. Secondary or associated defects are excess nasal air flow, articulatory distortions owing to loss of intraoral air pressure stolen by the nasal air leak, compensatory articulatory and phonatory substitutions, many of which are nonphonemic, articulatory distortions due to dental and palatal defects, and even dysphonia from compensatory vocal abuse.

In medical and speech pathology practice, hypernasality and nasal air emission and hyponasality have similar implications as dysphonia from laryngeal disease. That is, they signify structural, neurologic, or psychiatric pathologic conditions and, therefore, are essential to medical differential diagnosis, and they have developmental, educational, social, psychologic, and occupational handicaps that require treatment. The following dialogue illustrates these many factors involved in velopharyngeal insufficiency.

*   *   *

"Have you ever given a deposition before?"

"No, this is my first."

"Let me explain that a deposition is an official transcript of testimony in place of your appearance in court. We are the attorneys for Miss Alquist, who is suing the surgeon who removed her tonsils and adenoids. She claims as a result of that surgery her speech was so impaired that she was placed on indefinite leave of absence without pay from her teaching position. She also claims that when she swallows, fluids leak out her nose. So, we are taking testimony from specialists who have independently investigated Miss Alquist's complaints. I understand you are the speech pathologist who evaluated Miss Alquist's speech, and that the plastic surgeon and otolaryngologist who also saw her will be following you. This is the official stenographer who will take down your testimony. You will have a chance to read the transcript and make corrections before it is put into final form. Some of the questions I will ask may seem oversimplified, but remember, this testimony will go before a jury of lay individuals who have no technical knowledge of the subject. You have already stated your full name and address. What is your occupation?"

"I am a speech pathologist."

"I notice you are addressed as 'doctor.' Are you a medical doctor?"

"No. I hold a Ph.D. in Speech Pathology."

"Are you licensed to practice Speech Pathology?"

"In this state there are no licensure laws for speech pathologists."

"Will you tell the court what a speech pathologist is and does?"

"We identify, describe, diagnose, and treat people who have disorders of communication, that is, voice, speech, and language disturbances from organic or psychiatric illnesses. Where I work, speech pathologists consult to physicians of all specialties."

"Thank you. Now, do you know the plaintiff, and if so on what occasion have you conferred with her?"

"I evaluated Miss Alquist's speech on May 21 of last year. That evaluation took approximately one and one-half hours."

"Are these the clinical notes that you wrote as a result of your evaluation?"

"Yes, they are."

"Are these the audiotape and videotape recordings you made of the patient during your evaluation?"

"Yes, they are."

"When you evaluate a patient's speech, Doctor, what exactly do you do?"

"I ask the patient to perform different tasks that will provide me with an adequate sample of the patient's speech. I usually tape record the speech for more detailed analysis later. I might also make certain laboratory tests, such as airflow and spectrographic, that is, acoustic recordings of the patient's speech."

"Based on your analysis of Miss Alquist's speech, would you say her speech was abnormal?"

"Yes, I would."

"In what way, specifically?"

"She had hypernasality and nasal emission."

"Would you please explain the meaning of these words for the court."

"Hypernasality refers to excess resonation of speech sounds within the nasal chambers because of partial or complete failure of the soft palate to close off the nasal from the oral cavities, or from incomplete closure of the hard palate."

"You mean like cleft palate?"

"Yes. But she did not have a cleft palate."

"Doctor, please point out on this chart the parts of the speech mechanism you are talking about."

"This is a side view of the head and neck. This plate of bone separates the oral from the nasal cavity. It is called the hard palate. This flap of tissue is called the soft palate. It can lift upward and backward to contact the back wall of the throat. When it does, it seals off the oral from the nasal cavity."

"And, what if it doesn't?"

"As I explained before, then speech will be abnormally resonated in the nasal cavities. I would add that consonants will be heard as weak or absent if the opening is very large. People would then have trouble understanding what the speaker was saying."

"We will return to what you found out about the plaintiff's speech mechanism, but at this point, I would like you to explain more fully the implications of Miss Alquist's speech defect."

"As I said, she was hypernasal and had nasal emission of the airstream as she spoke. If I may, I would like to play a videotape of the patient so that you can hear and see what I'm talking about. . . As you can hear from the tape, her speech has a noticeable and distracting nasal quality, and some of her words are difficult to understand. Also, you can see she has a tendency to narrow her nostrils and wrinkle her forehead on many consonant sounds. This is a kind of compensation people with palatal insufficiencies develop. It is an attempt to constrict the nostrils so that less air will pass out through them."

"How would this disorder interfere with the patient's everyday life?"

"A speech defect is a personal matter. Two people with defects of the same type and severity often react differently, depending upon their personality and the importance of speech in their daily lives."

"And, how would you characterize the effect of Miss Alquist's defect on her?"

"Based on the psychologic and social history portion of my examination, Miss Alquist was devastated by her speech disorder."

"What is your evidence for that statement?"

"She broke down several times during the examination, especially during discussions of the effects of her disorder on her professional activities. She said her speech had always been important to her; that she used her speech to favorable advantage in the classroom, that she knew she had a good voice, would often dramatize segments of the curriculum through plays and storytelling, and that she taught singing. Outside of the classroom, she was active in teachers' organizations and was known as a good public speaker and debater."

"Has this changed as a result of her disorder?"

"It has, according to what she told me, turned her life around completely. Her students, she said, became inattentive. She began to notice derisive facial expressions of students and colleagues as she would speak. Some of the children made fun of her. Speaking tired her out—she had to exert much more effort to make herself understood."

"Has her speech disorder affected her in any other ways?"

"According to Miss Alquist, she was called into the principal's office and told that she would have to take a leave of absence until something was done about her speech. That was a year ago. She has not worked since. She says she has become withdrawn, has a fear of using the telephone, and has been seeing a psychiatrist for depression."

"Have any attempts been made to correct, treat, or rehabilitate her speech?"

"Not to my knowledge. No one recommended speech therapy in her locality."

"Doctor, let's get back to the physical examination of the plaintiff. What, in your opinion, was the reason she developed this disorder at this time in life? Why would anyone whose speech had been not only normal, but who was in fact a skilled speaker, suddenly acquire this kind of defect?"

"I would feel more comfortable if you asked the plastic surgeon and otolaryngologist that question, although I think we agree, having discussed the case in private, on the cause of the disorder."

"Nonetheless, the court is interested in your opinion; as an expert witness in your field, you are justified in commenting on the physical aspects of the case."

"Well, we have photographs of the patient's mouth and x-ray motion pictures of her soft palate during speech. These lateral motion picture studies clearly show that, although the soft palate is able to lift up, it is too short to make closure contact against the back wall of the throat; it elevates, but there is a considerable gap left between it and the posterior pharyngeal wall. During our examination, although the hard and soft palate looked all right when the patient opened her mouth, when we explored her hard palate we felt a notch at the back where the soft and hard palate join. This notch is called a submucous cleft. We also noticed, and we almost missed this because it was so subtle, that the little pendulum of tissue that hangs down from the middle of the soft palate, the uvula, was almost invisibly split; you could separate it with a tongue depressor, but most of the time the two halves stuck together so that it looked like solid tissue. You can see the split on this photograph."

"Would you give us the implications of all this?"

"We think Miss Alquist has had a lifelong condition of submucous cleft palate, a cleft in the bone and muscular tissue that is hidden under the mucosal tissue. In her case a speech disorder was not evident because she was able to attain adequate closure by contacting her soft palate against her adenoids. In other words, the adenoids were serving as an anatomic structure on the back wall of the throat and were helping to effect complete closure; when they were removed, the space created was too great for her soft palate to bridge. The adenoid removal unmasked the submucous cleft."

"Is this condition remediable?"

"A prosthetic device called a palatal lift would partially close the gap. More permanent would be a surgical procedure, a pharyngeal flap operation, in which a flap of tissue raised from the pharyngeal wall is sutured to the soft palate, or a sphincter pharyngoplasty."

"We want to thank you for your testimony. If we have any further questions, we'll arrange another appointment through your secretary."

*   *   *

Although hypernasality and nasal emission are only aesthetically displeasing when mild, when excessive, they diminish or even destroy intelligibility, producing serious occupational and psychologic disturbances. When hard palate or velopharyngeal port defects are present in infancy or eary childhood, they impede speech and language development and negatively influence the self-concept. Even when they occur for the first time in adulthood, as in the case just presented, they can produce profound psychologic and occupational maladjustments. One might ask, "Which would be more devastating—aphonia (whispered speech) from laryngeal disease or severe hypernasality and nasal emission from velopharyngeal or palatal insufficiencies?" Our first impulse might be to answer that the aphonia would have more profound consequences. In actual fact, loss of normal velopharyngeal closure can be much more serious, because without adequate intraoral pressure, most consonants lose their identity. This fact is amply illustrated in isolated paralyses of the soft palate; respiration, phonation, and articulation are normal, yet, speech is unintelligible solely on the basis of diminished intraoral pressure.

Classification and Definition of Nasal Resonatory Disorders

Nasal resonatory disorders can be classified into three main auditory-perceptual types.

1. *Hypernasality and nasal air emission*
   a. *Hypernasality.* Synonyms are *rhinolalia aperta, hyper-rhinolalia,* and *open nasality.* Defined as excess resonance of vowels and voiced consonants within the nasal cavities. The anatomic-physiologic basis is open coupling between the oral and nasal cavities due to incomplete closure of the hard palate and/or velopharyngeal sphincter.
   b. *Nasal air emission.* Defined as abnormal flow of air from the nares during the production of high-pressure consonants, it is measurable biophysically via airflow (aerodynamic) techniques. It is heard as friction noise accompanying or replacing the target consonant and may have a "gurgly" quality if there is coexisting nasal congestion. It is sometimes referred to as a *nasal snort.*
   c. *Nasal and/or facial grimacing.* Defined as occlusion of the nares by contracting the alae of the nose, with associated wrinkling of the forehead, during consonant production, a compensatory action in an attempt to impede the nasal flow of air.

2. *Hyponasality*
   Synonyms are *denasality, rhinolalia clausa,* and *closed nasality.* Defined as diminution or absence of normal nasal resonance of the nasal semivowels /m/, /n/, /ŋ/ and loss of normal assimilation nasality. Its physical basis is overclosure of the portal or obstruction between the oral and nasal cavities owing to space-occupying lesions within the nasopharynx or nasal cavities. Two subtypes are recognized.
   a. *Rhinolalia clausa, posterior.* A type of closed nasality in which the nasal semivowels lose their normal resonance because of an obstruction in the *posterior region* of the nasal cavities or the nasopharynx. The nasal phonemes /m/, /n/, and /ŋ/ are heard as oral stops /b/, /d/, and /g/.

   b. *Rhinolalia clausa, anterior.* A type of closed nasality in which all the vowels and nasals are produced with a hollow-sounding resonance owing to obstruction in the anterior region of the nasal cavities. It is also called *cul-de-sac* resonation.

3. *Mixed nasality*

   A synonym is *rhinolalia mixta.* Defined as simultaneous velopharyngeal insufficiency and nasal obstruction resulting in a hollow resonation of all vowels and voiced consonants.

Etiology of Nasal Resonatory Disorders

The etiologies of nasal resonatory disorders are outlined in Table 9–1. Their causes can be subdivided into *organic* and *psychogenic.* Organic causes of *hypernasality* and *nasal emission* are *anatomic defects,* such as clefts of the hard and soft palate, and *neurologic disease* producing paralysis of the velopharyngeal musculature. Psychogenic causes of hypernasality and nasal emission are *conversion reaction, immature personality development, poor motivation,* and *imitation.* Hypernasality is common in persons with severe, congenital sensorineural *hearing loss* owing to poor auditory feedback.

   Causes of *hyponasality* are primarily organic: *Space-occupying lesions,* such as tumors, inflammations, nasal polyps, and hypertrophied adenoid tissue, and *structural deformities,* such as deviated nasal septum.

   Mixed nasality is caused by coexisting velopharyngeal insufficiency and obstruction of the nasal passageways.

Table 9–1   Etiology of Nasal Resonatory Disorders

Hypernasality and nasal emission
  Organic
    Anatomic
      Overt cleft palate with or without cleft lip
      Submucous cleft palate
      Congenitally short soft palate or large nasopharynx
      Traumatic structural damage
    Neurologic (dysarthria)
      Lower motor neuron (flaccid)
      Unilateral upper motor neuron ("flaccid")
      Bilateral upper motor neuron (spastic)
      Mixed lower-upper motor neuron (flaccid-spastic)
      Hyperkinetic (dystonic-choreic)
  Psychogenic
    Conversion reaction
    Immature personality
    Poor motivation
    Imitative
Hyponasality
  Organic
    Hypertrophied adenoids
    Tumors
    Inflammations
    Postsurgical repair
    Patulous eustachian tube
    Nasal deformity
Mixed nasality
  Combinations of organic etiologies of hypernasality and hyponasality.

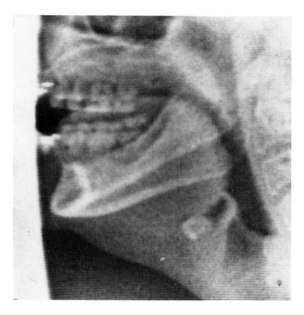

Figure 9–1 Lateral radiograph showing the hard and soft palate.

ANATOMY AND PHYSIOLOGY OF THE VELOPHARYNGEAL MECHANISM

Surface Anatomy

The anatomy that pertains to normal and abnormal nasal resonatory functions consists of the oral, nasal, and pharyngeal cavities bounded by muscles and their bony attachments. The x-ray in Figure 9–1 illustrates the separation of the oral from the nasal chambers by the bony *hard palate*. Suspended from its posterior edge is the resting *soft palate,* or *velum*.

Because a lateral view of the velopharyngeal port only affords a two-dimensional appreciation of this valve, vertical and anteroposterior views are needed, shown in Figure 9–2. The port is bounded anteriorly by the velum, and laterally and posteriorly by the lateral and posterior pharyngeal walls. Its eliptical-shaped opening hints at its pattern of closure, which is either sphincteric, similar to a drawstring or camera aperture, or eliptical.

Another view of the hard and soft palate is through the open mouth, although this approach affords limited information in comparison with x-rays. Figure 9–3 shows the soft palate with its two symmetric arches. Suspended from its midline is the *uvula*. Running down from the arches on either side of the soft palate are two folds of tissue. The one closer to the front of the mouth is the *anterior pillar of the fauces* and the one toward the rear is the *posterior pillar of the fauces*. Nestled between them are the *palatine tonsils*.

The roof of the mouth is bordered by the upper dental arch and is covered by ridged mucosal tissue under which lies a thick periosteal tissue covering. The anterior two thirds of the roof consists of the hard palate, and the posterior one third, the soft palate. It is difficult to see where one ends and the other begins, but their junction is easy to feel by running the index finger along the midline of the hard palate from front to back until the finger sinks into soft tissue marking the border between the hard and soft palate.

Bones

The velopharyngeal musculature is suspended from three bones: The hard palate, the sphenoid bone, and the temporal bone.

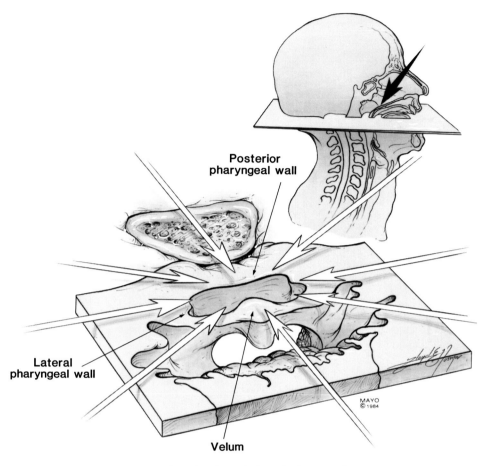

Posterior pharyngeal wall

Lateral pharyngeal wall

Velum

Figure 9–2   Three dimensional view of section through the velopharyngeal port.

HARD PALATE

The hard palate is formed by the *palatine processes of the maxillae* and the *horizontal plates of the palatine bones* (Fig. 9–4). It is covered by a dense *periosteum* surfaced by *mucous membrane*. When stripped to the bone, the hard palate reveals that it is divided by sutures. The *palatomaxillary suture* divides the more anterior, larger palatine process of the maxilla from the smaller, more posterior horizontal plate of the palatine bone. Its posterior margin serves as the attachment of the soft palate. At its midline is a sharp spicule of bone called the *posterior nasal spine*.

The two halves of the palatine processes of the maxilla are joined in the midline at the *intermaxillary suture*. The two halves of the horizontal plates of the palatine bone are joined in the midline at the *interpalatine suture*. The opening in the anterior hard palate is the *incisive fossa* and in the lateral portions of the palatine bone, the *greater palatine foramina*. Medial and posterior to these are the *lesser palatine foramina*.

SPHENOID BONE

The sphenoid bone lies at the base of the skull in front of the temporal bones and the basilar part of the occipital bone (Fig. 9–5). The *lateral pterygoid plate* and especially the *medial pterygoid plate* with its *pterygoid hamulus* are portions of the sphenoid bone directly concerned with the soft palate musculature.

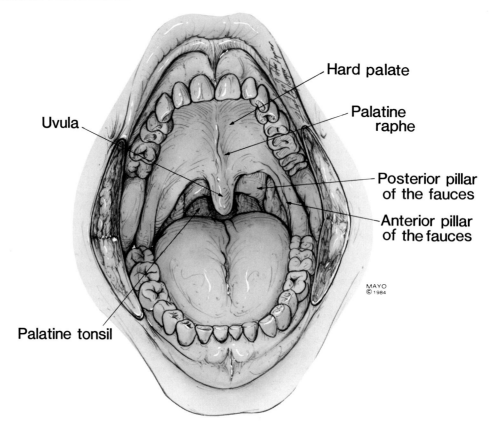

Figure 9–3   The soft palate and surrounding structures as seen on peroral examination.

TEMPORAL BONE

The temporal bones form the sides and base of the skull, the latter of which is a point of attachment for the soft palate musculature.

Blood Supply

The hard and soft palate are supplied by the *greater palatine artery*. It gives off *lesser palatine arteries* that supply the soft palate and tonsils. The greater palatine artery emerges on the oral surface of the palate through the greater palatine foramina, runs forward in a groove near the alveolar border of the hard palate through the incisive canal, and, linking up with the *sphenopalatine artery,* is distributed to the gums, palatine glands, and mucous membrane of the roof of the mouth.

Muscles

LEVATOR VELI PALATINI

This muscle arises from the *base of the skull* anterior to the carotid canal and descends anteromedially along the posteroinferior border of the eustachian tube. It inserts into the *palatine aponeurosis* of the middle third of the soft palate. Its fibers fan out and interweave with its mate of the opposite side and with the remaining muscles of the soft palate.

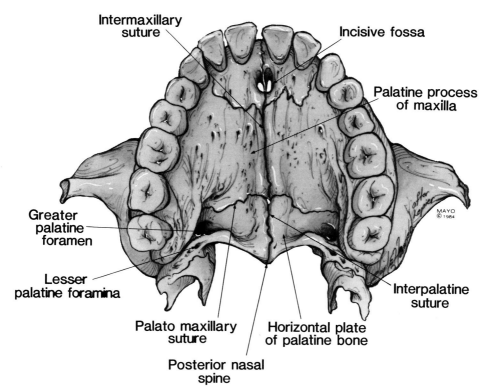

Figure 9–4   The hard palate. Inferior view.

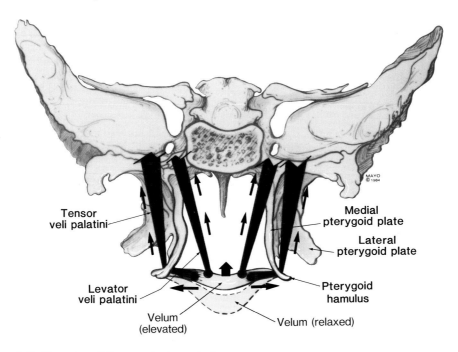

Figure 9–5   The sphenoid bone and schematic drawing of levator and tensor veli palatini muscles. Posterior view.

TENSOR VELI PALATINI

This flat, triangular-shaped muscle originates from the *base of the skull* between the spine of the sphenoid bone, the root of the *pterygoid process,* and the *eustachian tube.* The muscle ends in a tendon that makes a right-angle turn around the *pterygoid hamulus* and then runs horizontally into the *palatine aponeurosis* along with the other muscles of the soft palate.

PALATOGLOSSUS

The palatoglossus forms the *anterior pillars of the fauces.* It is a small, thin muscle that arises from the *palatine aponeurosis* and descends to insert into the *lateral border of the tongue,* infiltrating its transverse muscle fibers.

PALATOPHARYNGEUS

This muscle forms the *posterior pillars of the fauces.* It is larger than the palatoglossus muscle. It originates from the *back and side walls of the pharynx* and from the *thyroid cartilage* and ascends to the *posterior and lateral portions of the soft palate.* Some of its fibers insert into the tip of the medial cartilagenous wall of the eustachian tube and are considered by some anatomists to comprise a separate muscle, the *salpingopharyngeus.*

CONSTRICTOR PHARYNGIS SUPERIOR

The superior pharyngeal constrictor forms the lateral and posterior walls of the velopharyngeal port. It attaches to the *pterygoid process,* the *pterygomandibular raphé,* the *mandible,* and the *tongue.* Its most cranial portion, which attaches to the *medial pterygoid plate* and to the *pterygoid hamulus,* is most directly active in velopharyngeal closure.

MUSCULUS UVULAE

The paired uvulae muscle arises from the *posterior nasal spine* of the hard palate and the palatine *aponeurosis* and inserts into the *uvula.*

Velopharyngeal Biomechanics

Velopharyngeal *closure* is produced by contracting the *levator veli palatini, tensor veli palatini,* and *superior pharyngeal constrictor* muscles, actions schematized in Figure 9–5. The levator is the most important muscle of velopharyngeal closure during speech. It elevates the midportion of the soft palate in a superior-posterior direction. The tensor does not contribute directly to velar elevation and retraction during speech, although upon being pulled taut it may raise the velum to the level of the hard palate. It is alleged that it also depresses the anterior velum opening the eustachean tube during swallowing. The *superior pharyngeal constrictor* narrows the port further by moving its walls medially and anteriorly.

> Contraction of the superior pharyngeal constrictor sometimes produces a slight bulge or transverse fold in the posterior pharyngeal wall, called Passavant's ridge, first described in 1869 by Passavant as a discrete bar or protuberance that forms on the posterior pharyngeal wall during speech only. This prominence occurs in many normal speakers, in whom it may be of little importance, and in a much higher number of those who have velopharyngeal incompetence with and without cleft palate in whom it probably contributes toward closure.

Velopharyngeal *opening* is not completely passive and due only to muscular relaxation and gravity. It is not known for sure, but the soft palate may have an active antagonist, the palatoglossus, which pulls the soft palate downward and forward.

Although contraction of the *musculus uvulae* shortens the uvula, it is doubtful that this muscle seriously contributes to swallowing or speech, because many normal people are missing the uvula for congenital or surgical reasons without any untoward effects. However, congenital deficiency of the bulk of this muscle may be responsible for minor velopharyngeal insufficiency.

VIDEOFLUOROSCOPIC STUDIES

Static x-ray tomograms or radiographs cannot do justice to the ceaseless undulations of the soft palate as it opens and closes the port during contextual speech that alternates between nasal and non-nasal phonemes. But such photographs can allow for the beginning of understanding of the closure mechanism. In Figure 9–6a an x-ray tomogram of a normal person just beginning to produce the vowel /i/, the soft palate is beginning to rise. In Figure 9–6b the soft palate is elevated and retracted against the posterior pharyngeal wall. A basal view of this action shows the sphincteric configuration of this closure. From their multiview radiographic studies, Skolnick and colleagues (1969, 1970, 1973) have immeasurably enriched our understanding of velopharyngeal closure and concluded:

> We believe that concepts which view velopharyngeal closure as resulting from a combination of velar (flap valve) and lateral pharyngeal wall movement are only partially correct . . . It appears that the mechanism . . . is really a sphincteric one . . . poorly appreciated because of the difficulty in visualizing the velopharyngeal portal in the manner necessary to show the sphincteric movements.

Rather than conceptualizing soft palate and lateral and posterior pharyngeal wall movements as separate during closure, Skolnick showed radiographically that *all move as a single, functional unit,* and *there is no precise demarcation between the lateral aspects of the velum and the beginnings of the pharyngeal wall*. Although a lateral view is useful for demonstrating the vertical extent of the pharyngeal contribution to the sphincter, it is the basal view that permits a view of the port "en face" and gives us a true appreciation for the sphincteric concept of velopharyngeal closure.

ELECTROMYOGRAPHIC STUDIES

Another approach to the study of normal velopharyngeal closure is by electromyography (EMG). Studies do not fully agree on the extent to which each of the velopharyngeal muscles participate during closure (Bell-Berti, 1976; Benguerel et al., 1977; Cooper, 1965; Li and Lundervold, 1958; Lubker, 1968; Lubker and Curtis, 1966; Seaver, 1979). A representative study of closure in normal subjects was done by Fritzell (1969), who placed EMG electrodes in the velopharyngeal musculature and measured their potentials during speech. A sample of recordings from different muscles is shown in Figure 9–7. From his study he found:

1. The *levator veli palatini* was continuously active during speech.
   a. Activity began before onset of sound.
   b. Activity ceased before termination of phonation.

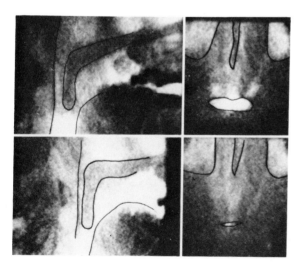

Figure 9–6 Videofluoroscopic frames showing lateral and base views of normal velopharyngeal closure. *From* Skolnick, M. L.: Videofluoroscopic examination of the velopharyngeal portal during phonation in lateral and base projections. Cleft Palate J., 7:803–816, 1970.

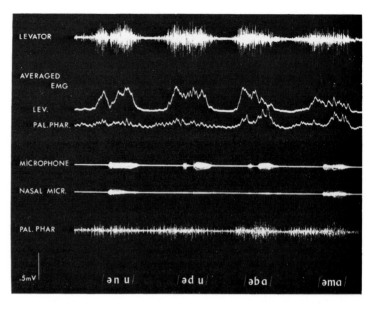

Figure 9–7 Electromyographic recording of the levator veli palatini and palatopharyngeus muscles during speech. *From* Fritzell, B.: The Velopharyngeal muscles in speech. Acta Otolaryngol, [Supp], 250: 1969, p. 13.

c. Degree of activity fluctuated during speech.

d. Little or no activity occurred during nasal semivowels.

2. The *tensor veli palatini* behaved with considerable intersubject variability and in many cases with little or no activity.

3. *Superior pharyngeal constrictor* muscle activity was similar to levator, i.e., active during all except the nasal sounds.

4. The *palatoglossus* produced bursts of activity preceding nasal semivowels but was weak or inactive for oral sounds. However, there is conflicting opinion on the validity of this finding.

5. The *palatopharyngeus* varied considerably among subjects; it always showed some activity but of low intensity.

Fritzell drew the following conclusions from his study:

1. The *levator* is the most important muscle of closure during speech.

2. The *tensor* is nearly silent and has no typical relationship to speech.

3. The *superior constrictor* has patterns similar to the levator.

4. The *palatoglossus* actively pulls down the velum; lowering is not due only to gravity.

5. The *palatopharyngeus* has little activity during speech.

6. A high positive correlation (0.76) exists between extent of EMG levator activity and extent of velar displacement.

7. Velar movement begins within 40 msec. after onset of EMG levator activity and speech follows about 300 msec. later, varying widely, depending upon the initial phoneme and speaking situation.

NASAL AIRFLOW STUDIES

The extent of nasal airflow can be measured by an instrument known as the heated pneumotachograph, which consists of a flowmeter and a differential pressure transducer. Airflow from the nose passes across a heated wire mesh screen. The resulting pressure drop is linearly related to the volume rate of airflow and is converted by a pressure transducer into an electrical voltage that is recorded on a direct writing instrument.

Pressure flow studies summarized by Warren (1964) have yielded the following important data:

1. Normal intraoral pressure for pressure consonants is between 3 and 7 cm H_2O.
2. Normal consonant intraoral pressure cannot be maintained if the velopharyngeal portal is open more than 0.02 cm^2 (Fig. 9–8).
3. Audible nasal emission and hypernasality occur when openings are between 0.1 and 0.2 cm^2.
4. Influencing the amount of nasal airflow are extent of oral airway opening, amount of nasal airway obstruction, and volume of the oral cavity.
5. Normal speakers have imperceptibly small amounts of nasal airflow during production of non-nasal phonemes.
6. Speakers vary in the duration of portal opening during production of nasal phonemes.

ACOUSTIC STUDIES

Hypernasality arises from coupling between the oral and nasal cavities. Acoustic studies of hypernasalized vowels produced by normal speakers show the following spectral distortions (Dickson, 1962; House and Stevens, 1956; Peterson and Barney, 1952; Smith, 1951):

1. Reduced intensity of the first vowel formant.
2. One or more loci of antiresonance, that is, a sharp drop in the intensity of a portion of the spectrum.
3. Extra resonances, contributed by the nasal cavities, that is, reinforced harmonics at frequencies at which energy is not normally expected.
4. A shift in the center frequencies of the formants.

ORGANIC AND PSYCHOGENIC HYPERNASALITY AND NASAL AIR EMISSION

Cleft Lip and Palate

Clefts of the hard and soft palate are the most serious of all causes of hypernasality and nasal emission. Because full coverage of this subject is not possible here, we especially recommend the selected readings at the end of this chapter.

DEFINITION AND CLASSIFICATION

Cleft lip and palate represent a failure of the lip and hard and soft palate segments to join during those stages of embryonic development when closure should have occurred. An infant with cleft palate at birth has a direct communication between the oral and nasal cavities. The airstream during speech passes, unchecked, into the nasal cavities and out of the nares. The speech effects are: (1) Hypernasality of vowels; (2) nasal emission of the airstream; and (3) weak pressure consonants due to loss of intraoral pressure. Communication may be further compromised by delayed articulatory and language development, hearing loss, and reactive psychologic and educational disturbances.

Several classifications of cleft lip and palate have been proposed. The most comprehensive is the American Cleft Palate Association's classification found in Table 9–2.

EMBRYOLOGY

The embryologic sequence of face and palate development is illustrated in Figure 9–9 and is described as follows:

1. *Face*
    a. *Fourth week (early): facial primordia* begin to appear surrounding the primitive mouth or *stomodeum.*
        (1) *Frontonasal prominence.* Forms the upper boundary of the stomodeum. Originates from proliferation of mesenchyme ventral to the brain.

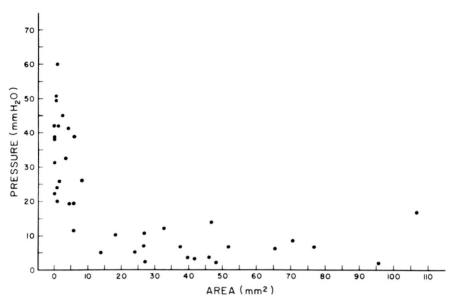

Figure 9–8 Relationship between velopharyngeal orifice size and intraoral pressure during consonant productions. *From* Warren, D. W.: Velopharyngeal orifice size and upper pharyngeal pressure-flow patterns in normal speech. Plast. Reconstr. Surg., 33:148–162, 1964.

Table 9–2 American Cleft Palate Associations's Classification of Cleft Lip and Palate

Clefts of prepalate		
Cleft lip	Unilateral	Right, left
		Extent in thirds
	Bilateral	Right, left
		Extent in thirds
	Median	Extent in thirds
	Prolabium	Small, medium, large
	Congenital scar	Right, left, median
		Extent in thirds
Cleft of alveolar process	Unilateral	Right, left
		Extent in thirds
	Bilateral	Right, left
		Extent in thirds
	Median	Extent in thirds
		Submucous right, left, median
Cleft of prepalate	Any combination of foregoing types	
	Prepalate protusion	
	Prepalate rotation	
	Prepalate arrest (median cleft)	
Clefts of palate		
Cleft soft palate	Extent	Posteroanterior in thirds
		Width (maximum in mm.)
	Palatal shortness	None, slight, moderate, marked
	Submucous cleft	Extent in thirds
Cleft hard palate	Extent	Posteroanterior in thirds
		Width (maximum in mm.)
	Vomer attachment	Right, left, absent
	Submucous cleft	Extent in thirds
Cleft of soft and hard palate		
Clefts of prepalate and palate	Any combination of clefts described under clefts of prepalate and clefts of palate.	

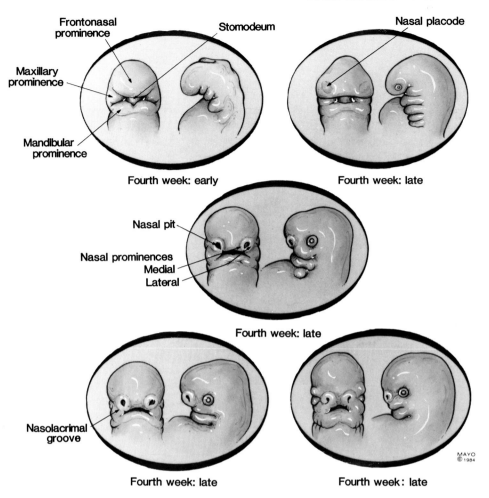

Figure 9–9a   Embryonic and fetal development of the face and palate.

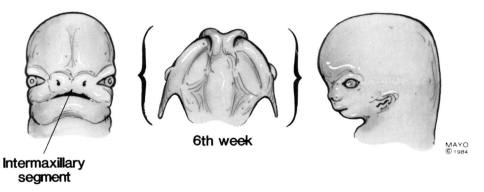

Figure 9–9b   Cont'd

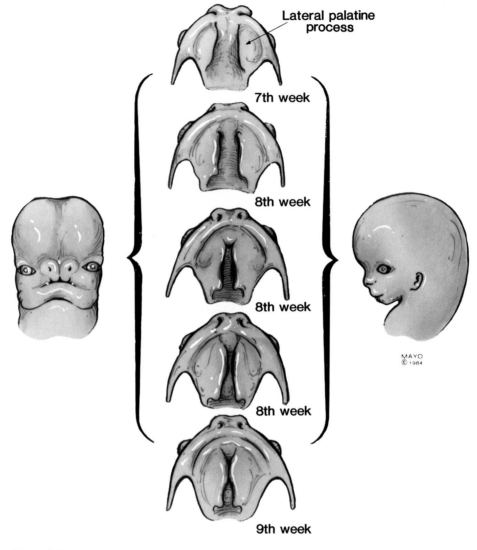

Lateral palatine process

7th week

8th week

8th week

8th week

9th week

MAYO
© 1984

Figure 9–9c

Cont'd

(2) *Maxillary prominences*. Form the lateral boundaries of the stomodeum. Originate from first branchial arch.

(3) *Mandibular prominences*. Form lower boundary of stomodeum. Originate from first branchial arch.

(4) *Mandibular prominences*. Form lower boundary of stomodeum. Originate from first branchial arch.

b. *Fourth week (late)*

(1) *Nasal placodes*. Bilateral oval-shaped thickenings develop from surface ectoderm in lower part of each frontonasal prominence.

(2) *Medial and lateral nasal prominences*. Horseshoe-shaped prominences at margins of nasal placodes develop from mesenchyme.

(3) *Nasal pits*. Depressions in the nasal placodes.

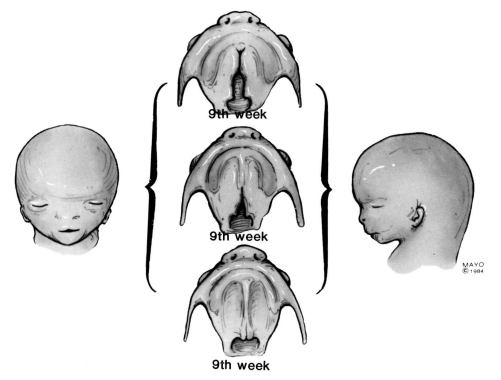

9th week

9th week

9th week

MAYO
© 1984

Figure 9–9d

    (4) *Maxillary prominences*. Grow toward each other and toward medial nasal promi-
        nences.
    (5) *Nasolacrimal groove*. Cleft or furrow separating lateral nasal prominence from
        maxillary prominences.
c. *Sixth and seventh weeks*
    (1) *Intermaxillary segment of upper jaw*. Formed by merging of medial nasal
        prominences. This segment gives rise to:
        (a) Philtrum; the middle portion of upper lip
        (b) Middle portion of upper jaw and gum
        (c) Primary palate
    (2) *Maxillary prominences*. Formed by lateral parts of upper lip, upper jaw, and
        secondary palate. Merge laterally with mandibular prominences reducing size of
        mouth.
    (3) *Primitive lips and cheeks*. Invaded by second branchial arch mesenchyme, giving
        rise to facial muscles.
    (4) *Frontonasal prominence*. Forms forehead and dorsum and apex of nose. Sides of
        nose (alae) derive from lateral nasal prominences.
    (5) *Final development of face*
        (a) Nose changes from flat to more mature form
        (b) Mandible more prominent
        (c) Forehead more prominent
        (d) Eyes move medially
        (e) Ears rise

2. Palate

The palate develops from two parts; the *primary* and *secondary palate,* between the fifth and the 12th week.

    a. *Fifth week (late)*

        (1) *Primary palate (median palatine process).* From innermost part of intermaxillary segment of upper jaw. Formed by merging of medial nasal prominences. Forms a wedge-shaped mass of mesoderm between maxillary prominences and developing upper jaw.

        (2) *Secondary palate.* Formed by two horizontal projections of mesoderm from inner surfaces of maxillary prominences called *lateral palatine processes.*

            (a) Initially project downward on each side of tongue

            (b) Later, grow toward each other and fuse

            (c) Also fuse with primary palate and nasal septum

            (d) Fusion begins *anteriorly* during *ninth week* and is completed *posteriorly* by the *12th week*

Cleft Lip.   Cleft lip is not a cause of hypernasality and nasal emission, but it is associated with clefts of the palate. They can range from a small notch in the vermillion border of the upper lip to a complete cleft into the floor of the nostril and through the upper alveolar ridge (Fig. 9–10).

    1. *Unilateral cleft lip.* Unilateral cleft lip represents a failure of the maxillary prominence on the affected side to fuse with the medial nasal prominence.

    2. *Bilateral cleft lip.* Bilateral cleft lip results from failure of the maxillary prominences to fuse with the medial nasal prominence. The clefts on both sides may be similar or have different degrees of defect.

    3. *Median cleft lip.* Median cleft of the upper lip is rare and represents a partial or complete failure of the medial nasal prominences to fuse and form the intermaxillary segment. Median cleft of the lower lip is also rare and represents a partial failure of the mandibular prominences to fuse.

Cleft Palate.   Cleft palate represents failure of the lateral palatine processes to fuse with each other, with the nasal septum and/or with the posterior margin of the median palatine process or primary palate (Figure 9–11).

Palatal clefts may be of the uvula only, or they may extend through the soft and hard palates, and through the alveolar process and lip bilaterally. They may be overt or submucous.

    1. *Clefts of the anterior (primary) palate.* These are clefts anterior to the incisive foramen.

    2. *Clefts of the anterior and posterior palate.* These are clefts that involve both the primary and secondary palate.

    3. *Clefts of the posterior or secondary palate.* These are clefts posterior to the incisive foramen.

Incidence.   The incidence of cleft lip and palate varies according to race, sex, geographic area and source of statistical reports. Ross and Johnston (Cooper et al., 1979), after reviewing many surveys and selecting only those that they believed were adequately performed, showed a distinct gradient in the incidence of cleft lip and cleft palate among various racial groups.

    1. The lowest incidence was among American blacks, ranging from 0.21 to 0.41 per 1000 live births.

    2. The highest was among Orientals, with a range of 1.14 to 2.13 per 1000 live births.

    3. In the intermediate group were American and Western European Caucasians, with an incidence between 0.77 and 1.40 per 1000 births.

Associated Anomalies.   Individuals with clefts show an increased incidence of associated malformations, the most common being positional foot defects, extremity malformation, circulatory defects, and malformed ears, micrognathia, hypertelorism, exophthalmia, and microcephaly. Clefts of the palate are common in several syndromes, among which are the Pierre Robin and Treacher Collins syndromes.

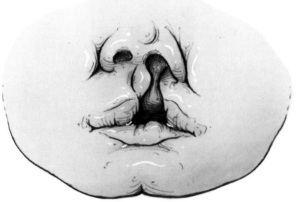

Left unilateral

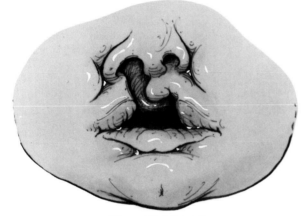

Bilateral R 3/3 L1/3

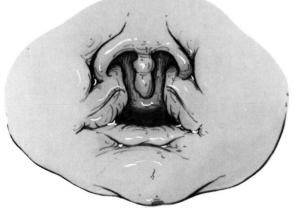

Bilateral

Figure 9–10   Varieties of clefts of the upper lip.

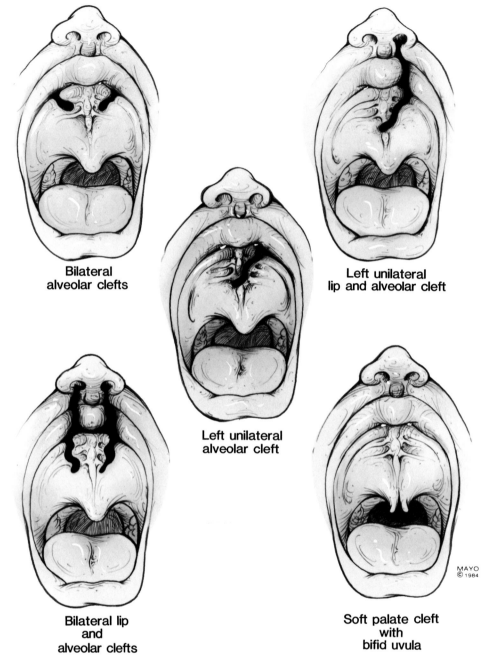

Bilateral
alveolar clefts

Left unilateral
lip and alveolar cleft

Left unilateral
alveolar cleft

Bilateral lip
and
alveolar clefts

Soft palate cleft
with
bifid uvula

MAYO
© 1984

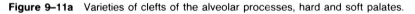

Figure 9–11a   Varieties of clefts of the alveolar processes, hard and soft palates.

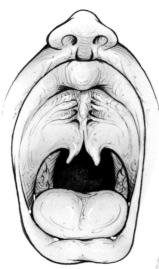

Soft palate cleft
with bifi uvula and
short soft palate

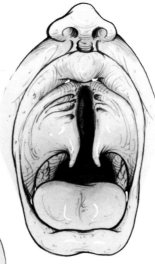

Soft and Hard
palate cleft

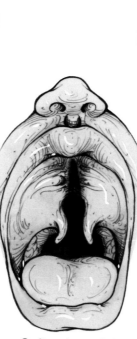

Soft palate cleft
and submucous
hard palate cleft

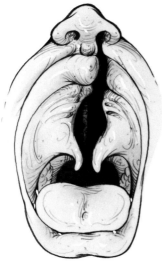

Left Unilateral
Complete cleft,
Lip and Palate

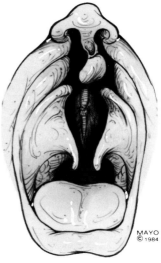

Bilateral complete cleft,
Lip and Palate

MAYO
© 1984

Figure 9–11b

ETIOLOGY

Heredity.   Heredity is the most important cause of cleft lip and palate. Two genetic groups that have been identified are: (1) *Cleft lip alone, or, cleft lip and cleft palate.* Both are more common in males. They have a positive family history in about 40 percent of cases. (2) *Cleft palate alone.* More common in females. There is a positive family history in about 20 percent of cases (Edwards and Watson, 1980).

The mechanism of inheritance is not clear. Cleft lip and palate pedigrees tend to show a recessive mode, although dominance does occur. Cleft palate alone shows simple dominance.

As yet, there is no way of predicting with accuracy whether a subsequent member of a family will have a cleft lip or cleft palate. The only exception to this is when a specific syndrome is recognized that lends itself to simpler patterns of inheritance. However, statistical tables for risk rates are available:

Risk rates for cleft lip (with or without cleft palate) (Fogh-Andersen, 1942) are as follows:

1. For siblings, one child affected, parents normal, 4 percent
2. For siblings, one child affected, one parent affected, 14 percent
3. For offspring, one parent affected, 2 percent

Risk-rate for cleft palate alone (Fogh-Andersen, 1942) is as follows:

1. For siblings, one child affected, parents normal, 2 percent
2. For siblings, one child affected, one parent affected, 17 percent
3. For offspring, one parent affected, 7 percent

Cleft palate (Fraser, 1970) rates are as follows:

1. When one parent has a cleft palate, each child has roughly 1 chance in 16 of being affected.
2. If the parents are unaffected but have a near relative with a cleft palate, the chances that their future children would be affected is about 1 in 15.
3. If the parents of a cleft palate baby are unaffected and do not have an affected near relative, the chance that they will have another child with a cleft palate is about 1 in 50 for each child.
4. If an affected parent has an affected child, then the risk for future children goes up to about 1 in 6.

In cleft lip with or without cleft palate, if two offspring are affected, the risk goes up for subsequent offspring from 4 to 9 percent. There is no change in risk with cleft palate alone.

Environment.   Sixty percent of cleft lip cases alone, or cleft lip and cleft palate, and 80 percent of cleft palate cases alone appear to be solitary occurrences with no family histories of clefts. Although intrauterine causes, e.g., anatomic and physiologic variations of the uterus, metabolic alterations, infections, drugs, diet, and x-radiation are suspected, no compelling evidence for exogenous causes in these solitary cases has been found. Incomplete family histories may account for some in this group, who really belong in the hereditary category.

SPEECH AND LANGUAGE DEFECTS

No two patients with cleft palate, with or without cleft lip, have the same type and degree of communicative disorder; the end product of these palatal defects depends upon several factors: extent and location of the palatal defect; dental abnormalities; hearing loss; intelligence; cultural environment; emotional stability; prior medical and surgical therapies. Following are the kinds of speech and language defects that can occur:

1. Hypernasality of vowels and voiced consonants
2. Nasal emission on pressure consonants
3. Weak pressure consonants
4. Nonstandard laryngeal, pharyngeal, and lingual sound substitutions for standard consonants, i.e., compensatory articulations

5. Delayed articulatory and language development
6. Articulatory defects secondary to dental defects
7. Articulatory defects secondary to hearing loss
8. Dysphonia
9. Nasal and facial grimacing associated with speaking.

Articulatory Defects.   These are inevitable in children with cleft lip and palate. Rarely does cleft lip alone produce defects of articulation unless its repair produces an exceptionally short, tight upper lip that prevents the lower one from reaching it for the bilabial sounds /p/, /b/, and /m/. Perceptually acceptable, although cosmetically distracting, are the child's compensatory attempts to approximate the upper incisors with the lower lip in order to make bilabial sounds, called labiodentalization.

The remaining articulatory defects in children with cleft lip and palate are from the following causes:

Reduced Intraoral Pressure.   Even when articulatory placements are correct, reduced intraoral pressure secondary to nasal air escape will cause consonant distortion. The greater the nasal air escape the less intraoral air available for pressure consonants. Somewhere along the intraoral pressure deficiency continuum, intelligibility begins to deteriorate, ending in unintelligibility.

Minor velopharyngeal insufficiency producing intraoral pressure loss that results in mildly weak consonants presents a different set of problems than large openings with correspondingly poor consonant precision. The mild or borderline insufficiencies cause more decision-making problems. Clinicians find themselves asking "Is he hypernasal or isn't he? Are the consonants weak or aren't they? Yesterday she sounded hypernasal, today she doesn't. She's hypernasal only when she's tired or talks fast. If she puts forth considerable exhalatory pressure she is less hypernasal." What these statements reveal is that the patient is on the verge of velopharyngeal insufficiency, and the slightest drop in effort during exhalation or velopharyngeal closure elicits the audible effects of the borderline velopharyngeal status.

A secondary consequence of nasal emission are audible noises from air passing through the nares, distorting and masking consonants and distracting the listener.

Compensatory Articulatory and Phonatory Substitutions.   Remarkably, children born with palatopharyngeal insufficiencies seem intuitively to grasp early in life the pressure physiology of their own speech mechanisms. Without instruction, they discover they can produce nonstandard sounds with the larynx, pharynx, velum, and tongue that simulate the *manner* of production of standard consonants, which they cannot make. The correct *place* of production is, however, often sacrificed. Those who acquire velopharyngeal insufficiency later in life have much less tendency to develop compensatory errors. The drawings in Figure 9–12 correspond to the following substitutions, derived from Trost's (1981) radiographic studies.

1. *The glottal stop.* An explosive-like grunt or glottal coup / ʔ /, made by tightly adducting the vocal folds, building up infraglottal air pressure, and suddenly releasing it by abducting the vocal folds. Glottal stop substitutions are used in place of the standard stop consonants /p/, /b/, /t/, /d/, /k/, and /g/. The glottal stop is often produced simultaneous with the correct articulatory placement for the sound (coarticulation).

2. *The glottal fricative.* A continuous friction noise made by approximating, but not fully adducting, the vocal folds. It is used as substitution for the standard fricative continuants /s/, /z/, / ʃ /, and / ʒ /.

3. *The pharyngeal stop.* A linguapharyngeal stop consonant substitution for /k/ and /g/. It can be simulated by first walking the tongue backward from the /k/ position downward against the posterior pharyngeal wall and then suddenly releasing air that has been built up below the level of the tongue.

4. *The pharyngeal fricative.* A continuous friction noise in place of standard fricative-continuants, formed by retraction of the tongue against the back wall of the pharynx.

5. *Velar fricative.* A continuous friction noise in place of standard fricative-continuants, formed by retraction of the tongue against the posterior palate.

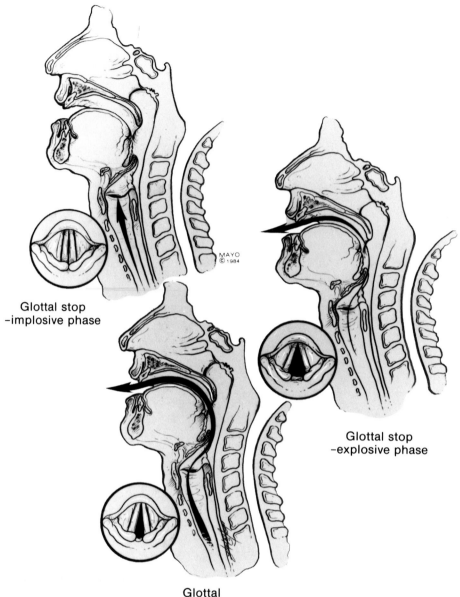

Glottal stop
–implosive phase

Glottal stop
–explosive phase

Glottal
fricative continuant

Figure 9–12a Compensatory, nonstandard articulatory substitutions in palatopharyngeal insufficiency.

6. *The posterior nasal fricative.* A velopharyngeal fricative produced by airway constriction as the soft palate approximates the pharyngeal wall, but which does not close the port. The air is then nasally released. The movement is sometimes aided by posterior posturing of the tongue. The sound is heard as an audible friction noise associated with nasal air escape. Radiographically, this velar articulation is seen as a blurring of movement called *velar flutter.* The posterior nasal fricative is used as a substitution for /s/, /z/, / ʃ /, and / ʒ /.

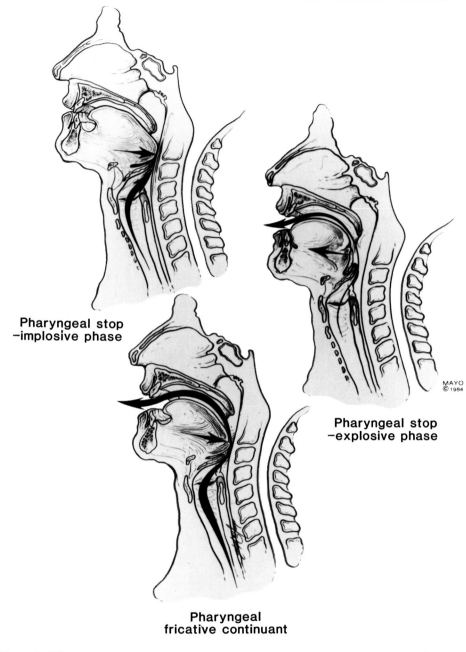

**Pharyngeal stop
—implosive phase**

**Pharyngeal stop
—explosive phase**

**Pharyngeal
fricative continuant**

MAYO
© 1984

Figure 9–12b   Cont'd

7. *The Mid-dorsum palatal stop.* A linguapalatal stop made by placing the tongue in the approximate position for the glide /j/. It is used as a replacement for /t/, /d/, /k/, and /g/.

The tendency for children with cleft palate to *posteriorize lingual placements* has been known for a long time. The tongue can exert an upward force on whatever soft palate tissue remains in an effort to seal off the port and, at the same time, impound air behind the tongue at this presumably more

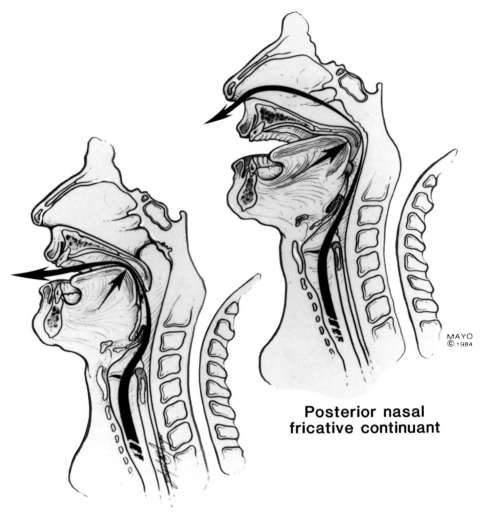

**Posterior nasal
fricative continuant**

MAYO
© 1984

**Velar
fricative continuant**

Figure 9–12c

Cont'd

advantageous location. Compensatory coarticulations or *atypical simultaneous articulatory maneuvers,* have also been observed, e.g., a glottal stop substitution for /b/ while at the same time approximating and separating the lips even though the air is released at the glottal and not at the bilabial level (Trost, 1951).

Bzoch (1979) made a useful comparison between the articulation errors of 120 children aged 3 to 6 without clefts who were considered "normal" in their articulatory development for their age range, and 60 matched children with cleft palate. Table 9–3, which contains normative information on mastery of articulatory skills based on data by Templin (1957) and Poole (1934), shows the differences between the normal and cleft palate children. Note the rampant glottal stop and laryngeal and pharyngeal fricative substitutions in the cleft palate population.

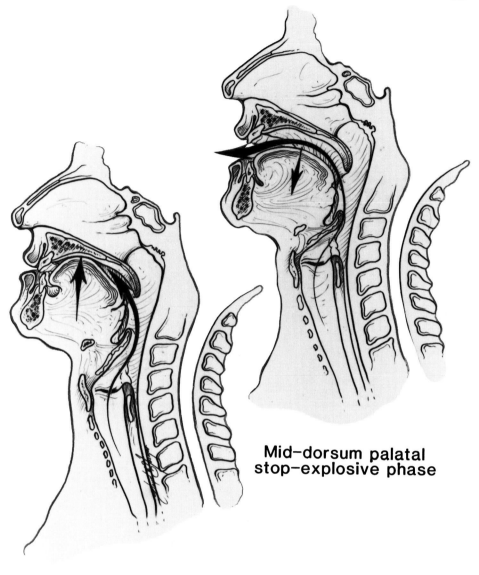

**Mid-dorsum palatal
stop-explosive phase**

**Mid-dorsum palatal
stop-implosive phase**

Figure 9–12d

Dental Abnormalities.   Most people with cleft palate have defects of dental and maxillary-mandibular relationship all their lives; missing teeth; malposed teeth; malocclusions; narrow, highly arched palates; scarred palates. Articulatory distortions arise from aberrant friction noise, or absence of friction noise, on sounds requiring that the airstream be deflected off of the anterior teeth. The anterior lingual consonants most affected are: /t/, /d/, /s/, /z/, / ʃ /, /ʒ/, /t/, and /d/. Interdentalization of these sounds is also common when the maxilla is abnormally small compared with the mandible, inducing a forward tongue carriage.

Table 9-3   Comparison of Articulatory Errors Most Often Found in
Preschool Children With or Without Cleft Palate

Speech Sound Element Tested	Templin Norm	Pool Norm	Errors of Control Subjects (N = 120, 3–6 yr.)	Errors of Cleft Palate Subjects in Order of Frequency of Occurrence (N = 60, 3–6 yr.)
/p/	3	3.5	None	ʔ/p, PF*
/b/	4	3.5	p/b	m/b, ʔ/b
/t/	6	4.5	d/t	ʔ/t, PF, k/t
/d/	4	4.5	t/d	ʔ/d, PF, n/d
/k/	4	4.5	t/k	ʔ/k, PF, t/k
/g/	4	4.5	k/g, d/g	ʔ/g, d/g, PF
/f/	3	5.5	p/f, b/f, s/f	ʔ/f, PF, p/f
/v/	6	6.5	b/v, f/v	b/v, ʔ/v, m/v
/θ/	6	7.5	t/θ, s/θ, f/θ	ʔ/θ, PF, t/θ
/ð/	7	6.5	d/ð	d/ð, ʔ/ð, PF
/s/	4.5	7.5	θ/s, t/s	PF, ʔ/s, t/s
/z/	7	7.5	s/z, θ/z, d/z	PF, ʔ/z, s/z
/ʃ/	4.5	6.5	s/ʃ, tʃ/ʃ	PF, ʔ/ʃ
/tʃ/	4.5	—	ʃ/tʃ, s/tʃ, t/tʃ	PF, ʔ/tʃ, ʃ/tʃ
/dʒ/	7	—	tʃ/dʒ, d/dʒ, ʒ/dʒ	PF, ʔ/dʒ, ʒ/dʒ
/l/	6	6.5	w/l	w/l, ʔ/l
/j/	3.5	4.5	ʔ/j	ʔ/j, w/j, l/j
/r/	4	7.5	w/r	w/r, j/r, PF
/w/	3	3.5	j/w	ʔ/w, l/w
/m/	3	3.5	b/m	PF, ʔ/m
/n/	3	4.5	m/n	ʔ/n, j/n
/ŋ/	3	4.5	n/ŋ	n/ŋ

*PF = either pharyngeal or velar fricative substitution.
From: Bzoch, K.R.: *Communicative Disorders Related to Cleft Lip and Palate*, Boston, Little Brown Inc., 1979, p. 166.

Conductive Hearing Loss.   Serous otitis media producing conductive hearing loss is practically universal in the cleft palate population because of defective aeration and equilibration with atmospheric pressure of the middle ear. The cause is failure of the eustachian tube to open during swallowing because of defective velar musculature. If hearing loss is severe, it may interfere with expressive language and articulatory development or, if mild, can produce phonemic distortions.

Delayed Speech and Language Development.   When research findings on articulatory and language development in children with cleft palate are collated, they provide convincing evidence that, as a group, these children are delayed. Differences in tests used and research methodology employed require that the following statements be interpreted cautiously.

1. Most children with cleft palate are slower than normal in articulatory development (Bzoch, 1956; Counihan, 1960).
2. They say their first words later than normal children (Bzoch, 1956).
3. They use shorter and less complex sentences than normal children (Spriestersbach et al., 1958).
4. They are delayed in language comprehension and usage (Philips and Harrison, 1969).
5. They are behind in expressive language (Smith and McWilliams, 1968).

Studies by Bzoch et al. (1973) pointed to an even more definitive picture of expressive language delay. In 23 of 25 infants, mean age 18 months, they found an almost consistent and significant delay in expressive language but, interestingly, not in receptive, despite histories of widespread conductive hearing loss. Swanson (1973) reported similar findings in 37 infants.

Voice Disorders.   It has been established that children and adults with cleft palate and associated hypernasality and nasal emission have disorders of phonation often associated with hyperplasia and hyperemia of the vocal folds (McDonald and Baker, 1951; Brooks and Shelton, 1963).

Breathy, husky voice quality commonly observed in children who have cleft palate has been attributed to an attempt to *compensate* for the loss of intraoral pressure (Bzoch, 1964) by overdriving the vocal folds in order to overcome reduced intelligibility of speech. McWilliams et al. (1969, 1973) found that 27 of 32 children with cleft palate were chronically hoarse and later developed bilateral vocal fold nodules. Again, compensatory laryngeal valving, overdriving the vocal folds, was blamed for these vocal abuse disorders. Bronsted et al. (1984) showed that more than half of the patients with cleft palate and velopharyngeal insufficiency were dysphonic. The incidence of structural changes of the vocal folds from hyperemia to vocal nodules is not difficult to understand in light of the fact that the use of glottal stops as compensatory plosives produce pressure, friction, and blunt trauma to the vocal folds.

Leder and Lerman (1985) hypothesized that adults, like children, with cleft palate and hypernasality also hyperadduct their vocal folds to produce a constriction below the velopharyngeal portal in an attempt to decrease nasal air leak. Based on acoustic spectrographic analyses, the authors concluded that the vocal folds were inappropriately hyperadducted in order to provide a constriction in place of the inadequately functioning velopharyngeal portal in an effort to eliminate nasal air leak, a causal factor for increased vocal nodules in the cleft palate population.

Congenitally Short Palate and Large Nasopharynx

Velopharyngeal insufficiency can exist without overt clefts of the hard or soft palate. The suspected causes are congenital short soft palate, large nasopharynx, or both, but in many cases neither can be anatomically established and the velopharyngeal insufficiency must be considered idiopathic. These conditions often remain undetected until adenoidectomy deprives the patient of mass tissue in the nasopharynx (Gibb, 1958; Green, 1957; Neiman and Simpson, 1975). A functionally short soft palate will often look normal on routine oral examination and may elevate well, but it does not contact the posterior pharyngeal wall (Figure 9–13).

Two anatomic defects sometimes associated with a functionally short soft palate are *submucous cleft* and *bifid uvula* (Figure 9–14). A submucous cleft can vary from a slight notch into the posterior border of the hard palate to a large U-shaped absence of bone. Bifid uvula, partial or total, may be a clue to occult embryologic palatal defects (Figure 9–15).

Injuries

Hypernasality and nasal emission can result from traumatic damage to the palatal or velopharyngeal anatomy.

1. Surgical removal of portions of the hard and soft palate for benign and malignant tumors.
2. Damage to the velopharyngeal musculature during *tonsillectomy* and *adenoidectomy,* producing scarring and stiffness of the muscles and restricting full sphincter motion.
3. Sequelae to *surgical removal of adenoids,* unmasking submucous occult velopharyngeal insufficiency.
4. *Traumatic accidents,* such as falling on hard or sharp objects in the mouth and other lacerations or penetrating wounds of the palate.

Neurologic Disease

Neurologic disease can cause hypernasality and nasal emission by producing weakness (paresis or paralysis) or incoordination of the velopharyngeal muscles. A concept already stated about neurologic voice disorders is also true of nasal resonatory disorders: *Hypernasality and nasal emission due to neurologic velopharyngeal insufficiency are components and signs of a more generalized dysarthria and, although such resonatory disorders can occur in isolation, they are most often embedded in a complex of associated respiratory, phonatory, and articulatory dysarthric signs.* Hypernasality and nasal air emission can be among the first indicators of

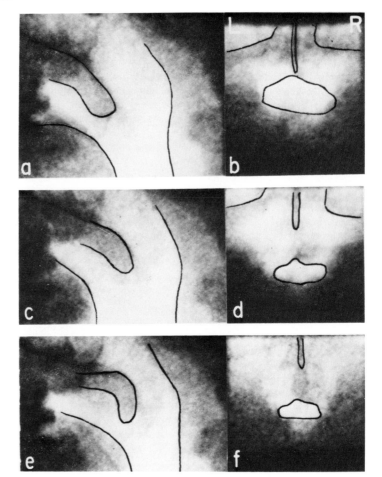

Figure 9–13 Videofluoroscopic frames showing congenital velopharyngeal insufficiency in a six-year-old child at rest and during speech. *From* Skolnick, M. L.: Videofluoroscopic examination of the velopharyngeal portal during phonation in lateral and base projections. Cleft Palate J., 7:803–816, 1970.

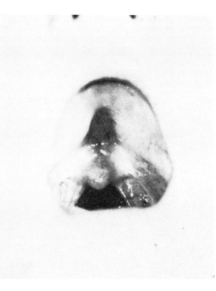

Figure 9–14 Congenital submucous cleft. *From* Luchsinger, K., and Arnold, G. E.: Voice-Speech Language. Belmont, Cal., Wadsworth Publishing Co., 1965.

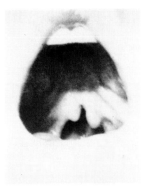

Figure 9–15 Bifid uvula and submucous cleft. *From* Massengill, R.: Hypernasality. Charles Thomas, 1972.

neurologic disease. The following types of dysarthria commonly manifest hypernasality and nasal emission from velopharyngeal weakness or incoordination:

- Unilateral or bilateral lower motor neuron (flaccid) dysarthria
- Unilateral upper motor neuron ("flaccid") dysarthria
- Bilateral upper motor neuron (spastic) dysarthria
- Mixed lower-upper motor neuron (flaccid-spastic) dysarthria
- Hyperkinetic (choreic-dystonic) dysarthria

In Chapter 5 on neurologic voice disorders, the velopharyngeal insufficiency component of the dysarthrias is discussed. Unlike phonatory and articulatory dysarthric signs, that have individual characteristics depending upon site of lesion, thereby giving a clue to location of the lesion, there is nothing perceptually distinctive about the hypernasality and nasal emission of one dysarthria compared with another. An exception may relate to constancy or intermittency of hypernasality, depending upon whether the dysarthria is of the continuous or fluctuating type, a distinction that will be made shortly. It is, however, important for the diagnostician to know which dysarthric types produce hypernasality and which do not. For example, a patient suspected of Parkinson's disease who has hypernasality and nasal emission in addition to a hypokinetic dysarthria, should be suspected of harboring a lesion in another area of the nervous system in addition to the basal ganglia, because pure hypokinetic dysarthria does not include velopharyngeal insufficiency.

FLACCID HYPERNASALITY AND NASAL EMISSION: XTH (VAGUS)
NERVE LESIONS

The muscles of velopharyngeal closure for speech are innervated by the Vth, IXth, Xth, and XIth cranial nerves. Specifically:

1. The levator veli palatini by the pharyngeal branch of the Xth (vagus) nerve.
2. The tensor veli palatini, which contribution to closure is uncertain, by the motor division of the Vth (Trigeminal) nerve.
3. The pharyngeal muscles by the IXth, Xth, and XIth cranial nerves (pharyngeal plexus).

In Chapter 5, Figure 5–2 and Table 5–1 show that damage to the pharyngeal branch of the Xth nerve, or above that level, up to the nucleus ambiguus in the medulla, produce *unilateral or bilateral flaccid paralysis of the soft palate*. Figure 5–3 shows how a *right unilateral lesion* of the vagal nucleus produces weakness of the soft palate on the same side of the lesion. Key points concerning this locus of lesion are:

1. The paralyzed right side rests lower in the mouth than the normal side
2. On phonation, or upon stimulation of the gag reflex, the soft palate pulls upward toward the normal side

The same figure shows the effects of a *bilateral lesion* of the vagal nucleus:

1. Both sides of the soft palate rest low in the mouth
2. On phonation or stimulation of the gag reflex both sides move sluggishly or not at all

Absence or reduction of a gag reflex, also called an *hypoactive gag reflex,* is exclusively a sign of flaccid lower motor neuron paralysis. However, it is, infrequently, also a psychogenic sign.

Neurologic diseases that commonly damage the nucleus ambiguus or the Xth nerves as they exit the base of the skull are: tumors, vascular diseases, cerebrovascular accident, infectious diseases, bony malformations of the base of the skull, and degenerative diseases. Myasthenia gravis, when of the bulbar type, can affect the pharyngeal branch of the vagus nerve at the myoneural junction (see Chapter 5). Hypernasality and nasal emission are prominent signs of this disease.

"FLACCID" HYPERNASALITY AND NASAL EMISSION: UNILATERAL UPPER MOTOR NEURON LESIONS

A unilateral cortical or subcortical lesion of the pyramidal tract (upper motor neuron) often produces *unilateral paralysis of the soft palate on the side opposite the lesion.* The classic case is the patient who sustains a left frontal cerebral hemisphere lesion and becomes hemiparetic, dysarthric, and apraxic. These patients typically have a unilateral upper motor neuron dysarthria that consists of mild articulatory imprecision from unilateral facial and tongue weakness on the side opposite the lesion. The effects of the unilateral soft palate paresis may not be heard because of its mildness, but it can be seen on oral examination. Evidently the tongue, lower face, and soft palate are not as well endowed with ipsilateral corticobulbar fibers as the larynx, which has no such unilateral paresis from unilateral corticobulbar tract lesions.

The asymmetric appearance of a unilateral upper motor neuron paresis of the soft palate at rest is indistinguishable from a unilateral lower motor neuron paresis; in both, phonation and stimulation of the gag reflex cause the soft palate to pull up toward the normal side.

SPASTIC (PSEUDOBULBAR) HYPERNASALITY AND NASAL EMISSION: BILATERAL UPPER MOTOR NEURON LESIONS

Typically, hypernasality and nasal emission are components of spastic dysarthria. However, the muscular physiology is not one of paralysis, as in flaccid dysarthria, but slowness of velopharyngeal movement due to disinhibition of antagonist muscles producing dyssynchronous movements and incomplete closure. Attesting to the intactness of its innervation is either a *normal* or *hyperactive gag reflex;* upon stroking the faucial arches or back wall of the pharynx with a tongue depressor, the gag is easily elicited; the soft palate thrusts upward bilaterally and the pharyngeal walls briskly move medially.

MIXED FLACCID-SPASTIC HYPERNASALITY AND NASAL EMISSION: LOWER PLUS UPPER MOTOR NEURON LESIONS

The most severe cases of hypernasality and nasal emission are found in patients with mixed flaccid-spastic dysarthria owing to their cumulative effects. The classic example is *amyotrophic lateral sclerosis (ALS).* However, *any* lesion that can affect both upper and lower motor neurons simultaneously can produce this same form of velopharyngeal insufficiency. In ALS, the most common disease seen in clinical practice producing this mixed dysarthria, hypernasality and nasal emission are mild in the early stages. As the dysarthria progresses, hypernasality and nasal emission worsen until there is virtually no movement of the velopharyngeal muscles. The soft palate hangs low in the mouth, immersed in ropy saliva, and remains immobile during phonation or stimulation of the gag reflex. The paralysis is not always symmetric; even though both sides of the soft palate are usually paralyzed, one side may be more than the other.

HYPERKINETIC (CHOREIC-DYSTONIC) HYPERNASALITY AND NASAL
EMISSION: BASAL GANGLIA LESIONS

Fluctuating during the course of contextual speech are the hypernasality and nasal emission of the choreic and dystonic movement disorder dysarthrias. The dysarthrias of dystonia, choreoathetosis, and chorea all have periodic velopharyngeal insufficiency, whether the movement disorder is the congenital or early acquired "cerebral palsy" or of later onset. Common to all are spontaneous, uncontrolled velopharyngeal movements, more prominent in the dystonias than the choreas because of the slowness of the dystonias and longer duration of velopharyngeal opening.

PALATOPHARYNGOLARYNGEAL MYOCLONUS

Discussion of the slow (1 to 4 Hz) rhythmic myoclonic-like movements of the soft palate and lateral pharyngeal walls in palatopharyngolaryngeal myoclonus is somewhat paradoxical here, because these movements rarely produce hypernasality or hyponasality even though each time the soft palate elevates myoclonically it touches the posterior pharyngeal wall, and, when it pulls away it opens the velopharyngeal port. The moment of closure is so brief that its perceptual effects escape the ear. For clinical purposes, then, palatal myoclonus is a visual, not an auditory sign. *But, its importance in neurologic diagnosis cannot be overstated. It is easily overlooked because of its subtle movements, yet its presence indicates a brainstem lesion.*

Psychogenic Factors

The incidence of nonorganic hypernasality and nasal emission in clinical practice is low, but a group of patients comprise what is sometimes called "functional" hypernasality. These are children and adults who sound hypernasal but who have normal palatal structure and function as demonstrated on the oral examination and videofluoroscopy. The etiologies of nonorganic "velopharyngeal insufficiencies" are:

1. Conversion reaction
2. Reduced effort to produce normally vigorous speech owing to poor self-image, sometimes combined with borderline organic velopharyngeal insufficiency
3. Reduced speaking effort as a sign of "path of least resistance" in physically ill, debilitated patients
4. Imitation of relatives or friends with whom the person strongly identifies

ORGANIC HYPONASALITY

Hyponasality, or denasality, is the opposite of hypernasality. It is the reduction or absence of nasal resonation on the normal nasal semivowels and during normal assimilation nasality. It is due to velopharyngeal overclosure or to obstruction. In common everyday terms it is called "adenoid speech," or speaking with a "stuffy nose." Curiously, many professional people in medicine and allied health fields confuse hypernasality and hyponasality; when they hear hyponasality sometimes they not only use the term "hypernasality" or "nasal speech" instead, but they also infer velopharyngeal insufficiency instead of nasal or nasopharyngeal obstruction. It is an easy mistake to make by the untrained listener, because both types are so closely associated with the nasal cavities.

Official terminology for disorders of nasal resonance from nasal cavity obstruction follows:

1. *Rhinolalia clausa* (closed nasality)
   a. *Rhinolalia clausa, posterior:* A perceptually distinctive type of hyponasality from obstruction of the posterior nasal cavities or nasopharynx.
   b. *Rhinolalia clausa, anterior:* A perceptually distinctive type of hyponasality from obstruction of the anterior nasal cavities.

The normal speaker can simulate both types. *Posterior:* Say a sentence having nasal semivowels with the *velopharynx continuously closed*. For example, "Many men marched and sang at night." Note that the only phonemes adversely affected are the nasals /m/, /n/, and /ŋ/, which shift toward /b/, /d/, and /g/. Patients who have hypertrophied adenoids, tumors, or polyps in the nasopharynx are, in effect, speaking as if in a state of continuous velopharyngeal closure. *Anterior:* Say the same sentence with *normal velopharyngeal action* but while *pinching the nares closed,* producing the effect of an anterior nasal cavity obstruction. Now a hollow, muffled resonation on the nasal semivowels is heard for the reason that, although the nasal cavities are resonating the sound, the far end is closed, a condition called *cul-de-sac* resonation.

A secondary effect of nasal obstruction is *mouth breathing*. If nasal airflow during inhalation is reduced, the only way of maintaining adequate oxygen intake is orally. The child or adult whose mouth is always open and who has hyponasal speech is likely to have nasal obstruction that ought to alert the clinician to the need for investigation of its cause.

Nasal obstructions are most often due to *inflammations* of the nasal turbinates from upper respiratory infections or allergies, benign and malignant *tumors, enlarged tonsils* that can push the velum against the pharyngeal walls, and *surgical overclosure of the velopharyngeal port* secondary to pharyngoplasty for velopharyngeal insufficiency. Because such operations, exemplified by the pharyngeal flap, cannot be "fine tuned," often the flap is made too wide for the nasopharynx. The patient enters surgery hypernasal and emerges hyponasal. Often this is just temporary from edema that disappears, leaving an adequate nasal airway, but sometimes it is persistent because the flap is too wide. If the obstruction is complete or nearly so, the following complications may occur:

1. Habitual mouth breathing
2. Snoring
3. Reduced sense of smell with loss of appreciation for food
4. Halitosis from susceptibility to microorganisms in the nasal cavities and drying of the oral mucosa
5. Drying of gingival tissues around the anterior teeth which, according to some dentists, can lead to periodontal disease
6. Danger of choking on food

The only recourse is to modify the flap surgically.

A pharyngeal flap operation after a child or adult becomes *hypernasal following tonsillectomy and adenoidectomy (T and A)* can be premature. Many people with normal velopharyngeal function who become hypernasal, sometimes for a few months, following T and A, if left alone, will spontaneously adapt to loss of adenoid tissue and will recover normal velopharyngeal closure. Thinking that the hypernasality is a sign of permanent organic velopharyngeal insufficiency, surgery is sometimes performed, and then complete function of the musculature returns, with the effect of overclosure and consequent hyponasal speech and secondary obstructive effects.

Patulous Eustachian Tube

A most unusual and little discussed cause of hyponasality is a syndrome called patulous eustachian tube. It is worthy of discussion because it is easily missed and misdiagnosed. Its symptoms are:

1. A roaring sound in the ears synchronous with respiration, known as *autophony*
2. A feeling of fullness in the ears
3. Irritability, depression, anxiety, and preoccupation with the symptoms
4. A change in speech, as if the person were talking with a cold in the nose, i.e., *hyponasality*
5. Disappearance of symptoms when lowering the head between the knees or when lying down

The reason for patency of the eustachian tube is the loss of tissue mass surrounding its orifice or from a change in velopharyngeal muscular tonicity.

The subjective sensation of voice amplification is due to the fact that the voice is resonated in the middle ear cavity, having traveled up the open eustachian tube, which is supposed to remain closed except upon swallowing. Autophony may have been first described by Johannes Müller who wrote in his *Handbook of Physiology* that he could produce a snapping sound in his ears when he contracted his palatine muscles and elevated his soft palate. He said: "If immediately afterwards I emit a humming vocal tone while my mouth is either closed or slightly open, this tone has an extraordinary resonance" (Perlman, 1939).

Specific causes of chronic opening of the eustachian tubes are:

1. Significant loss of weight, for example from morning sickness during the first trimester of pregnancy or from debilitating diseases, such as cancer
2. Loss of tissue fluids from the use of diuretics
3. Radiation therapy to the nasopharynx
4. Administration of estrogen hormones to females

Hyponasality as a sign and symptom of this syndrome (Landes, 1957), has an interesting purpose, chiefly protective; *the patient keeps the velopharyngeal port closed in order to prevent the voice from reaching the eustachian tube,* which opening lies above the level of the velopharyngeal sphincter. The reason the symptoms disappear with the head lowered or when the patient is lying down is that venous engorgement of the area surrounding the opening closes the eustachian tube.

Treatment consists of (1) patient education as to the causes of the disorder, (2) weight gain, or (3) injection of Teflon at the orifice of the tube to close it. Anxiety, depression, and the general impression of psychoneurosis improves noticeably in patients treated with Teflon. Crary et al. (1979) found that nine of 10 patients so treated said that they felt much better, had improved concentration, had increased enjoyment of life, and, on the Minnesota Multiphasic Personality Inventory showed a decrease in the neurotic triad of hypochondriasis, depression, and hysteria.

MIXED NASALITY

Mixed nasality, also called *rhinolalia mixta,* may seem paradoxical; simultaneous velopharyngeal insufficiency and nasal obstruction without one cancelling out the other. A mixture of hyponasality of nasals and hypernasality of vowels nevertheless does occur in patients who have coexisting obstruction in the anterior or posterior nasal cavities simultaneous with organic or nonorganic velopharyngeal insufficiencies.

CLINICAL EXAMINATION

The following primary questions need to be answered about the patient suspected of a nasal resonatory disorder:

1. Does, in fact, a nasal resonatory disorder *exist?* If so,
2. What *type* is it? (hypernasality, hyponasality?)
3. How *severe* is it?
4. What is its *cause?*
5. How should it be *treated?*
6. With what *physical, psychologic,* and *educational* deficiencies is the resonatory disorder associated and what are their interactions?
7. How can they be *reduced* or *eliminated?*

In order to answer these questions, the following data are necessary:

1. *History* of the primary and associated disorders
2. *Perceptual* examination as to presence, type, and extent of the nasal resonatory disorder
3. *Examination of the speech anatomy and physiology* via direct observation and indirect biophysical measurement
4. *Articulation* analysis

5. *Language* evaluation
6. *Psychometric and psychologic* evaluation
7. *Social work* evaluation
8. *Allied health specialist* consultative evaluations and recommendations

Perceptual Examination

Judgment as to the presence and severity of a nasal resonatory disorder lies within the ear and mind of the speech pathologist and not a mechanical or electronic instrument, although such devices can support the clinical impression.

CONTEXTUAL SPEECH IMPRESSION

Have the patient simulate everyday speech as closely as possible. Depending upon age and cooperativeness, two kinds of connected speech samples can be obtained, simultaneously *audiorecorded* for confirmational analysis later: *conversational speech* and *oral reading*. As the patient speaks, the clinician should try to answer the following questions:

1. Do I hear *normal, excess,* or *insufficient nasal resonation?*
2. How *distracting* is the resonatory disorder as I try to grasp the content of the patient's speech?
3. Are *consonant pressures low* so that the sounds are difficult or impossible to identify?
4. Are *vowels hypernasal?*
5. Are *nasal semivowels hyponasal?*
6. Do I hear *nonstandard sound substitutions?*
7. Do I hear *standard sound substitutions?*
8. Does *language development sound delayed?*
9. What is the level of *overall speech intelligibility?*
10. Is a *voice (laryngeal) disorder* also present, and if so, what are its perceptual features?
11. Does the patient's behavior suggest a *hearing loss?*
12. Does general behavior suggest *intellectual, personality, or emotional disturbances?*
13. What is the impression given by the patient's *physical appearance?*
14. Do *facial grimaces* or other habit patterns accompany contextual speech?

Semiobjective Tests for Hypernasality and Hyponasality.   Suppose, after listening to contextual speech, the clinician suspects *hypernasality, nasal emission,* or *hyponasality*. Additional arguments for, or against, their presence can be obtained by means of the following practical tests:

1. *Mirror-clouding test*
   a. Hypernasality and nasal emission
      (1) Place a hand mirror or cold shiny metal object under the patient's nares.
      (2) Ask the patient to repeat a sentence that is *free of all nasal semivowels,* e.g., "We see three geese" or "The big black dog caught the stick." People who have normal palatal and velopharyngeal closure *should not leak air* out the nose during such phrases. *Fogging of the mirror under one or both nares indicates velopharyngeal insufficiency.*
   b. Hyponasality
      (1) Ask the patient to repeat a sentence containing ample nasal semivowels, e.g., "Many men sang at noon"
      (2) People with normal velopharyngeal opening *should leak air out* the nares during the nasal sounds, fogging the mirror. *Little or no fogging indicates nasal obstruction*
2. *Nasal vibration test*
   a. Hypernasality and Nasal Emission

(1) While the patient repeats a sentence free of nasal sounds, such as "We see three geese," with thumb and index finger lightly straddle the cartilagenous portion of the nose: *If vibration can be felt, nasal resonation is likely*

(2) Have the patient repeat the sentence, but this time pinch the nares shut: *If cul-de-sac resonation can be heard, excess nasal resonation is likely*

b. Hyponasality

(1) While the patient repeats a sentence rich in nasal sounds, such as "Many men sang at noon," straddle the nose with thumb and index finger: *If vibration cannot be felt suspect nasal obstruction. If pinching the nares during the production of nasal sounds does not produce cul-de-sac resonation, also suspect nasal obstruction*

3. *Consonant differential pressure test for hypernasality and nasal emission*

a. Have the patient repeat a sentence free of nasal sounds and rich in pressure consonants, such as "The paperboy saw a baseball." The first trial should be produced while the examiner listens carefully to consonant sharpness and sentence intelligibility

b. The second trial should be produced while the examiner pinches the nares shut and listens for any change in the consonant sharpness and intelligibility. *A noticeable rise in audible consonant pressure or sharpness and intelligibility with the nares pinched indicates grossly the extent of the insufficiency. It also provides an impression of what the patient's speech could be like with successful surgical or prosthetic treatment of the insufficiency*

4. *Nares occlusion test of exhalatory efficiency*

a. With *nares open* ask the patient to inhale as deeply as possible and then on exhalation count to as high a number as possible until all breath is exhausted. (First demonstrate a rate of about two numbers per second.) Repeat this three times and take the average maximum number attained on the three trials.

b. While the examiner pinches the *nares shut,* the patient repeats the same three trials of counting, again taking the average of the three trials. *Patients who have normal velopharyngeal closure produce little or no differences between the maximum number attained on counting with nares open versus nares occluded. Patients who have hypernasality and nasal emission will produce a noticeably lower maximum number with the nares open versus closed, giving evidence of the extent of nasal air wastage*

These practical tests can be done in the office without special equipment. Quantification of nasal airflow and intraoral pressures by electronic instruments can yield similar results but are not essential for clinical purposes.

Examination of the Speech Anatomy

Once the clinician has identified a nasal resonatory disorder by the methods just discussed, the next step is to find a physical explanation for the hypernasality and nasal emission or hyponasality. For this portion of the examination, the following equipment is required:

1. A quiet room
2. A chair for the patient that will enable the examiner to look into the patient's mouth at different angles; a dental chair is ideal
3. An excellent source of light. Although a good flashlight will suffice, natural lighting, dental or surgical lighting, or light reflected from a head mirror are even better
4. Tongue depressors
5. Dental mirror

The physical examination begins by asking the patient to sit upright, relaxed and comfortable.

1. While the patient is breathing quietly, the clinician should be thinking of the following questions:
   a. Are there *friction noises* that suggest nasal or oral obstruction?
   b. Is the patient a *mouth breather?*

    c. Are there unilateral, bilateral, or midline *clefts of the upper lip?*

    d. Is there *evidence of surgical repair* of clefts of the lip?

    e. Does the upper lip appear *thin or contracted?*

    f. Does one or both sides of the *nose appear flattened or distorted?*

    g. Does the *maxilla appear abnormally small?*

    h. Does the *mandible appear incongruously large,* protruding beyond the maxilla?

    i. Does the *mandible appear incongruously small* in comparison to the maxilla?

2. *Voluntary lip movements*

    a. Does the patient have difficulty *approximating the upper and lower lips?*

    b. Does the patient have difficulty *rounding, retracting, and protruding the lips?*

3. *Voluntary mandibular movements*

    a. Does the patient have *difficulty depressing, lateralizing, protruding, or elevating the mandible?*

    b. On occluding the teeth, *does the mandible protrude beyond the maxilla?*

4. *Dental configuration*

    a. Are *teeth missing* in the upper or lower dental arch?

    b. Are teeth *improperly formed or positioned* within the dental arch?

    c. Is there *malocclusion* between the upper and lower teeth?

    d. Do *extra teeth* (supernumerary) crowd the dental arch?

5. *Hard palate configuration*

    a. Is there a *unilateral or bilateral cleft* of the hard palate?

    b. Is there an *alveolar cleft?*

    c. Is there a *notch in the posterior hard palate on palpation?*

    d. Is there a *palatal fistula* present?

    e. Is the hard palate *abnormally high and narrow?*

    f. Is the *hard palate scarred* from previous surgeries?

    g. Have *teeth erupted from the hard palate?*

6. *Soft palate configuration*

    a. Does the soft palate appear *abnormally short* at rest?

    b. Is the soft palate *asymmetric at rest?*

    c. Is the soft palate *scarred?*

    d. Are the palatine *tonsils enlarged?*

    e. Is the *uvula absent?*

    f. Is the *uvula bifid or split?*

    g. Is the soft palate *thin and translucent?*

    h. Does the soft palate *elevate asymmetrically* on phonation of /a/?

    i. Does the soft palate *fail to elevate bilaterally on phonation?*

    j. Does the soft palate *fail to elevate bilaterally on stimulation of the gag reflex?*

    k. On cineradiographic, videofluoroscopic, endoscopic, or nasendoscopic examination:

        (1) Does a lateral view show that the soft palate *fails to contact the posterior pharyngeal wall* on non-nasal sounds?

        (2) Does a lateral view show that the *soft palate is short?*

        (3) Does a lateral view of the soft palate *fail to show a knee-angle during phonation?*

        (4) Does a lateral view show the soft palate contacting a *Passavant's ridge on phonation?*

        (5) Does a lateral view show *adenoids present,* providing a point of contact by the soft palate on non-nasal sounds?

        (6) On basal view, does the *velopharyngeal sphincter fail to close?*

        (7) On frontal view, is there a *reduction or absence of medial pharyngeal wall movement?*

Articulation Analysis

Articulatory analysis is done for three reasons in patients with palatopharyngeal insufficiency: To determine the presence or extent of deviant articulatory development; to identify distortions secondary to orofacial and dental anomalies; and to identify compensatory, nonstandard articulatory substitutions and distortions. These objectives are separate and distinct. It is important to objectify the presence of impaired articulatory development, which may, or may not, be caused by the palatopharyngeal insufficiency. It may be due to mental retardation, hearing loss, or environmental deprivation. The second and third reasons for articulation testing are that cleft palate and other palatopharyngeal insufficiencies produce their own special articulatory defects. For example, dental, maxillary, and mandibular anomalies markedly interfere with normal articulation, and, because no two individuals have the same anatomic abnormalities, their articulatory acoustics are never identical. Hence, no standard nomenclature or precise phonetic symbols exist to indicate the peculiarity of a given individual's distortions caused by anomalous oral architecture. The same can be said for the compensatory glottal, pharyngeal, and lingual stops and fricatives so common in children and adults with cleft palate. In short, the ordinary developmental or descriptive articulation test for assessing general articulatory development needs to be supplemented to document the articulatory defects in this population that extend beyond delayed development.

Addressing the special needs of the cleft palate population, Bzoch (1979) designed an Error Pattern Diagnostic Articulation Test (Fig. 9–16). In addition to *simple substitutions, omissions,* and *distortions* this test adds recording space for *gross substitutions,* such as glottal stops, and pharyngeal fricatives, and for *nasal emissions* of sounds. The clinician should also describe in detail the location of the error, particularly the nonstandard distortions and substitutions produced by atypical labial, dental, lingual, pharyngeal, or laryngeal movements.

Language Evaluation

Children with cleft lip and palate are known for their delayed language in addition to delayed articulatory development. Confronting the clinician is the need to establish *whether* language is delayed and *why,* a more than usually complicated question within the context of cleft palate, for such delay often has multiple causes. Consequently, evaluation must consider not only documentation of language developmental milestones, but audiologic, familial, social and psychologic history as well. The clinician who works with children with craniofacial anomalies needs to be aware of the physical, environmental, and psychologic disturbances that can contribute to delayed language development. For example:

1. *The cleft itself.* Inability to generate intraoral pressures within the first two or even three years of life, a period having implications for pressure-consonant development, in itself probably delays not only articulation but intelligibility.
2. *Dental anomalies.* Missing and malpositioned teeth and malocclusions have the same effect of depriving the child of normal anatomy for speech development.
3. *Trauma.* Oropharyngeal pain from surgical procedures.
4. *Emotional deprivation.* Rejection by parents and siblings.
5. *Language deprivation.* Reduced language stimulation because of hospitalizations and family disruptions.
6. *Hearing loss.* From serous otitis media and middle ear infections.
7. *Mental retardation.* As an associated disorder not stemming from environmental factors per se.
8. *Self-consciousness.* Reduced willingness to speak in order to minimize conspicuousness.

Therapy for nasal resonatory disorders and cleft palate rehabilitation have not been included in this chapter owing to their extensiveness and complexity. This subject is covered in references under Suggestions for Additional Reading.

BZOCH ERROR PATTERN DIAGNOSTIC ARTICULATION TESTS   1978-A

Name _____ Birth _____ Age ____ Sex _____ No. _____

Examiner _____ Date _____ Stimulus _____

C = correct,   T = indistinct from nasal emission alone,   D = distortion (.5 error),   SS = simple substitution (1.0 error),
GS = gross substitution (1.5 error),   O = omission (2.0 error).

		C	T	D	SS	GS	O		C	T	D	SS	GS	O		C	T	D	SS	GS	O
PLOSIVES																					
/p/	Pencil							aPPle							cuP						
/b/	Ball							baBy							tuB						
/t/	Table							mounTain							boaT						
/d/	Dog							canDy							beD						
/k/	Cat							chiCKen							booK						
/g/	Gun							waGon							piG						
FRICATIVES																					
/f/	Fork							elePHant							kniFE						
/v/	Vase							shoVel							stoVE						
/θ/	THumb							tooTHbrush							mouTH						
/ð/	THis							feaTHer							baTHE						
/s/	Sun							bicyCle							houSE						
/z/	Zipper							sciSSors							noSE						
/ʃ/	SHoe							diSHes							fiSH						
/ʒ/	XXXXX							televiSion							garaGE						
AFFRICATIVES																					
/ʧ/	CHair							maTCHes							waTCH						
/ʤ/	Juice							briDGes							oranGE						
ASPIRATES																					
/h/	Horse							grassHopper							XXXXXX						
GLIDES																					
/w/	Window							sandWich							XXXXXX						
/l/	Lion							baLLoons							doLL						
/y/	Yarn							onIOns							XXXXXX						
/r/	Rabbit							aRRow							caR						
NASALS																					
/m/	Man							haMMer							druM						
/n/	Nail							baNana							traiN						
/ŋ/	XXXXXX							haNGer							swiNG						
BLENDS																					
	SPider							STar							neST						
	STRawberries							SKirt							boX						
	SLide							SMoke							SNake						
	PLiers							BLock							beLT						
	worLD							CLown							FLag						
	PResent							BRoom							TRuck						
	DRess							heaRT							swoRD						
	CRy							GRapes							coRK						
	FRog							THRead							aRM						
	dropPED							inseCT							siFT						
	WHeel							teNT							haND						

Figure 9–16 Error pattern diagnostic articulation test. *From* Bzoch, K. R.: Communicative disorders related to cleft lip and palate, Boston, Little Brown and Co., 1979, p. 169.

SUMMARY

1. Hypernasality and nasal emission interfere with the aesthetics of speech and can seriously compromise intelligibility, producing serious psychologic, educational, and occupational consequences.

2. Hypernasality and nasal emission are caused by cleft palate, congenitally short palate or large nasopharynx, and nasopharyngeal trauma and by neurologic diseases that cause weakness and dyssynchronous movements of the velopharyngeal sphincter.

3. Hyponasality, or denasality, is caused by obstruction of the nasopharynx or nasal passages.

4. Normal velopharyngeal closure is produced primarily by sphincteric action of the levator veli palatini and the superior pharyngeal constrictor muscles and not solely by elevation and retraction of the soft palate.

5. Clefts of the palate involve the primary (lip and alveolus) palate only, the secondary palate only, or primary and secondary palates combined.

6. Speech defects common in cleft palate are hypernasality and nasal emission, weak pressure consonants, nonstandard substitutions of laryngeal, pharyngeal, and lingual sounds, deviant and/or delayed articulatory and language development, articulatory problems due to dental defects, and to hearing loss, and dysphonia.

7. Neurologic velopharyngeal insufficiencies are associated primarily with flaccid, spastic, and hyperkinetic dysarthrias.

8. In a small percentage of cases, hypernasality and nasal emission can be psychogenic.

9. Clinical examination should answer questions as to type, severity, and cause of the resonatory disorder. Associated psychoeducational, physical, physiologic, articulatory, voice, and language functions also require investigation.

SUGGESTIONS FOR ADDITIONAL READING

Cooper, H.R., Sr., Harding, R.L., Krogman, W.H., Mazahari, M., and Millard, R.T. (Eds.): Cleft Palate and Cleft Lip. Philadelphia, W.B. Saunders Co., 1979. A comprehensive textbook covering all aspects of cleft lip and palate.

Fritzell, B.: The velopharyngeal muscles in speech: An electromyographic and cineradiographic study. Acta Otolaryngol. [Suppl] (Stockh), 250:1969. A comprehensive electromyographic study that shows the timing and extent of velopharyngeal muscle activity in closing and opening of the velopharyngeal portal during speech.

Hirschberg, J.: Velopharyngeal insufficiency. Folia Phoniatr. 38:221–276, 1986. This extensive article should be read for its historical and technical review of the entire subject of velopharyngeal insufficiency from Hippocrates to the present, including the anatomy and physiology of velopharyngeal closure, etiologic classification of velopharyngeal insufficiency, diagnosis, physiologic measurement, surgery, and speech therapy.

McWilliams, B.J., Morris, H.L., and Shelton, R.L.: Cleft Palate Speech, Philadelphia, B.C. Decker, 1984.

Moore, K.L.: The Developing Human. Philadelphia, W.B. Saunders Co., 1977. A lucid depiction of the embryology of the maxillofacial anatomy.

Pulec, J.L., and Hahn, F.W.: The abnormally patulous eustachian tube. Otolaryngol. Clin. North Am., 3:131–140, 1970. An excellent review of a highly uncommon cause of hyponasality that will elude the unwary clinician.

Ross, R.B., and Johnson, M.C.: Cleft Lip and Palate. Baltimore, Williams & Wilkins Co., 1972. A detailed discussion of the incidence, etiology, and genetics of cleft lip and palate; especially suitable for the researcher.

Ruscello, D.M.: A selected review of palatal training procedures. Cleft Palate J., 19:181–193, 1982.

Skolnick, M.L.: Videopharyngography in patients with nasal speech, with emphasis on lateral pharyngeal motion in velopharyngeal closure. Radiology, 93:747–755, 1969.

Skolnick, M.L.: Videofluoroscopic examination of the velopharyngeal portal during phonation in lateral and base projections—a new technique for studying the mechanics of closure. Cleft Palate J., 7:803–816, 1970.

Skolnick, M.L., McCall, G.N., and Barnes, M.: The sphincteric mechanism of velopharyngeal closure. Cleft Palate J., 10:286–305, 1973. These three references represent pioneering radiologic work that has changed our conception of velopharyngeal closure from a two-dimensional to a three-dimensional one.

Trost, J.E.: Articulatory additions to the classical description of the speech of persons with cleft palate. Cleft Palate J., 18:193–203, 1981. A radiographic study that clarifies the anatomy of the articulatory compensations made by cleft palate speakers.

Trost, J.E.: Differential diagnosis of velopharyngeal disorders. In Bradford, L.J., and Wertz, R.T. (Eds.): Communicative Disorders, an audio Journal for Continuing Education. New York, Grune & Stratton, 1981. An instructive tape-recorded lecture on velopharyngeal disorders with illustrative examples of the effects of velopharyngeal insufficiencies on speech.

REFERENCES

Bell-Berti, F.: An electromyographic study of velopharyngeal function in speech. J. Speech Hear. Res., 19:225–240, 1976.

Bengueral, A.P., Hirose, H., Sawashima, M., and Ushijima, T.: Velar coarticulation in French: A fiberscopic study. J. Phonet., 5:149–158, 1977.

Bronsted, K., Liisberg, W.B., Orsted, A., et al.: Surgical and speech results following palatopharyngoplasty operations in Denmark, 1959–1977. Cleft Palate J., 21:170–179, 1984.

Brooks, A., and Shelton, R.: Incidence of voice disorders other than nasality in cleft palate children. Cleft Palate Bull., 13:63–64, 1963.

Bzoch, K.R.: An investigation of the speech of pre-school cleft palate children. Ph.D. Dissertation. Evanston, Ill., Northwestern University, 1956.

Bzoch, K.: The effects of a specific pharyngeal flap operation upon the speech of 40 cleft palate persons. J Speech Hear. Disord., 29:111–120, 1964.

Bzoch, K.R., Morley, M., Fex, S., Laxman, J., and Heller, J.: Development of Speech and Language in Cleft Palate Children. In Proceedings of the 2nd International Congress on Cleft Palate, 1973.

Bzoch, K.R.: Communicative Disorders Related to Cleft Lip and Palate. Boston, Little, Brown and Co., 1979.

Cooper, F.S.: Research techniques and instrumentation: EMG. American Speech and Hearing Association Reports, No. 1. Conference on Communication Problems in Cleft Palate, 1965, pp. 153–168.

Cooper, H.K., Sr., Harding, R.L., Krogman, W.M., Mazahari, M., and Millard, R.T. (Eds.): Cleft Palate and Cleft Lip. Philadelphia, W.B. Saunders Co., 1979.

Counihan, D.: Articulation skills of adolescents and adults with cleft palates. J. Speech Hear. Disord., 25:181–187, 1960.

Crary, W.G., Wexler, M., and Berliner, K.: The abnormally patent eustachian tube. Arch. Otolaryngol., 105:21–23, 1979.

Dickson, D.R.: An acoustic study of nasality. J. Speech Hear. Res., 5:103, 1962.

Edwards, M., and Watson, A.C.H.: Advances in the Management of Cleft Palate. Edinburgh. Churchill Livingstone, 1980.

Fraser, F.C.: The genetics of cleft lip and palate. Am. J. Hum. Genet., 22:336–352, 1970.

Fogh-Andersen, P.: Inheritance of Cleft Lip and Palate. Copenhagen, Nordisk Forlag, Arnold Busck, 1942.

Fritzell, B.: The velopharyngeal muscles in speech: An electromyographic and cineradiographic study. Acta Otolaryngol. [Suppl] (Stockh) 250:1, 1969.

Gibb, A.G.: Hypernasality (rhinolalia aperta) following tonsil and adenoid removal. J. Laryngol. Otol., 72:443, 1958.

Green, M.C.L.: Speech of children before and after removal of adenoids. J. Speech Hear. Disord., 22:361, 1957.

House, A.S., and Stevens, K.N.: Analog studies of the nasalization of vowels. J. Speech Hear. Disord., 21:218, 1956.

Landes, B.A.: Hyporhinolalia associated with eustachian tube dysfunction. Laryngoscope, 77:244–246, 1957.

Leder, S.B., and Lerman, J.W.: Some acoustic evidence for vocal abuse in adult speakers with repaired cleft palate. Laryngoscope, 95:837–840, 1985.

Li, C.L., and Lundervold, A.: Electromyographic study of cleft palate. Plast. Reconstr. Surg., 21:427, 1958.

Lubker, J.F., and Curtis, J.F.: Electromyographic-cinefluorographic investigation of velar function during speech production. J. Acoust. Soc. Am., 40:1272, 1966.

Lubker, J.F.: An electromyographic-cineradiographic investigation of velar function during normal speech production. Cleft Palate J., 5:1–18, 1968.

McDonald, E., and Baker, H.K.: Cleft palate speech: An integration of research and clinical observation. J. Speech Hear. Disord., 16:9–20, 1951

McWilliams, B.J., Bluestone, C.D., and Musgrave, R.H.: Diagnostic implications of vocal cord nodules in children with cleft palate. Laryngoscope, 79:2072–2080, 1969.

McWilliams, B.J., Lavarto, A.S., and Bluestone, C.D.: Vocal cord abnormalities in children with velopharyngeal valving problems. Laryngoscope, 83:1745–1753, 1973.

Neiman, G., and Simpson, R.: A roentgencephalometric investigation of the effect of adenoid removal upon selected measures of velopharyngeal function. Cleft Palate J., 12:377–389, 1975.

Perlman, H.B.: The eustachian tube: Abnormal patency and normal physiologic state. Arch. Otolaryngol., 30:212–238, 1939.

Peterson, G.E., and Barney, H.L.: Control methods used in a study of the vowels. J. Acoustic. Soc. Am., 24: 175, 1952.

Philips, B., and Harrison, R.: Language skills in preschool cleft palate children. Cleft Palate J., 6:108–119, 1969.

Poole, I.: Genetic development in articulation of consonant sounds in speech. Elementary English, 2:159, 1934.

Seaver, E.J.: A Cinefluorographic and Electromyographic Investigation of Velar Movement During Speech. Doctoral Dissertation. Iowa City, University of Iowa, 1979.

Skolnick, M.L.: Videopharyngography in patients with nasal speech, with emphasis on lateral pharyngeal motion in velopharyngeal closure. Radiology, 93:747–755, 1969.

Skolnick, M.L.: Videofluoroscopic examination of the velopharyngeal portal during phonation in lateral and base projections—a new technique for studying the mechanics of closure. Cleft Palate J., 7:803–816, 1970.

Skolnick, M.L., McCall, G.N., and Barnes, M.: The sphincteric mechanism of velopharyngeal closure. Cleft Palate J., 10:286–305, 1973.

Smith, S.: Vocalization and added nasal resonance. Folia Phoniatr., 3:165, 1951.

Smith, R.M., and McWilliams, B.J.: Psycholinguistic abilities of children with clefts. Cleft Palate J., 5:238, 1968.

Spriestersbach, D., Darley, F., and Morris, H.: Language skills in children with cleft palates. J. Speech Hear. Res., 1:279–285, 1958.

Swanson, J.F.: Language-development in young cleft palate children. M.A. Thesis. Gainsville, University of Florida, 1973.

Templin, M.C.: Certain language skills in children, their development and interrelationships. Institute of Child Welfare, Monograph. Series 26. Minneapolis, University of Minnesota Press, 1957.

Trost, J.E.: Articulatory additions to the classical description of the speech of persons with cleft palate. Cleft Palate J., 18:193–203, 1981.

Warren, D. W.: Velopharyngeal orifice size and upper pharyngeal pressure-flow patterns in normal speech. Plast. Reconstr. Surg., 33:148–162, 1964.

SECTION II

Chapter Ten

INDIRECT LARYNGOSCOPY

    Mirror Laryngoscope
    Right-Angle Telescope
    Fiberscope

DIRECT LARYNGOSCOPY

RADIOGRAPHY

    Tomography
    Laryngography

VOICE EVALUATION

    Preliminary Considerations
    Phase I. History of the Voice Disorder
    Phase II. The Voice Evaluation
    Phase III. Interpretation of Findings
    Phase IV. Making Decisions

CLINICAL EXAMINATION OF VOICE DISORDERS

Rien ne vaut une oreille attentive.

—Passy

L'oreille est bien plus sensible qu'une analyse expérimentale du timbre.

—Husson

The laryngologic examination and voice evaluation are inseparable and interdependent. The laryngologist correlates the sound of the voice with visual clues of laryngeal disease. The speech pathologist must know the extent to which the abnormal voice is congruent with the physical findings. An expert ear is indispensable for detection and description of abnormal voice, and experience with correlation of history and physical findings is needed for interpretation of its meaning. In short, diagnosis of voice disorders is an art.

The first step in the voice evaluation is a thorough history and examination of the interior of the larynx; the oral, pharyngeal, and nasal cavities; and the head, neck, and chest.

INDIRECT LARYNGOSCOPY

Indirect laryngoscopy derives its name from the technique of viewing the interior of the larynx indirectly via a mirror or some other optical instrument rather than with the naked eye. Alternative methods are available.

Mirror Laryngoscope

In this traditional method of viewing the vocal folds, the physician faces the upright patient, wraps the tongue in gauze to protect the frenum from the lower incisors, and, with thumb and middle finger, draws the tongue out of the mouth (Fig. 10–1). The mirror, slightly warmed and tested against the dorsum of the hand, is introduced into the mouth, the examiner carefully avoiding contact with the tongue. The mirror, guided posteriorly by pushing the uvula upward and backward, is positioned in the oropharynx. Gagging can be inhibited by encouraging the patient to breathe through the mouth and to keep the eyes open. Otherwise, a topical anesthetic agent is sprayed into the oropharynx. Mild sedation is sometimes offered. If the patient still cannot tolerate the procedure, which is common in children and infants, a direct laryngoscopic examination under general anesthesia may be necessary. With the laryngeal mirror properly positioned, the clinician reflects a light beam off a head mirror onto the laryngeal mirror to see the laryngeal interior. In Figure 10–1, the letter *R* and *L* illustrate reversal of the reflected image; what appears to be the left vocal fold in the mirror is actually the right, and vice versa. The vocal folds seen in the mirror correspond with the actual folds. What is different is that the anterior commissure is directed posteriorly in the mirror, whereas in actuality, the commissure always points anteriorly.

With the mirror, the laryngologist inspects the base of the tongue, the anterior surface of the epiglottis, the valleculae, the pharyngeal walls, the pyriform sinuses, the posterior border of the epiglottis, the aryepiglottic folds, and the mucosa of the posterior commissure. The vocal folds are viewed during quiet breathing and while the patient sustains the vowel /e/ or /i/. The effort to

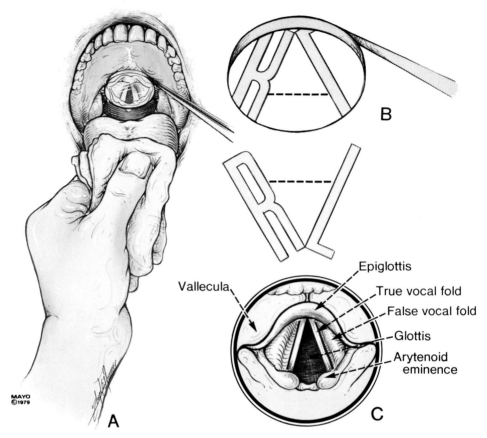

Figure 10-1 Mirror laryngoscopy illustrating mirror reversal of vocal folds and key anatomic landmarks.

produce these vowels causes the larynx to rise in the neck, affording a clearer view of the vocal folds. The examiner searches for symmetry of glottal opening and closing, normalcy of color, presence or absence of mass lesions, or inflammation.

Right-Angle Telescope

An alternative to the mirror laryngoscope is the right-angle telescope. Its use requires less skill than mirror laryngoscopy. While the patient protrudes the tongue, the objective end of the telescope is glided gently posteriorly over the base of the tongue, bringing the larynx into view. One investigator reported completion of 500 consecutive telescopic laryngoscopies without topical anesthesia (Klein, 1975).

Fiberscope

In this technique, a flexible fiberoptic bundle is threaded through the nasal passages, the tip of the scope providing its own light source and magnifying the laryngeal image. This technique is the only one by which the clinician can view the vocal folds while the patient is speaking.

DIRECT LARYNGOSCOPY

Direct laryngoscopy—necessary for examination of infants and young children, whose larynges are difficult to see indirectly and who do not tolerate the indirect examination well—provides a truer, more detailed view of the interior of the larynx. The technique is also used in conjunction with surgery of the vocal folds and the surrounding anatomy. It may be used when the patient is either topically or generally anesthetized, the latter being selected for the more apprehensive patient. With the patient supine, the laryngoscope is introduced along the right side of the tongue and is guided down to the level of the vocal folds, the examiner inspecting structures along the way.

RADIOGRAPHY

Radiographs of the larynx in frontal (anteroposterior) and lateral projections reveal the presence, position, size, and shape of virtually all laryngeal lesions.

Tomography

Still x-ray photography of the larynx without the use of contrast media enables the viewer to distinguish between air and tissue. The air surrounding the laryngeal tissues affords a sufficient density differential.

Laryngography

Laryngographs are x-ray spot films of the larynx. The surfaces of the larynx are coated with an oily contrast material, giving them a sharper outline. After the oropharynx is sprayed with topical anesthetic agent, contrast medium is dripped onto the base of the tongue, whereupon it flows down and coats the interior surfaces of the larynx. The result is a sharper outline of the supraglottic, glottic, and infraglottic regions.

Additional techniques for laryngologic diagnosis are high-speed motion picture studies, video-fluoroscopy, cinefluorography or cineradiography, and stroboscopy. They are used primarily for the study of laryngeal movements rather than structure.

VOICE EVALUATION

Preliminary Considerations

Ordinarily, by the time the speech pathologist sees the patient for voice evaluation, the patient will already have had an ear, nose, and throat examination. Although the laryngologic examination may not have been performed, this should not prevent voice evaluation.

However, it is strongly recommended that the speech pathologist view the vocal folds of patients undergoing examination for voice disorders in order to know whether or not the type and severity of the abnormal voice is congruent with the structure and movement of the vocal folds. This information is of prime importance in judging the extent to which the voice disorder is organic, psychogenic, or both. Without such knowledge, the patient can neither be accurately or convincingly informed nor can therapy be rationally planned. If possible, the speech pathologist should try to be present during the laryngoscopic examination in order to view the vocal folds along with the laryngologist. Such contact among speech pathologist, laryngologist, and patient has other advantages. It gives the patient a feeling of mutual cooperation among the specialists who are trying to help and contributes to the continuing education of both laryngologist and speech pathologist. Decision-making is also smoother. Standards of practice vary extensively throughout the country, and communication between speech pathologist and laryngologist may be close, minimal, or nonexistent.

Referrals.   By whom patients with voice disorders are referred to speech pathologists and the reasons for their referral depend upon the organizational setting in which the speech clinician works, the speech pathologist's qualifications, and the physician's philosophy of patient care. The reasons for referral are (1) voice therapy, (2) assistance in differential diagnosis, (3) presurgical and postsurgical baseline purposes when the physician is concerned about the medicolegal implications of the voice, and (4) research documentation. In addition to physicians, patients are referred by other speech pathologists or classroom teachers. They may also be self-referred or discovered during voice disorder surveys.

Patients who refer themselves or who are referred by nonphysicians for therapy need to have laryngologic examinations either prior to voice evaluation or shortly thereafter. The physician, usually a laryngologist, rules out treatable illnesses or performs medical and surgical therapies to eliminate and correct laryngeal pathologic conditions. Typical referrals are patients who have had surgery of the vocal folds for the removal of benign or malignant lesions or those who have vocal fold paralyses. Some patients are referred because the laryngologist believes that they should be treated only with voice therapy in lieu of medical or surgical treatment, e.g., in cases of vocal nodule and contact ulcer. Patients with psychogenic voice disorders represent the largest group of referrals from laryngologists, who rarely treat these disorders. The physician has a deeply vested interest in the patient who has a voice disorder and does not wish to treat or rule out organic laryngeal disease, removing the threat of serious illness, only to see the patient leave the laryngologist's office with a bad voice. The speech pathologist becomes an important colleague of that physician in completing the treatment plan according to the total care philosophy.

The following are typical referral notes written from members of a department of otolaryngology to those of the department of speech pathology in a major medical clinic and hospital.

- Singer, speaker—says hoarseness for four months. Negative laryngeal examination.
- Voice therapy. Whispering after upper respiratory infection.
- Contact ulcer granuloma. Speech pathology evaluation.
- Weak voice for 17 years. Etiology? Therapy?
- Vocal nodules, large.
- Voice recording out. For Teflon injection.
- Voice evaluation. Hoarseness.
- Hysterical aphonia. Diagnosis and therapy.
- Dysphonia.
- Evaluation of increasing hoarseness and loss of voice when he speaks for a long time or attempts to sing.
- Paralyzed vocal cord.
- Evaluation and therapy. Patient had severe hypertrophic laryngitis. Quit smoking. Vocal cords have been stripped. Surgically looks good, but she still seems to be using false cords.
- Voice problem. Needs your advice and counsel.
- See ENT history. Laryngeal injury. Bowing of vocal cords. Psychogenic overlay?
- Dysphonia. Hysterical?
- Vocal cord nodules. Habitual throat-clearing in a 10-year-old boy.
- Speech pathology and therapy. Bilateral vocal cord nodules. Is preacher and sings loudly. Would appreciate your seeing him and therapy as necessary.
- Voice recording and consultation prior to vocal cord surgery for removal of polyp via direct laryngoscopy.
- Whispering. Please evaluate and therapy.
- Singer with pain in neck. Sounds like cramp. Vocal rehabilitation.
- Opinion re voice. Primary amyloidosis.
- Voice assessment and threatment. Eighteen-month history of stridorous breathing, hoarseness, apparent hyperventilation attacks. Dysphagia without weight loss. Negative bronchoscopy. Normal laryngologic examination.
- Child with hoarseness.
- Recording of her voice. Diplophonia. She has an established right vocal cord paralysis. We are investigating cause. Just wanted a record for teaching file.
- Fading voice.
- Voice therapy. Post-Teflon injection of vocal cord. Whispering. Had good voice on operating table after injection.

- Voice recording. Would like to present her case at rounds with photos and voice recording. She has had bilateral arytenoidectomies.
- Delightful lady with mild voice change. Needs many questions answered. Can you also discuss and advise?

Note that most of these referrals not only request voice therapy, but also ask for clarification of unexplained voice disorder findings, illustrating the demands that can be made on the voice specialist's diagnostic as well as therapeutic acumen.

Differential Diagnosis.   In medical centers that rely on subspecialty consultation, i.e., medical clinics, hospitals, and small group practices, where a close professional relationship between the speech pathologist and the laryngologist exists, the speech pathologist can help clarify the diagnostic significance of abnormal voice when the physician cannot find a cause. Because of a knowledge of the relationship between voice disorders and illness, the speech pathologist who has specialized in voice disorders can suggest certain diagnostic entities to the referring laryngologist or internist that will help them arrive at more accurate diagnoses.

Baseline Recordings.   Laryngologists are concerned about the medicolegal aspects of diagnoses and treatment of patients with laryngeal disease and may want to obtain preoperative and postoperative audio-recordings of the voice as documentation of changes due to medical, surgical, and voice therapies.

In his discussion of the legal pitfalls in laryngology, von Leden (1988) warned about the importance of documenting the voice before and after treatment.

> I have made it a rule to *record* the patient's *voice* before each elective surgical intervention. Weeks and months later patients and relatives often forget how hoarse the voice really was and a playback of the tape serves to refresh their memory. Simple acoustic measurements, such as the pitch range and the maximum phonation time, can be performed without any special equipment before and after the surgery.

Many laryngologists, either alone or in collaboration with speech pathologists, do research on voice that requires acoustic and biophysical voice studies. The speech pathologist refers voice patients to other specialists as well as receiving them, for example, patients who have not yet had a laryngologic examination or who, after voice evaluation, are found to need further medical or psychologic consultation.

Specialists in Medicine and Speech Pathology should take full advantage of referrals, communicating with one another as much as possible. Face-to-face discussions are best, telephone contact is next, and letters can be used as a last resort. The interdisciplinary teaching value of such consultations cannot be overstated. Collaborative workups and clinical case presentations at conferences in which medical and speech pathology examination results are integrated increase everyone's knowledge with ultimate benefits to the patient.

The Clinician's Mental Set.   A clear distinction needs to be made between *data collection* and *interpretation of findings*. Both are important, but one without the other will result in a less adequate examination. The order of evaluation procedures described next is not inviolable, but beginning clinicians ought to progress in an orderly fashion, perhaps using a checklist.

For differential diagnosis of voice disorders of unknown etiology, the speech pathologist needs to develop skepticism and independent thinking. The clinician must not take others' opinions for granted and should not be satisfied until the voice evaluation results are congruent with findings from medical and allied medical examinations. One should enter the clinical situation with an open mind, a "show-me" attitude. Although another clinician may have said "functional voice disorder," regardless of that person's reputation, one should never take the diagnosis for granted. *Misdiagnoses of voice disorders are common.* Clinicians who work in this field should be forewarned of this pitfall. During the evaluation, as many different etiologies as possible should be considered. One should try not to think of the voice disorder as an isolated phenomenon. For some reason voice specialists want to interpret everything that occurs during the examination in terms of just the voice or larynx, ignoring the possibility that the voice may be only a prominent sign of a more widespread involvement of the speech mechanism or of the entire organism. Before evaluation or therapy, the following checklist might be consulted.

- Are you ready for any contingency? Or is your mind already made up about the nature of the problem before you have investigated it? Are you prepared to meet any type of diagnostic unknown, simple or complex?
- Is your index of suspicion set at maximum sensitivity?
- Are you ready to challenge what others have said about the patient, based on your own findings?
- Are you in a flexible, creative state of mind, ready to try new things should you fail with the old?
- Is your office presentable and efficient?
- Is your electronic recording equipment ready to go?
- Do you have in mind a logical plan of action?
- Have you recently reviewed basic information on diagnosis of and therapy for voice disorders to refresh your memory regarding the meaning of discrete signs and symptoms?
- Have you read the medical record and other accompanying data for a total picture of the patient and the problem?
- Do you have a list of associates in Speech Pathology, Laryngology, and other medical specialties for purposes of referral or consultation, if necessary? Critical items on your checklist might be:
- Accepting other peoples' opinions too easily and missing an organic, particularly neurologic, dysphonia because you thought it was psychogenic.
- Failing to recognize a psychogenic voice disorder because you were prematurely convinced that it was organic.
- Emphasizing the voice aspects in diagnosis and therapy at the expense of background history, especially psychogenic factors.
- Failing to allow the patient sufficient opportunity to talk about feelings, attitudes, and experiences relating to the voice disorder.

Documenting Information.   Gaining control over the mechanics of data gathering can make the difference between a successful and a frustrating examination.

1. *Note-taking.* Developing a shorthand—writing down key items for later expansion—is probably the best way of preserving information. Writing places a barrier between patient and clinician, however. An alternative is to note routine data and stop writing when discussing personal matters, relying later on memory to record the details.

2. *Audiotaping.* An excellent way of acquiring patient data and accurately reproducing it later is to record part or all of the examination on audiotape. The main advantages of this technique are that it frees the clinician from note-taking to give full attention to the patient and affords the opportunity to review the evaluation later at leisure. Few patients object to continuous audio-recordings. The audio system should be in full view.

3. *Videotaping.* Videotape recordings can be valuable if visible signs accompany the voice disorder. Videotapes are excellent teaching media in speech pathology and medical school curricula. It is also valuable for clinician and patient to view them during therapy in order to obtain greater objectivity. However, unlike audio-recordings, patients are sometimes sensitive about being videotaped, and their permission should be explicitly asked. Many institutions require patients to sign permission forms. Videotape recordings should never be shown indiscriminately; the patient's rights of privacy must be protected as fully as possible.

The voice evaluation can be carried out in different ways; the following is not sacrosanct.

Phase I. History of the Voice Disorder

Familiarization Period.   A friendly relationship with the patient needs to be established from the point of initial contact. From early impressions, the clinician perceives the patient's reaction to a new situation and may find signs of tension, anxiety, or depression through facial expression, posture, gestures, and handshake. At the same time, the patient makes important judgments about the clinician: How interested the clinician is in seeing the patient; how secure, at ease, and skillful the clinician is in the interpersonal situation; in short, the kind of person with whom the patient is dealing. If confidence is generated early, the patient will find it easier to discuss personal history.

Basic Data.   Basic information consists of the following: patient's name; address; date of interview; telephone number; sex; birthdate; responsible party; place of birth; education; occupation; parent or guardian; siblings; martial status; spouse's name; name of referring agency; family physician; laryngologist; other concerned professionals. Such information can be obtained either during the initial phase of the interview or by completing a questionnaire prior to it.

Onset of the Voice Disorder.   "When and how did the voice trouble begin?" Patients find it difficult to establish precise onset of their voice disorders because most begin gradually rather than abruptly. Patients who give vague answers should be pressed as firmly as possible to think back to the month, or even time of day, when the voice disorder began. The most important question having to do with onset has considerable differential diagnostic importance: "Did the voice disorder begin *suddenly* or *gradually?" A change from normal voice to dysphonia or aphonia within minutes or hours almost invariably means a conversion voice disorder*. The only other possibility is stroke, but then the voice change will be almost invariably accompanied by dysarthria, apraxia, aphasia, or other neurologic signs. In contrast, organic voice disorders due to mass lesions of the vocal folds, degenerative neurologic diseases, musculoskeletal tension, and vocal abuse develop more gradually.

"Was the voice disorder accompanied by swallowing difficulties or nasal regurgitation of solids or fluids?" An affirmative answer raises suspicion of a neurologic etiology.

Previous Voice Disorders.   A history of previous dysphonia or aphonia having similar characteristics, history, and absence of laryngologic findings with spontaneous remissions, probably indicates nonorganic disease.

Time Course of the Voice Disorder.   "Has the voice disorder been present from the time of onset? Or have there been periods during which the abnormal voice returned to normal?" *Patients with nonorganic voice disorders due to musculoskeletal tension or conversion reactions will often report periods lasting from minutes to days when the voice returned to normal, only to worsen again. In contrast, patients with organic voice disorders due to either mass vocal fold lesions or neurologic disease will usually report continuously abnormal voice from time of onset, either remaining constant in severity or worsening gradually or precipitously*. Motor neuron degenerative diseases, such as amyotropic lateral sclerosis, are noted for this pattern of voice deterioration. In myasthenia gravis, worsening of the voice is related to prolonged speaking during which dysphonia and hypernasality may develop, only to improve after rest.

Two points need to be made concerning continuous deterioration versus periodic return of normal voice: (1) All voice disorders, regardless of etiology, worsen during physical fatigue and emotional stress. Therefore, the clinician should not presume that because of these fluctuations, the voice disorder is automatically psychogenic. (2) The clinician must be careful to elicit an exact statement about such episodes of "normalcy." What many patients originally describe as *normal* voice, upon further inquiry prove to be episodes of *improvement* only.

Events Associated with Onset.   (1) "Did the voice disorder begin with physical complaints of swallowing difficulty, nasal regurgitation, unusual changes in articulation, or flu-like episodes?" This question may determine the possibility of an acute or subacute neurologic episode. Abnormal voice can also be a sign of debilitation, fatigue, or anxiety resulting from general illness.

The clinician should be alert to the following trap: A history of laryngitis during upper respiratory infection which later disappeared leaving the dysphonia or aphonia. *Conversation voice disorders often begin with actual upper respiratory infections such as laryngitis or flu*. The laryngitis caused by the infection provides the psychologic rationale and trigger for the conversion voice disorder.

(2) *"Did the voice disorder begin in association with emotional problems?"* The importance of

this question transcends all others. A positive answer should arouse suspicion of either muscoloskeletal tension or a conversion voice disorder. This question needs to be asked of *every* person with a voice disorder, children and adults alike, and of their parents and relatives. Even when the ear, nose, and throat examination firmly establishes an organic voice disorder, the possibility of an intensifying psychogenic factor must be entertained.

Most people with primary psychogenic voice disorders or with secondary ones superimposed on organic disorders are notoriously unaware of causative emotional stress or interpersonal conflict. The mechanism of repression or denial is responsible, and clinicians beginning training in voice disorders need to be warned in advance of this common tendency. It is often responsible for bland emotional histories. Here are three common reactions to questions pertaining to emotional stress: (1) The patient steadfastly denies emotional or interpersonal problems associated with onset of the voice disorder. In such cases, the clinician should abandon the subject and return to it either later in the interview or following symptomatic voice therapy, perhaps saying, "It is often difficult for people to remember or to be aware of emotional problems, so we'll give you some time to think about it and return to it later." The probability that the patient will disclose a voice-related personal problem later in the interview or following therapy is high, so the clinician should not be discouraged by an early negative response. (2) Another type of patient, openly aware of definite emotional problems accompanying the voice disorder, immediately and sometimes eagerly produces a flood of pertinent emotional data. (3) A third is the patient who, despite repeated encouragement, vigorously and even angrily may deny any personal or emotional problems at all during interview and therapy. The meaning of this consistent denial is that either there are no problems or the patient's resistance and lack of insight are overwhelming. Later disclosure is unlikely.

The portion of the interview that has to do with investigation of personal problems, and, later, helping patients to understand the relationship between those problems and the voice disorder, requires counseling abilities. Because of its indispensability to the evaluation and treatment of voice disorders, a separate chapter on psychologic interviewing and counseling appears later in this book.

Events associated with onset of voice disorders suggesting progressive neurologic or systemic illness warrant further discussion. A finite number of organic illnesses begin insidiously with a voice change, and a few pointed questions can help include or exclude the possibility of their presence.

1. *Myasthenia gravis.* The following questions might help to elicit information as to the presence of this disease, discussed previously in the chapter on neurologic voice disorders. "Does your voice become noticeably worse after unusually brief periods of continuous speaking?" "Does your speech sound nasal or do you find it harder to move your lips, tongue, or jaw with prolonged talking?" "Have you noticed any double vision, drooping of your eyelids, or easy fatigability after exercise?" "Do you have an unusual feeling in your throat on swallowing, as if food gets stuck?" The complaint of uncomfortable swallowing raises an important differential diagnostic issue. Already noted is that the feeling of tightness and other discomfort in the throat, including swallowing, is common in the musculoskeletal tension accompanying psychogenic voice disorders. What is potentially confusing is that this complaint is also common in patients with bulbar myasthenia gravis. Consequently, tightness in the throat on swallowing in neurologic disease limited to dysphonia is often misdiagnosed as a psychogenic, functional, or conversion voice disorder. Tightness in the throat, then, is not automatically "globus hystericus."

2. *Motor neuron disease.* Because dysphonia can be the first sign of degenerative motor neuron diseases, such as amyotrophic lateral sclerosis, the clinician should ask about nasal regurgitation and difficulty in swallowing as well as in articulating.

3. *Endocrine disease.* Another insidious illness that can manifest itself initially through dysphonia is hypothyroidism or myxedema. Because this disease is so subtle that it can be missed by consecutive examiners, the clinician should inquire whether the voice disorder came on in association with: feeling continuously cold; keeping the temperature at home higher than before; needing to wear a sweater; complaint of change in facial configuration, namely puffiness around the eyes and a darkening of skin color; dryness of skin; loss of frontal hair; tiredness; increased sleeping during the day or at night; and possible mental confusion or slowness. Mild changes in articulatory precision should also be investigated. The clinician should inquire about the coincidental onset of any general illness that may have directly or indirectly caused general fatigue, and a dysphonia secondary to that fatigue. Any suspicion of a voice disorder related to systemic illness should be carefully noted, and arrangements should be made for patient referral for a general medical examination.

Vocal abuse is another important area of inquiry, especially if a laryngologic diagnosis of vocal nodule or contact ulcer has been made. However, even patients who do not have vocal fold lesions should be questioned, because their dysphonia may be in the early stages when the vocal folds are either free of lesions or only slightly inflamed. Children with vocal nodules should be interviewed alone if old enough to discuss their habits of voice use and questioned about frequency of yelling or screaming, or continuous talking at home, in the classroom, or on the playground. Because children with vocal nodules have a high incidence of associated personality, family, or school problems, investigation of the psychosocial aspects of the child's life is important. The same rule holds for adolescents and adults, although there is a higher incidence of vocal abuse secondary to singing in these age groups. However, even vocal nodules can occur for the first time in singers as a result of emotional stress. The clinician needs to know whether there had been any change in the patient's singing or speaking style prior to development of the vocal nodule. One might discover that during this period the patient had undergone emotional stress or physical fatigue.

Adult males with contact ulcer also should be questioned about vocal abuse; whether the style of voice use changed roughly coincidentally with the onset of the voice problem, and whether emotional stress was present. Patients who have vocal fold lesions secondary to vocal abuse often abuse their vocal folds in other ways, such as by inhalation of tobacco smoke, use of chemical irritants, alcohol consumption and esophageal reflux. Some laryngologists believe that the caffeine in coffee or tea has a drying-out effect on the vocal fold mucosa, contributing to irritation. Questions and observations about excessive coughing and throat clearing are important because of the mechanically damaging effects that these habits have on the vocal folds. A lesion, such as a vocal nodule and, especially, a contact ulcer, creates a feeling of a foreign body in the throat, prompting the patient to clear it out by coughing or throat clearing, thereby perpetuating the primary lesion.

For singers who have vocal nodules, concerns include the presence of loud musical accompaniment and singing at excessively high frequencies, inappropriate to the physical capabilities of the vocal folds. Whether or not patients with a contact ulcer use excessively low pitch for purposes of conveying greater authority should be determined.

Questions about style of voice use often reveal the patient's concept of how he or she ought to sound, i.e., the vocal self-image. Those who use their voices professionally often believe in the need for a deep, full, authoritative voice, and they phonate with a sharp glottal attack.

The following case study excerpt illustrates how the mechanics of voice use and abuse cannot be separated from the personality and life-style of the individual and how proper diagnosis and treatment are dependent upon understanding both.

* * *

A 27-year-old attorney began having increasing problems with hoarseness after assuming his responsibilities as district attorney for a metropolitan city. The ear, nose, and throat examination disclosed nonspecific laryngitis secondary to vocal abuse. His afternoons were spent talking across a noisy courtroom without a microphone using a low-pitched authoritative voice. "I don't exactly shout but I use my voice as a weapon. I've found that the more aggressive I am the more convictions I get. Friendliness toward the defense attorney or his client is definitely counterproductive. By the weekend, I'm completely exhausted and almost without a voice."

* * *

It is clear from this synopsis that the patient's concept of his role in the courtroom is actualized through his voice and that therapy will require teaching him that there are other ways of being intimidating than shouting down the opponent.

Phase II. The Voice Evaluation

Objectives of the voice evaluation are: (1) To describe the type and severity of the voice disorder for baseline purposes and reports. (2) To identify and interpret the abnormal voice for acoustic differential diagnosis. (3) To determine if the patient is a voice therapy candidate.

Audiotaping is usually sufficient for recording the voice, although videotape recordings are helpful for clinical teaching and for heightening patient awareness during therapy. The following acoustic and biophysical techniques usually are reserved for research purposes: acoustic spectrography, pneumotachography, respirometry, and electromyography. The trained ear and mind are, at present, the most useful instruments.

Voice Tests.   The following content is recorded:

1. *Contextual speech.* The patient reads a standard paragraph aloud into the microphone of the tape recorder. The clinician judges the overall severity of the voice disorder, rating aesthetic and intelligibility factors.

2. *Vowel prolongation.* The single most revealing voice test is to ask the patient to sustain the vowel /a/ as long and as steadily as possible. After repeatedly listening to vowel prolongations, the clinician rates the basic voice parameters: Quality, pitch, loudness, and steadiness. It is possible that all parameters will be normal. The voice may be breathy, giving the impression of rapid airflow through the glottis. It may have a certain quality of hoarseness. The voice may be strained, giving the examiner the impression that it is being forced through a constricted glottis. Loudness may be either reduced or excessive. The pitch may be excessively high or low. The clinician should determine the lowest pitch to which the voice is capable of descending, for some patients with organically low pitch have gotten into the habit of phonating at a slightly higher level to avoid revealing the lower pitch. Therefore, the patient should be asked to prolong vowels down to the lowest pitch possible. On vowel prolongation, rhythmic fluctuations or interruptions, as well as their frequency, should be noted. The patient's ability to sustain the vowel for a maximum period of time should be determined, and duration should be recorded in seconds as a measurement of either respiratory or glottal efficiency.

3. *Cough and sharp glottal attack.* One of the most useful tests for adductor vocal fold strength, especially in patients suspected of unilateral or bilateral vocal fold paralysis, is to have them cough as sharply as possible, and produce a vowel using the sharpest glottal attack possible (glottal coup). Patients who have normal adductor strength will produce these sounds with a sharp or abrupt onset. Patients who have mild true cord weakness will produce a normal or nearly normal explosive cough, because the false, as well as the true, vocal folds are contracted during this gross action, obscuring mild true vocal fold weakness. But, the glottal coup in such cases will reveal the weakness, because only the true vocal folds are adducted. In moderate to severe adductor vocal fold weakness both the cough and glottal coup will range from a slight loss of sharpness to "mushiness" to complete absence of momentary interruption of the airstream.

4. *Pitch range.* The patient should be asked to sing a scale as high up as possible and down as low as possible to determine if the pitch range has become restricted.

5. *Endurance.* In order to determine the capacity for maintenance of the muscular strength of the respiratory, phonatory, resonatory, and articulatory systems, the patient is asked to count vigorously to at least 100, with the clinician noting any appreciable deterioration of phonation, velopharyngeal closure, or articulation.

6. *Motor speech examination.* A routine motor speech evaluation of the entire peripheral speech mechanism should be performed for the detection of dysarthria, of which the dysphonia in question may be a component.

7. *Musculoskeletal tension testing.* Four criteria should be used to determine the presence of dysphonia-related musculoskeletal tension.
   a. Pain. In Figure 13–1a are several anatomic points on the larynx and hyoid bone that are either unilaterally or bilaterally painful in response to pressure or kneading, indicating chronic laryngeal muscle tension. The patient may also volunteer that pain radiates up to the ears or down to the sternum and upper chest.
   b. Elevation of larynx and hyoid bone. The thyroid cartilage and hyoid bone are elevated in

Voice Severity: 1   2   3   4   5   6   7

Yes _____   No _____

Length of sustained "ah" _____

<table>
<tr><td>LARYNGEAL CAVITY
PITCH
HIGH</td><td>RESONATING CAVITY
NASALITY
HYPERNASAL</td></tr>
</table>

```
              LARYNGEAL CAVITY              RESONATING CAVITY
                    PITCH                        NASALITY
                    HIGH                         HYPERNASAL

                     B                              C

                                                   + 4
                    + 3                            + 3
                    + 2                            + 2
A open  − 4  − 3  − 2     1   + 2   + 3 closed       1
                    − 2                            − 2
                    − 3
                    LOW                         HYPONASAL
```

Constant _____ Rate   Intensity   Vocal Range

Variable _____ − 2 1 + 2   − 2 1 + 2   − 2 1   + 2
                   Slow   Fast   Soft   Loud   Monotone   Variable
                                                             Pitch

Figure 10–2 The voice profile. (*From* Wilson, F.B., The voice-disordered child: A descriptive approach. Language Speech and Hearing Services in Schools, No. 4, 1970.)

the neck, and the width of the thyrohyoid space is diminished. The tongue musculature may be elevated while the patient holds the mouth open with the tongue at rest. Another indicator of tension or rigidity of the larynx and hyoid bone is resistance to displacement either laterally, superiorly, or anteroposteriorly.

   c. Voice improvement. As the clinician works the larynx and hyoid bone downward in the neck while kneading painful areas, the voice improves. (Figure 13–1b)

8. *Optimum pitch.* Certain patients are dysphonic because they are unconsciously or consciously making an effort to lower their voice pitch. The "Umhum" test (Cooper, 1973) was designed to determine the presence of excessively low pitch by asking the patient to make this utterance as spontaneously as possible, as if casually signifying agreement. The pitch of the voice will rise, dysphonia will clear, and "amplification," or increased resonance in the nasal area, will be felt and heard if, in fact, the voice pitch has been excessively low.

The Voice Profile.   A simple method of documenting abnormal voice in children and adults was devised by Wilson (1970) and is called the Voice Profile (Fig. 10–2).

Severity Rating.   In the section called "Voice Severity," in the upper right-hand corner, a rating of "1" means that the problem is barely perceptible; a "7" means that it significantly interferes with communication. This judgment has an effect on the decision to provide therapy and on the determination of progress during therapy.

Sustained /a/. The length of time that an individual can sustain this tone is related to laryngeal efficiency, provides an acceptable measure of air loss during phonation, and can indicate an obstruction of vocal fold closure.

In the figure, the horizontal line "A" deals with the open and closed positions of the vocal folds. At the extreme left, −4 means that the folds are totally open: The glottis is nonrestrictive of the airflow, and the individual produces little, if any, friction noise, i.e., aphonia. To the extreme right of line "A," +3 represents extreme tension, hyperadduction, or obstruction, the individual being unable to sustain normal vocal fold vibration, e.g., adductor spastic dysphonia. Between these extremes, moving from left to right, −3 represents a step toward narrowing of the glottis. Breathiness is represented by −2, and generally is characterized by turbulence and some friction. A normal voice is represented by 1, or the center point of line "A." The +2 side represents a voice characterized by much tension. The individual maintains vibratory motion, but has voice characteristics that give the listener the impression of vocal strain.

Laryngeal Cavity. The vertical line "B" labeled "Laryngeal Cavity" deals with pitch. Neither end of line "B," marked +3 at the high side and −3 at the low side, represents a fixed pitch. Rather, they denote those pitches that are sufficiently deviant to cause the individual to lose sexual identity, if this judgment is made on voice alone. Pitch levels at these extremes are rarely heard in children. The −2 and +2 represent deviations of pitch that cause concern primarily on the part of the critical listener, usually the speech clinician. They rarely cause the person social anxiety.

Resonating Cavity. Under the section "Resonating Cavity," Line "C," −2 represents the voice that lacks nasal resonance during the production of normally nasalized sounds. One represents normal, +2 represents assimilation nasality, +3 represents nasalization of vowels, with some shading of a nasal nature to the consonants, and +4 represents nasality of all sounds, with frequent nasal distortions of consonant sounds.

At the bottom of the figure, there are three additional components of voice: *rate, intensity,* and *vocal range.* In addition, at the bottom left-hand side, the clinician should check "variable" or "constant," referring to the existence of the deviation over time and under differing conditions.

Another method of documenting the results of the voice evaluation is to use the Buffalo Voice Profile (Wilson, 1979) (Fig. 10–3).

The skilled clinician learns not to go on a "fishing expedition" or to use the "shotgun approach," bombarding the patient with every question and test ever devised. Such a frontal attack on the voice disorder is a phase through which everyone passes before learning to isolate important clues and to follow them directly to the correct diagnosis. The efficient and knowledgeable clinician structures the interview and examination in such a way as to obtain the most information in the shortest time.

Phase III. Interpretation of Findings

After case history and voice examination data have been accumulated, they must be interpreted. The following list is not exhaustive.

1. *The type and severity of abnormal voice should be congruent with the size and position of vocal fold lesions or paralyses.* If such is the case, the dysphonia, in all likelihood, is purely organic. However, if the dysphonia is of greater severity or different in character than warranted by the lesion, a psychogenic component is strongly suspected. For example, a patient who has small bilateral vocal nodules should not be severely breathy or aphonic.

2. *The patient who neither phonates nor articulates in all likelihood has a conversion voice disorder.*

3. *The patient who whispers with or without transient laryngeal noises in whom the remainder of the peripheral speech mechanism is normal in all likelihood has a conversion reaction.* An important confirmatory sign is the patient's *ability to produce a sharp cough or glottal coup*

Name_____ Birth Date_____ Age_____ Sex_____

Rater _____ Date _____ Time of Day _____ Place _____

1. *Laryngeal Tone*							
Normal							
Breathy							
Harsh							
Hoarse	1	2	3	4	5	6	7
2. *Laryngeal Tension*							
Normal							
Hypertense							
Hypotense	1	2	3	4	5	6	7
3. *Vocal Abuse*							
No							
Yes	1	2	3	4	5	6	7
4. *Loudness*							
Normal							
Too loud							
Too soft	1	2	3	4	5	6	7
5. *Pitch*							
Normal							
High							
Low	1	2	3	4	5	6	7
6. *Vocal Inflections*							
Normal							
Monotone							
Excessive	1	2	3	4	5	6	7
7. **Pitch Breaks**							
None							
Amount	1	2	3	4	5	6	7
8. **Diplophonia**							
None							
Amount	1	2	3	4	5	**6**	**7**
9. *Resonance*							
Normal							
Hypernasal							
Hyponasal	1	2	3	**4**	**5**	**6**	**7**
10. *Nasal Emission*							
No							
Yes	1	2	3	**4**	**5**	6	7
11. *Rate*							
Normal							
Fast							
Slow	1	2	3	4	5	6	7
12. *Overall Voice Efficiency*							
Adequate							
Inadequate	1	2	3	4	5	6	7

Circle the appropriate descriptive term under *each* item. For each item *not* normal or adequate, circle a number on the scale for that item. Do *not* mark between numbers.
Key: 1 = slight deviation   4 = moderate deviation   7 = severe deviation
COMMENTS:

Figure 10–3 The Buffalo Voice Profile. (*From* Wilson, D.K., Voice Problems of Children, 2nd ed. Baltimore, Williams & Wilkins, 1979, p. 68.)

voluntarily or spontaneously, showing fundamentally normal adductor strength for glottal closure. As discussed in the chapter on neurologic voice disorders, patients having neurologic lesions of the Xth cranial nerve above the branching of the superior laryngeal nerve are also aphonic, but instead of a sharp cough or glottal coup, theirs is *weak or absent.*

4. The patient whose voice is breathy may have either an organic or a psychogenic dysphonia. *Incongruously severe breathiness in the presence of normal vocal fold adduction on examination and on coughing suggests psychogenic dysphonia.* The absence of motor speech signs elsewhere in the peripheral speech mechanism is further support of a psychogenic etiology. However, peripheral nerve disease can surface in the form of breathiness. The clinician should be particularly suspicious of myasthenia gravis and should administer the stress test of counting, listening for worsening of the dysphonia. Other motor speech signs, specifically hypernasality and articulatory imprecision, may also appear. At the point of maximum deterioration after stressful speaking, the cough or glottal coup is weakest. The voice improves with the administration of Tensilon (edrophonium chloride).

5. *A strained hoarse or harsh voice quality can be due to either a mass lesion, neurologic* *diseases, or psychogenicity.* Motor speech signs elsewhere in the peripheral speech mechanism may indicate pseudobulbar (spastic) dysphonia as a component of dysarthria. Intermittency, or waxing and waning of the strained-strangled hoarseness in the absence of other motor speech signs, may indicate one of the following.

a. One form of adductor spastic dysphonia, in which case vowel prolongation is likely to be clear, especially at higher pitches.

b. The essential (voice) tremor syndrome in which, on vowel prolongation, there are rhythmic voice arrests or interruptions within the range of 5 to 12 c/sec.

c. A dystonic or choreic movement disorder of which intermittent strained-strangled voice quality can be a component; however, associated motor speech signs are usually present.

6. Patients who have hypoadduction of the vocal folds for either organic or psychogenic reasons, manifesting breathiness to aphonia, will have an attendant reduction in the loudness of the voice. The same is true for patients who have hyperadduction of the vocal folds, which are squeezed together so tightly that voice is diminished. Reduced loudness of voice in and of itself, therefore, is not differentially diagnostic. However, parkinsonism should always be considered in patients with diminished loudness.

7. *Excessive loudness* of voice is uncommon and may be a sign of either sensorineural hearing loss or severe ataxic dysarthria.

8. *Excessively high pitch* is most commonly a psychogenic voice sign associated with musculoskeletal tension, conversion reaction, or mutational falsetto. The voice quality of mutational falsetto is different from that found with musculoskeletal tension or a conversion reaction. It is thin and breathy, possibly with elements of hoarseness, and has a low volume. The voice will break to a normally low pitch on phonation when using a sharp glottal attack.

9. *Excessively low pitch* is most often found in organic voice disorders. In structural or mass lesions, excessively low pitch and hoarseness occur together. Low pitch is also common in patients with unilateral vocal fold paralysis, pseudobulbar dysphonia, organic voice tremor, or the mixed dysarthria of amyotrophic lateral sclerosis.

10. *Rhythmic voice tremor or rhythmic voice arrests* on vowel prolongation, not always evident in contextual speech, can be a sign of an essential (voice) tremor. Intermittent, momentary voice arrests on vowel prolongation, not usually heard during contextual speech, may be a sign of laryngeal myoclonus, a component of the palatopharyngolaryngeal myoclonus syndrome. They occur at a rate of 1 to 4/sec. Rhythmic movements of the larynx, soft palate, pharynx, and sometimes of the tongue, at rest, are further manifestations of this syndrome.

11. *Shortened vowel prolongation or short phrases* during contextual speech can be due to hypoadduction of the vocal folds for either organic or psychogenic reasons, causing breathy air escape and an increased volume/velocity of airflow. Reduced vital capacity due to neurologic or pulmonary disease also requires an increased frequency of respiration in order to produce speech.

Severe hyperadduction of the vocal folds often requires such a great physical effort to force air through the constricted glottis that some patients will exhale suddenly after an initial try at phonation, thus reducing the phonation time.

12. *Weak cough or glottal attack* on a vowel is usually a result of unilateral or bilateral adductor vocal fold paralyses or paresis, worse when bilateral than unilateral.

13. *Inability to traverse the musical scale,* although common in normal voices, can signify cricothyroid muscle weakness. Monopitch in pseudobulbar dysarthria, in hypokinetic (parkinsonian) dysarthria, and, to varying degrees, in the remaining dysarthrias is common.

14. *Extreme, uncontrolled fluctuations in pitch* are rare. They can occur in mutational falsetto, musculoskeletal and conversion voice disorders, and sometimes in cases of uncontrollable respiratory-phonatory movements associated with ataxic dysarthria.

15. *Pain in the region of the larynx and hyoid bone in response to digital pressure, or mentioned by the patient, is strongly indicative of a psychogenic voice disorder caused by either musculoskeletal tension or a conversion reaction.* Other clues are an elevated position of the larynx and hyoid bone; difficulty in moving the larynx laterally, superiorly, inferiorly, or anteroposteriorly; and audible improvement in voice with downward pressure and kneading in the region of the larynx and hyoid bone. Spontaneous complaints of pain localized to one or both sides of the larynx, radiating up to the ears or down to the chest, or of a feeling of a lump or ball in the throat (globus) are signs of increased laryngeal musculoskeletal tension.

A final note on the interpretation of abnormal voice in a clinical environment: The voice during clinical diagnosis is usually not representative of the voice in the real world. Immensely susceptible to psychologic stress and physical fatigue, the severity of voice signs can fluctuate widely in daily life. Such knowledge will aid in realistic diagnosis and assessment of the effects of therapy.

Phase IV. *Making Decisions*

After completing the case history, voice evaluation, and data interpretation, the speech pathologist needs to decide on a course of action. The following are components of the decision-making process.

Consult. When in doubt about unexplainable or unclear findings, one should consult colleagues in Speech Pathology, Medicine, and Psychology.

Write. A complete written report for the speech pathologist's files is necessary. When appropriate, a concise letter to the referring physician describing the findings should be written.

Confer. Following the evaluation, a conference with the patient and family should be held.

1. Unless he is a young child who would be unable to understand, the patient wants and has a right to know the cause of the voice disorder prior to therapy. Adults initially fear that their voice disorder is caused by malignancy, and reassurance by the laryngologist, reinforced by the speech pathologist, that such is not the case relieves these anxieties.

Patients who have musculoskeletal or conversion voice disorders are the most difficult to convince that their disorder is psychogenic. To them, their severe dysphonia or aphonia, and especially the feelings of tension, pain, and obstruction, seem to argue for the presence of some kind of lesion. Reassurance that the ear, nose, and throat examination disclosed no such disease is necessary. The problem for the speech clinician then becomes one of explaining to the patient the effects of emotion on muscle tension and control. Many patients accept such explanations. Others do not, not because they disbelieve that the larynx is structurally normal, but because they cannot accept the idea that their voice disorders develop from emotional causes.

2. Discuss therapy plans. Once patients understand the mechanism of the voice disorder, some express interest in obtaining help, whereas others do not. The degree of their concern is roughly proportional to the severity of the voice disorder. There are, however, patients with mild voice disorders who are intensely concerned about therapy, but others with severe disorders are not. The utility of the voice in everyday life and degree of ego investment in the voice are usually determining factors.

The patient should be told what, if anything, can be done to improve the voice, and the outlook for partial or total recovery. Information concerning the duration, frequency, and cost of therapy should be given. Frequently, patients will ask what exactly is done in therapy. Clear, straightforward answers to these questions will benefit both clinician and patient. Patients with voice disorders should never be pressured into therapy. Once they have the information, they should be told that they have the right to accept or reject the therapy, and that it is not necessary to decide during the interview. Where children are concerned, parents should realize that they, too, will have to be involved.

Referral to Other Specialists.   Initiation of therapy may be premature if, in the clinician's judgment, the patient needs to be seen by other consultants in order to resolve unanswered questions or problems. For example, therapy for patients with unilateral vocal fold paralysis may need to be deferred until a decision has been made about the value of Teflon injection of the vocal fold.

One should not hesitate to refer patients to other speech pathologists or to consult with them. Voice disorders is a field in which considerable experience is necessary before the specialist begins to feel comfortable with all cases. Continuing education about voice disorders is necessary, and a valuable educational experience is to spend time at the elbow of an otolaryngologist observing ear, nose, and throat examinations as often as possible, matching abnormal voices with the laryngoscopic findings, discussing cases with the laryngologist, reading laryngologic textbooks and journals, and attending laryngology conferences. One should learn the vocabulary of Laryngology and understand the problems that confront the laryngologist in daily practice. Only through these activities will one feel comfortable with voice disorders. The speech specialist should realize that he or she has an important contribution to make to voice diagnosis and rehabilitation, and that the laryngologist also wants the best voice possible for the patient.

> The surgeon's voice on the telephone, usually well-modulated, could not conceal his concern. In his office was a patient on whom he had performed a thyroidectomy, who now had unilateral vocal fold paralysis, and who required voice therapy. Could he send the patient to my office? What he had not told me was that the patient, the president of an engineering firm, was furious. A large man, 67 years old, he had red hair and a freckled face, a ruddy complexion, and was obviously in excellent physical condition. When I asked him to tell me about his voice trouble, he let loose with a tirade of disgust over his voice. No one had told him that this could happen! How could he conduct board meetings? He could barely be heard at cocktail parties! People looked at him peculiarly! Worst of all, he feared losing his pilot's license because of not being understood during radio communications with air traffic controllers. Perhaps, he said, he ought to sue. Finally, he calmed down, looked up and grinned, "Now what can you do about my voice?"

SUMMARY

1. Mirror laryngoscopy is the most common method of examining the interior of the larynx. Direct laryngoscopy, radiography, laryngography, and videofluoroscopy are used for more specialized studies.

2. The voice evaluation is performed in order to determine whether the patient is a candidate for voice therapy, to assist the laryngologist in differential diagnosis of the voice disorder, for baseline recordings, and for research documentation.

3. The voice evaluation should be conducted according to an organized but flexible plan and should be undertaken with an open mind. The evaluation can be divided into several phases: (1) history of the disorder, (2) voice evaluation, (3) interpretation of findings, and (4) making decisions.

4. In taking a history, the clinician obtains information on the duration of the voice disorder, rate of onset, time course, and physical and emotional illness that may have been associated with its onset.

5. The actual voice evaluation should include tape recordings of the voice during contextual speech and vowel prolongation. Testing for musculoskeletal tension is indispensable in the voice evaluation. Abnormal vocal parameters are rated by the examiner.

6. When interpreting findings, the clinician must determine whether the voice disorder is congruous with the laryngologic examination, and the extent to which it is consistent with either an organic, psychogenic, or mixed etiology.

7. Following the examination, the clinician consults with others, writes reports, and confers with the patient and family concerning impressions of the voice disorder, recommendations for therapy, or referral to other specialists.

SUGGESTIONS FOR ADDITIONAL READING

Markus, J.F., and Konrad, H.R.: The right-angle laryngeal telescope in undergraduate medical education. Arch. Otolaryngol., 108:344–346, 1982.

McFarlane, S.C., and Lavarato, A.S.: The use of video endoscopy in the evaluation and treatment of dysphonia. Commun. Disord., 9:No. 8, 1984.

Wilson, D.K.: Voice Problems of Children. Baltimore, Williams & Wilkins, 1979.
    See section on evaluation of the child's voice.

REFERENCES

Cooper, M.: Modern Techniques of Vocal Rehabilitation. Springfield, Il., Charles C Thomas, 1973.
Klein, H.C.: Routine telescopic laryngoscopy. Am. Family Physician, 11:86–89, 1975.
von Leden, H.: Legal Pitfalls in Laryngology. J. Voice, 2:330–333, 1988.
Wilson, D.K.: Voice Problems of Children. Baltimore, Williams & Wilkins, 1979.
Wilson, F.B.: The voice-disordered child: A descriptive approach. Lang. Speech Hear. Serv. Sch., 1:1970.

Chapter Eleven

RATIONALE

THE SPEECH PATHOLOGIST AS A PERSON

INDICATORS OF PERSONALITY GROWTH

RECOGNITION OF PSYCHOPATHOLOGY

The Obsessive Patient
The Hysterical Patient
The Depressive Patient

PSYCHOLOGIC INTERVIEWING AND COUNSELING FOR VOICE DISORDERS

A quiet hour spent in discussing the problems of the patient will help much to remove anxieties and restore vocal function.

—Brodnitz

RATIONALE

During the question-and-answer period following the presentation of a paper on voice therapy for transsexualism at a national convention, the speaker had emphasized how, in addition to changing the patient's pitch, inflection, and vocabulary, she found it necessary to provide psychologic support for the identity problems that vexed her patient, who was going through a profound life change. A young student's hand tentatively rose, and with a voice and frowning expression that clearly communicated her perplexity, she asked, "But . . . are . . . we . . . psychologists?" In that single question dwelt all the ambiguity, ambivalence, and uncertainty that has characterized the profession's stance on the question of the responsibility for knowing and practicing psychologic interviewing and counseling with patients who have communicative disorders. The predominant school of thought has been to avoid the subject, narrowly defining the clinician's field of practice as the retraining of vocal habit patterns. The other believes it impossible to treat people who have voice disorders without weaving into therapy the personal and technical skills of the psychiatrist, psychologist, and social worker. Any in-depth study of voice disorders forces us to conclude that so long as clinicians obtain privileged information from patients; so long as people have voice problems because of life stress and interpersonal conflict; so long as voice disorders produce anxiety, depression, embarrassment, and self-consciousness; so long as patients need a sympathetic person with whom they can discuss their distress, will speech pathologists need to consider their training incomplete *until they have learned the basic skills of psychologic interviewing and counseling.* Most psychogenic voice disorders, particularly of the conversion type, are unlikely to improve without a proper balance between direct voice therapy and psychotherapeutic discussion.

As a psychiatrist, Kolb (1971), wrote:

> Today the interview is used by members of all the professions directly concerned with sustaining or improving mental health . . . All are confronted with the abnormal from time to time. All elicit information concerning personality traits and symptoms that are distressing to the patient. All, too, must conduct themselves in such a way as to establish the compassionate understanding of the problem revealed to them by the person being interviewed.

Speech pathologists who treat patients with voice disorders require interviewing and counseling skills to aid them in determining the presence of emotional factors and the extent to which they are instrumental in causing or perpetuating voice disorders. They must recognize patients who are in need of professional psychodiagnostic and psychotherapeutic help when their emotional problems overshadow their voice disorders or when the emotional aspect needs to be managed before the voice disorder can be treated. If the speech pathologist has neither the skills to bring out the voice

259

patient's troubles nor enough knowledge to recognize serious emotional illness, a disservice is done to the patient. Stated clearly and unequivocally, speech pathologists are not being advised to conduct psychotherapy except for obtaining background information and relieving acute distress by providing psychologic support. Its purpose is the *diagnosis of voice disorders, and the identification and referral* of voice patients to psychiatrists, psychologists, and other mental health specialists.

In a study by Butcher et al. (1987) an attempt was made to determine the value of the speech pathologist functioning as a psychotherapist in collaboration with the clinical psychologist in patients who were unable to respond to speech therapy alone. The authors concluded that psychotherapy as a treatment for psychogenic voice disorders was able to achieve a 50 percent success rate in patients for whom voice therapy alone had been unsuccessful, and that a psychotherapeutic model for patients with psychogenic voice disorders with the speech pathologist and the psychologist working as co-therapists was highly workable in treating psychogenic voice disorders that had not responded to traditional approaches. They discovered that speech pathologists using psychotherapeutic techniques in patients who had psychogenic voice disorders achieved in their patients improved voice and positive psychologic changes.

After discovering a considerable divergence of training, attitudes, and practice in the treatment of patients with psychogenic voice disorders in the United Kingdom, Elias et al. (1989) decided to survey 244 practicing speech clinicians to determine their current opinions and practices in the diagnosis and treatment of psychogenic voice disorders and whether or not they thought they were properly educated to deal effectively with this population. In their survey they paid particular attention to preparation in psychology and psychiatry and their experiences in relating to these professions within the framework of voice disorders. What they found was that:

1. About 75 percent of speech clinicians surveyed said they always treated psychogenic dysphonia or aphonia when patients were referred to them.
2. Asked how confident they were in their understanding and treatment of these disorders, 4 percent said they always were, 58 percent that they usually were, 33 percent said some of the time, and 5 percent never.
3. About 75 percent of the clinicians said that their patients usually improved.
4. A variety of treatment techniques was used by the population surveyed, the main ones being relaxation, voice exercises, and counseling. A minority of clinicians used a diversity of psychologic techniques.
5. The clinicians expressed the opinion that they could expect more improvement from psychogenic dysphonic patients than aphonic ones.
6. Although voice exercises, breathing, and relaxation methods were taught at the undergraduate level, psychologic techniques were more likely to have been learned subsequently.

The observation that counselling was much more freely advocated than taught corresponded with comments that it was important, and not as extensively taught as needed. About 70% would still welcome further training in the treatment of voice disorders from a clinically involved psychologist or psychiatrist, and a number of respondents felt that more post-qualification courses should be available than there are at present.

7. Over 75 percent of the respondents considered their undergraduate course in psychology and psychiatry as "mainly theoretical."
8. Only 15 percent rated their psychology lectures as related to their voice disorders lectures, the remainder equally divided between those who perceived little relationship and none at all.
9. Referral of patients with psychogenic voice disorders to a psychologist or psychiatrist was practiced by 74 percent of the respondents, of whom 42 percent felt uncertain as to when to refer. Over 75 percent would have liked better access to a psychologist or psychiatrist but indicated that a barrier to cooperation with these professions was their limited interest in voice disorders.

Based on their survey, the authors concluded that there is no reason to dispute the textbook advice that patients with psychogenic aphonia and dysphonia should be treated by speech pathologists and that improvement usually follows. They expressed their support for the concept that therapy for psychogenic voice disorders should not be addressed solely to the voice itself, quoting Greene (1972):

Recovery of voice, however, is not the sole aim of treatment. Therapy must aim at removing or alleviating the cause and obtaining better adjustment of the patient to his difficulties by gaining some insight into the connection between the voice symptom and the precipitating factors.

In their discussion of the results of this survey the authors concluded:

It is, therefore, important that any speech therapist* treating psychogenic voice disorders, which are not uncommon, should have psychological skills, and a clear idea when cooperation with, or referral to, a different specialist would be the best course. In this context it is disappointing that . . . education in psychology and psychiatry is perceived as remote from everyday practice. Moreover, many speech therapists have found it necessary to acquire important psychological skills after qualification.

The education of speech therapists should always incorporate counseling and other relevant psychological skills. These are already taught in some centres. This would provide a welcome application of the theory and an appropriate preparation for current practice. Speech therapists should be prepared before qualification for undertaking joint therapy with a psychologist or psychiatrist, since this is not a rare undertaking when there is an interested person available. Post-qualification courses are essential to enable therapists already in practice to acquire the psychological skills they have found they require.

It is difficult to convince others how deeply voice disorders strike at the heart of the patient's total being and how special voice is in the average person's emotional and intellectual life. Always impressive is how chronic voice disorders can jar loose even the most stable personality. The following letter was written by a college professor who had had recurrent laryngeal nerve resection for adductor spastic dysphonia. She was having intermittent difficulties during the postsurgical voice stabilization period, and she wrote this letter to a fellow patient with similar voice adjustment problems.

*   *   *

I was reliving a night about 15 months after my surgery when I read of your recent frustrations. I had been getting along beautifully off and on but then I had about four or five days in succession when my voice sounded like a scratchy whisper. I just *knew* that the worst possible was happening—that my remaining vocal cord was giving out and that I would become voiceless. [This was her erroneous interpretation of the facts.] I was actually crying one night at 9:00 p.m., filled with fear and the phone rang. My husband answered. The call was for me. It was [the speech pathologist] calling to check how I was getting along. Can you imagine getting a call at that hour? Well, I poured out my fears to him and a very noticeable softness and quietness became evident in *his* voice. He told me that he had never heard of anyone losing the use of the second vocal cord. In that quiet voice that sounded as if he were suffering with me because of my fears, he gave me a great amount of strength by telling me not to worry about it—that he didn't know what I was experiencing what I was going through but that he felt sure that within a short time my voice would be back to what it had been in the weeks before this very frightening period. The assurance, the calming effect, the knowing that he was *concerned* about me after so long a time was the best medicine that I could have had. And do you know what? The very next morning my voice was back! I can't explain it. Unless the horrible fear of truly losing the ability to speak caused the voice to be worse than it really needed to be.

I think we must both be concerned too much with how we *sound* to others. Even yet I am very self-conscious of how I sound to others much of the time. I *am* getting better. Sometimes I actually forget about my voice quality, but most of the time I hear my voice as something less than what I would desire if I had a chance. But I am so thankful for what I have that I don't know why I can't do as you suggest—talk as I do with what I have and forget about what people think about it.

My voice has been strong for the most part during the Christmas holidays. But today it is thick, as though there is a fog within me. I dreaded answering the phone a while ago. Frustrating. I don't know *why* our voices fluctuate so. Frankly, I do not believe that you should quit your job. You see, since I teach, I have three months in the summer when I don't teach. *My voice has the same periods of fluctuation then as it has when I teach.* I think *life* itself causes our bodies to change. For a normally healthy person without the voice problem that we have, these changes are not evident as they are in us. And in the summer when I am not working and under no stress

---

*"Speech therapist" is the official term used in the United Kingdom.

and strain, I will have my days of *bad voice.* On my bad days my voice sounds thick, sort of gravelly, and has very little volume. When I try increasing the volume, some of my sounds come out as air instead of audible sounds. Frustrating? I can't tell you how very much. And of course that just makes it all the worse. But why wouldn't I be frustrated when I am lecturing to college students and my voice comes out in a stupid-sounding way. But the point is that it happens on weekends, in the summer, during Christmas vacation, etc.

Does your voice carry in a large supermarket? Does your voice perform normally in any large area? Mine doesn't. I need walls for the voice to bounce off of, it seems. My voice is always much better in a small room. Nearly all my classes are conducted in rooms that can accommodate 30 people. When I teach in a larger room, I have to work harder. However, I found out just very recently that even when my voice seemingly has very little volume, it has something that causes it to "carry" much better than one would have reason to hope for. But in a noisy large area such as a supermarket, a listener has to come quite close to me to hear what it is I am saying. And I have a lot of trouble talking to the supermarket clerk when I am being checked out. When they talk to me and ask me something, I answer, but they have problems hearing me. I feel very embarrassed, hurt and frustrated at such times.

Now, after all that complaining, I must quickly say that I am so *thankful* for having had the surgery, for having the ability to talk *without that horrible strain* that I had prior to surgery, for being able to function well enough to be able to keep my teaching job. It still is the best thing that ever happened to me.

* * *

The reasons that the speech pathologist should be trained in psychologic interviewing and counseling are the following.

1. The high incidence of psychologic causes and effects of voice disorders requires that these factors be investigated so that they may be understood and dealt with.

2. Improvement or even disappearance of the voice disorder is common during the patient's disclosure of interpersonal problems.

3. Parcelling out the patient with a voice disorder to psychological personnel in order to obtain basic personal data and to manage less critical emotional problems is impractical.

4. Patients who have psychogenic voice disorders relate better to a psychologically oriented speech pathologist (one not officially defined as a mental health specialist), during the initial phases of evaluation and therapy than to a psychologist or psychiatrist because voice patients tend to reject such referrals. The speech pathologist leads the patient into areas of psychologic sensitivity and gradually educates the patient about the need for professional counseling. Such an approach has salvaged many patients who otherwise would have become offended and who would have rejected premature referral to mental health personnel.

5. Many voice disorders are caused by mild, transient interpersonal problems and not by life-long psychoneuroses. These patients are not a danger to themselves or to others. They can be safely and conveniently managed by speech pathologists trained in psychologic interviewing and counseling.

6. In clinics in which speech pathologists have easy access to laryngologists, psychiatrists, and psychologists, the risk of encountering trouble dealing with the emotional problems of voice patients is practically eliminated.

7. The interviewing and counseling skills learned by speech pathologists increase their self-understanding and their understanding of others. It teaches how to ask questions and how to deal effectively with people in trouble.

THE SPEECH PATHOLOGIST AS A PERSON

The most important ingredient in successful interviewing and counseling is the speech pathologist as a person. Clinicians who communicate best with people with problems have the following traits.

1. *The clinician whose orientation to life and to others is one of equanimity and acceptance.* Voice patients come from different cultural, educational, and economic backgrounds, talk differently, look different, and harbor beliefs and habits of unimaginable varieties, many contrary to the clinician's. If one is by nature hypercritical and threatened by such behaviors, although not verbally disapproving, it will nevertheless be communicated in other ways. Consequently, we must learn to accept patients' habits and ideas as belonging to them, separate from our own, and we must deal with patients within a framework of their life orientation.

2. *The clinician who responds to personal information with understanding and encouragement;* one who provides an atmosphere in which the patient perceives that the clinician is interested and concerned.

3. *The clinician who knows how to ask questions.* The speech pathologist must ask questions that will encourage the patient to free-associate. "Tell me about your family, your work, your relationships." Speech pathologists should interrupt only when the patient seriously strays off the track or skirts personal data, reciting names, dates, and places, thereby avoiding disclosure of personal information. The clinician's objective is to elicit how the patient *feels,* not just a recitation of events.

4. *The clinician who knows how to listen.* We must learn to become attentive listeners and to refrain from giving advice. This rule has exceptions, but in general we want to help patients solve their own problems by allowing them to rely on their own resources.

5. *The clinician who is perceived as sympathetic and trustworthy.* As such, patients will find it easier to confide in us. To witness the superficial, defensive, organ-oriented patient give up facades and become more human, reacting on a more personal level, using more personal language, is a satisfying accomplishment. Tears well up in their eyes. They apologize for losing emotional control; the clinician reassures them that it is proper and desirable for them to express themselves. Full expression of emotion in interviewing and counseling for voice disorders is tension relieving. Such an abreaction has untold clinical importance. During such release, "functional" voice disorders, or organic disorders with "functional" components, often disappear, convincing clinician and patient alike that the voice problem was wholly or in part related to the emotions, a point the patient often resists up until this breakthrough. With emotional release, patients suddenly find themselves free to discuss situations openly that they have been guarding. The speech pathologist is often the first individual to whom they have disclosed this private information, and they feel tremendous relief after having done so. *What often begins as a "voice disorder" ends as a larger problem that demands a solution; the voice disorder was only the "tip of the iceberg."* We must recognize and accept that many voice disorders are substitute solutions for patients who cannot solve larger problems. Our job in such cases is to help them recognize that the voice is only a surface sign and that they need to face and solve primary problems before a normal voice will be attainable. Many voice disorders occur because of interpersonal conflicts in which the patient has suffered an injustice for which he has not had his "day in court." To have one's "day in court" is to be able to express one's need for justice, something these patients have been unable to do.

6. *The clinician who is willing to set aside adequate time* for the psychologic aspects of the examination and therapy. Psychologic interviewing and counseling take time. No matter how knowledgeable the clinician, if a special block of time is not set aside for leisurely discussion, rarely will the patient open up. Rushing is antithetical to good counseling.

* * *

It is 3:30 in the afternoon on a Friday. One ought not be distracted by thoughts of the coming weekend's diversions, but one is, nevertheless. This is the last patient of the day, and I wish for something simple. The history is as follows. The patient was referred to speech pathology by a clinic otolaryngologist. She had been referred to him in turn by her clinic internist because of dysphonia and throat pain. Her general health was good. Her main reason for coming to the clinic was back pain, neck pain, and hoarseness. She feared cancer. For her low back pain, she had seen a clinic psychiatrist, who had prescribed relaxation exercises and who told her to lose weight. No etiology of her pain had been formulated along the way, and she was being treated symptomatically.

The laryngologist found her larynx to be clean as a whistle—not a shred of evidence of a lesion or paralysis, and he reassured her that she did not have laryngeal cancer. She had pain and tenderness, especially on the right side of her neck just beneath the jaw, level with the hyoid bone, and the area was sensitive to pressure. The laryngologist injected lidocaine into the region, which numbed the pain temporarily, but her dysphonia remained. He then sent her for evaluation and treatment of her voice disorder.

She was a neatly dressed, ruddy-faced woman of 56 years from Saskatchewan where she and her husband farmed, apparently prosperously. This was her second marriage and had lasted 15 years. There were no children. She described the marriage as happy, and she denied life problems associated with her voice disorder. Gradually, three years ago, she became aware of both a tightness in her throat and episodes of hoarseness, which became chronic. The throat pain began during her dysphonia.

On examination, her voice was hoarse and strained, resembling adductor spastic dysphonia, except that the hoarseness did not fluctuate; it was continuous. It did not have quite the proper configuration for spastic dysphonia. Her entire neck musculature felt rock stiff to the touch, and she winced and withdrew when I touched her neck just below the angle of the mandible.

Did she abuse her voice, I asked? How much, and under what circumstances? Not very much, she shrugged. Once in a while she would shout across a field to her husband, but she was not a talker. I wondered if she felt isolated living on such a large farm with few neighbors. But, she was content.

The discussion fell off into silence. She gazed at the wall and frowned. "Come to think of it," she said, "I have had to raise my voice in talking to my husband. He seems to be getting hard of hearing. It's irritating. I say something and he asks me to repeat it; it gets tiring. No, he has never had his hearing tested." We talked about the possibility that voice strain and general muscular tension might have been brought on by her having to speak in this way to her hard-of-hearing husband. I encouraged her to get her husband to see an otologist to determine the cause and treatment of his hearing loss.

By now it was 4:30 and I wished for an ending to this evaluation. But I felt irritated with myself as I lifted half off the chair to extend my hand to say goodbye. The next words came as if from some other jurisdiction in my head. I dropped back into my chair. "There's one more question I'd like to ask, if you'll permit me. How is your sexual relationship with your husband?" For the first time in over an hour, she looked me dead in the eyes. There was a long moment of silence. Then she turned her head so that I would not see her face. She turned back, eyes closed, head down. A tear rolled down each cheek and cascaded onto her lap. She could not speak but answered with a negative shake of her head. When she had regained her composure, she explained that during the past few years her husband's sexual interest had declined to nearly complete inactivity. Until then, their relationship had been good. Then she found that she would have to initiate any relations, and most of the time he would decline, saying that he was too tired or wouldn't be able to perform. How did she feel about this, I asked. Tears again welled up in her eyes, and she said that she guessed she'd have to accept the situation, but hadn't quite anticipated such an early sexual demise. She said that she felt guilty for having brought up the subject because she loved her husband and, with that, cried out bitterly. We talked about her husband for a while, that he was only 58, still relatively young. Perhaps, she thought, his growing obesity might have something to do with his declining sexual interest.

By 5:15, at least 50 percent of her hoarseness had disappeared. We talked about marital counseling, and she was certain that their family doctor could help them find a counselor closer to home. We both sat in wonder at how the voice reveals pent-up emotions and how the throat pain came from suppression of crying, which she admitted doing. As she left, she thanked me for bringing her problem into the open; nobody else had, she said.

*   *   *

7. *The clinician who is patient and persistent.* Previously noted was the tendency for patients with voice disorders to deny emotional problems. Because patients skirt main issues, which they are either unconscious of or unwilling to divulge, the clinician must be prepared to wait. One must not be afraid to press gently for information when one feels that he is obtaining sterile information and that he can detect something beneath the surface which the patient is concealing. With patients who have voice disorders, the completely nondirective approach is not quite the right one. The optimum falls somewhere between the directive and the nondirective.

8. *The clinician who is authentic.* Many professionals have the idea that professionalism is equated with formality, rigidity, and even coldness. They entrench themselves behind their desks. Their posture, the architecture of the room, and uncomfortable lighting restrict verbal and emotional intimacy. The clinician should get out from behind the desk; sit closer to the patient; look the patient in the eyes. There is nothing wrong with touching the person on the arm or hand during more sensitive discussions to signify understanding. He should enter into the mood of the discussion with his own facial expression and bodily movements. It is important to try to feel what the patient is feeling; one should not be afraid to agonize with the patient. If the clinician has difficulty in expressing emotions, he or she is going to have difficulty doing so with patients. The world is cold and impersonal, and people do not display their feelings easily. It is rare for patients to meet someone who behaves humanly. They are grateful for it.

9. *The clinician who is honest.* Patients respect professionals. They imbue them with more knowledge than they deserve. There is a dangerous temptation for the clinician to erect a facade of superiority and authority. Patients ask many questions about the causes of and therapy for their voice disorders. Could it be caused by this pollution, that postnasal drip, or some incident that happened years ago? At such times, there is a temptation to appear more knowledgeable than reality justifies. If we don't know, we should say so. Patients have to learn to accept our fallibility as well as their own. Nonetheless, we are being consulted for our knowledge and, therefore, should communicate technical information as clearly and efficiently as possible. For this reason, thorough knowledge of voice disorders and related fields is imperative. We must be as well read as possible, and if we don't know the answers to certain questions, we should find out for ourselves and for the patient.

10. *The clinician who helps the patient form his or her own conclusions.* When it comes to helping patients realize the relationship between a psychogenic voice disorder and events in their lives, we must encourage them to speculate whether there might be such a connection, and we must not make the interpretations for them. People who arrive at their own conclusions believe them more firmly than if they are told. The process is called *insight*. It is a coming together, a Gestalt, a realization of the interrelationships among things.

INDICATORS OF PERSONALITY GROWTH

Patients with voice disorders of primarily psychogenic origin are experiencing a failure to express their "selves." We must help that person learn a greater freedom of verbal self-expression. There is no magic to this kind of therapy. It is nothing more or less than giving the patient encouragement to achieve what he or she has wished for many years: to express the self at any level with a feeling of freedom.

Rogers (1961) has analyzed the process of change from lesser to greater communication with the self and the outside world as a result of psychotherapy.

The process is one of change from fixedness to "flowingness."

Stage I
1. Unwillingness to communicate with the self.
2. Feelings and personal meanings neither recognized nor owned.
3. Rigid personal constructs. Communicative relationships construed as dangerous.
4. No problems recognized by the patient.
5. No desire for change.
6. Considerable blockage of internal communication.

Stage II
1. Expression begins to flow on the subject of nonself topics.
2. The patient perceives problems as being external to the self.
3. No sense of personal responsibility for those problems.
4. Language indicates that patient does not "own" ideas expressed, and he does so in the past tense.
5. Feelings expressed are unrecognized and unowned.
6. Experience is bound by the structure of the past.
7. Contradictions are expressed with little recognition by the patient that they are contradictions.

Stage III

1. Freer flow of expression about the self as an object.

Stage IV

1. Expresses more intensive feelings.
2. Greater expression of feelings in the present tense.
3. Loosening of the matter with which experience is intertwined.
4. Greater feeling of self-responsibility for problems.

RECOGNITION OF PSYCHOPATHOLOGY

Patients who have voice disorders are often in need of help because of psychopathology either related or unrelated to their voice disorders. Recognition and referral for psychiatric consultation may or may not be productive. The following material has been abstracted from *The Psychiatric Interview* by MacKinnon and Michels (1971), which is strongly recommended reading.

Psychopathology is concerned with emotional disorders—neuroses and psychoses. Behavior and character disorders are included; they interfere with the patient's ability to function properly at home, at play, at work, and in affectional relationships.

The distinction between neurotic and character traits is that neuroses consist of compromises between repressed wishes and unconscious fears in which the individual is trying to deal not only with the real world but with inner anxieties. The neurotic is aware of something foreign in his or her makeup and wishes to be free of it whether it be depression, anxiety, phobias, obsessions, compulsions, or conversion reactions. Character traits, on the other hand, are more basic to the individual's personality, and the individual feels relatively comfortable with them. Nevertheless, such people may be irresponsible, impulsive, aggressive, and mistrustful. The following are common clinical syndromes found in patients with voice disorders.

The Obsessive Patient

The main character traits of the obsessive personality are punctuality, conscientiousness, tidiness, orderliness, and reliability, stemming from a fear of violating the rules of social conduct. Parsimony with time and money is characteristic, as is exaggerated concern about proper social codes and competitiveness. Intellect is used to avoid confrontation with the emotions; the obsessive is a cerebral individual. Vocabulary and theoretical constructs are highly developed, and the language used in communicating with others is often confusing rather than clarifying. An over-reliance on detail often masks the major point of the commentary.

The interview is characterized by a tendency for the obsessive to control the interviewer and the interviewing situation in order to avoid the expression of deeper feelings. Definitions, terminology, and other intellectual aspects of behavior are chosen by the patient for discussion rather than underlying feelings and emotions. Sometimes the obsessive overcontrols the interview to such an extent that the roles of interviewer and interviewee appear reversed. In order to avoid disclosure of underlying feelings, the patient may show characteristic speech patterns, particularly in the voice. Loudness may be low or speech articulated so poorly that the interviewer will not be able to hear what the patient is saying. Silence often occurs; it is another technique used to avoid emotional contact.

The Hysterical Patient

The hysterical personality is warm, imaginative, charming, and exuberant. Such patients are often attractive physically, as well as in personality. Verbal communication is characterized by the expression of inner feelings of emotion in relating experiences. Exaggeration is a common quality of their language. Overdramatization is at the core of their communications.

The reason that these traits are considered pathologic is that they are superficial, and the patient is often devoid of any real feeling of affection, love, or intimacy. Although in outward appearance the patient may seem at ease and confident, beneath may lie anxiety and insecurity.

Female hysterics are often seductive and are possibly a trap for the male clinician, but the purpose of this behavior is to obtain approval and admiration rather than sexual intimacy. Helplessness and dependency may pervade the clinical relationship, with the patient attempting to maintain a childlike relationship with the clinician.

In contrast to the obsessive patient, the hysteric lacks orderliness and punctuality. Ordinary daily tasks are boring and avoided. Thinking is impulsive and intuitive. Commonly, there are marital or sexual problems because of the fear of emotional expression. *Apropos to voice disorders, patients with hysterical personalities frequently develop conversion voice disorders as well as other somatic complaints.*

Although interviewing hysterical patients is often personally and socially pleasant, such patients can produce sterile interview results because of their inability to discuss deeper feelings. Overdramatization and role-playing become irritating to the clinician attempting to get beneath the surface. The language of the hysteric impedes communication of the true self, as does the obsessive's overintellectualization. In the hysteric, the language is different, however; it is one of overdramatization, exaggeration, and distortion. The clinician gets the uneasy feeling of a lack of congruence between the patient's language and what the patient is actually feeling or the facts the patient is disclosing about his or her background and experience.

The Depressive Patient

Sadness, helplessness, and reduced self-esteem are mild signs of depression with which all humans must contend. Clinically depressed patients lose interest in life, however, and have diminished appetite and little enthusiasm for the general pleasures of life. Such people are preoccupied with themselves, ruminating about the past. Anxiety can be part of the syndrome, and so can anger. Overall, the depressed patient is slow of thought and movement, is preoccupied with bodily complaints and health, has difficulty in sleeping, awakens early, is fatigued, and has loss of appetite. Although many depressions stem from life-long family pathologic conditions, others are considered constitutional or biologic. Many individuals become depressed over the loss of friends or relatives through death or separation. Paradoxically, certain people become depressed after promotion or other forms of recognition which threaten to expose incompetence, either real or imagined, or because success is equated with hostile aggression.

Patients with voice disorders are usually depressed. It is either a cause of the voice disorder or a result of the voice disorder's interfering with their enjoyment of life. If the depression is the effect of the voice disorder, voice improvement often resolves the depression. Otherwise, psychiatric consultation and therapy are necessary. Often, patients with voice disorders are depressed because they are under the misconception that they have "caused" the disorder. Their depression is often alleviated when they are reassured that such is not the case; clinicians have an important educational function in this regard. In addition, the hope that can be generated from voice therapy, as well as the encouragement of the speech pathologist, can contribute considerably to the alleviation of depression. Information and reassurance go a long way in helping the patient with a voice disorder to attain a happier frame of mind.

Which of the abovementioned personality types do you recognize in the following histories?

* * *

A 30-year-old mother of three children has been under stress from several sources: She works at a supermarket full time to supplement the family income while having to maintain her household. She is dominated by her mother, who is hypercritical of how the patient manages her life. The patient and her husband disagree on many matters, and communication between the two is very poor because both have emotional problems. She has had several previous episodes of aphonia and dysphonia, but on interview her voice is nearly normal. Laryngologic examination was normal.

C: Your voice sounds fairly normal to me. Is this the problem that you came to the clinic for?
P: Well, I've had trouble off and on for about the last two years.
C: Do you actually lose your voice completely so that you have to whisper?
P: Back on the 18th of September, I could hardly get it up at all. I felt as if I was dragging everything right on out. But usually it is mostly a whisper.
C: What is the longest period of time that you have lost it?

P: Well, I wouldn't say that I've completely lost it, except for this last time on the 18th of September. But it's always been hoarse . . . almost gone.

C: How long a period of time had you lost it starting with the 18th of September?

P: Well, it sounded like I had laryngitis for about a week before. And then it just left.

C: Did you go around whispering then?

P: Well (laughs), I could hardly do even that. I mean, I felt like I was pulling everything right on out. My husband called the doctor and he gave me some medicine. It took about 24 hours before it took hold.

C: And did you lose it again?

P: It got hoarse, but I never lost it again.

C: Then why did you come here?

P: My doctor sent me here to see this guy (laryngologist) that looked down my throat, and he referred me to you.

C: Did anything happen on or about September 18th that might have upset you?

P: I wouldn't say it's any one thing. I can go back several years. I work, and I was hired to work three days a week. Well . . . it so happens that I think the first time it happened was I got left alone—we usually have three girls working—and I handled the whole burden plus three children at home, housework. Ever since then I have been carrying more of a load. They've been quitting, coming and going, and now we've been one gal short since . . . last of March, and this hoarseness has been pretty steady since then. So I think it's an emotional thing.

C: Why do you say it's emotional?

P: Well, I think it's nerves . . . I'm trying to do too much. You know, putting in five days a week, eight and a half hours a day, plus taking care of a home, children.

C: As you tell this to me, you seem to be on the verge of crying. (Mention of this brings tears to the patient's eyes.)

P: Nerves. (Smiling, holding back tears.)

C: How about people who are close to you at home and at work? Are you having any problems with any one individual?

P: Hmmm . . . not now, not since this one gal quit. She wanted a job. She had to have a job to get out of the house because she was tending to be an alcoholic, but she didn't really want to work and I was more-or-less carrying her load and my load both. Well, she was getting on my nerves. Other than that, I don't know . . . my kids get on my nerves.

C: How about your husband? (Note at this point her unawareness or her unwillingness to divulge the problem of her husband as a major source of her unhappiness and how it comes to the surface later in the interview.)

P: Very seldom.

C: How about your relatives.

P: (Laughs) My mother.

C: What about your mother?

P: (Patient gives a long sigh.) Well . . . oh, she keeps trying to run our lives, I guess . . . telling me what to do and what I shouldn't do, sometimes running me down.

C: How does she try to run your lives?

P: Well, I don't known. SInce we've been first married, well, I don't know, she says my husband hasn't got a good enough job, or I don't call her often enough. She has never approved of the doctor we go to, and (long sigh) she's started in on the dentist I go to, and I don't know, I never keep my house clean enough. She seems to think I am not strict enough with the kids, training them, you know, to say "thank you" or "please" . . . I don't know, it's a lot of things in general (close to tears again). I guess I let too many people bother me, I think.

C: What else?

P: Gee, I don't know . . . I don't know if there is anything else. My husband and I are perfectly happy, we don't have very many arguments. I know we don't see eye to eye on a lot of things.

C: Like what?

P: But I try not to contradict him, I let him have his own way.

C: What kinds of things don't you see eye to eye on?

P: Politics, a few things at church (laughs, long pause). We-l-l-l, we've been rivals through high school (becoming mildly indignant). Now, this is a silly thing. Every year at this . . . (becomes more tearful, voice beginning to quaver), he runs down my school, talks up his, every time sports start—especially basketball (laughs).

C: Does he do it good-naturedly, or does he do it maliciously?

P: Well, I'm always wrong. No matter what I say, he runs it down.

C: Everything you say?

P: Other things, too.

C: So, there is some problem between you and your husband.

P: Hm. I suppose you could say that. Let him have his way. Don't argue with him. What's there to do? Instead of causing an argument, I keep my mouth shut. . .

C: Has this been going on since you were married? Or has it been more recently?

P: Well, I don't know. When he used to listen to his ball games, I used to walk out of the house. He used to get on my nerves.

C: Why?

P: I don't know. He sits there telling me all of the faults of what they are doing or what they should have done, and it don't interest me. And if I tell him I don't want to hear about it, well, then he gets mad. I mean, if there is times when I want to talk to him, if the sports news is on or a political thing or something (closer to tears) he wants to watch, I've got to keep my mouth shut, but if there is something I want on and he wants to talk, I've got to sit there and listen or he gets mad.

C: Is he a short-tempered person?

P: I am. I don't know, he is more calm (crying now). But it seems like he's got to have more of his way. Not really his way, I don't know just how to put it. If he wants help with something, you just have to jump to it right away or else he gets mad. When I do things, I just go ahead and do it. I don't stop and ask whether I should do it this way or do it that way or do it all. But, with him he's got to discuss every little detail. If he should do it, or how it should be done. So often he's got to have help with everything.

C: Is he a perfectionistic person? It sounds as if he wants things to be done just so.

P: I'm more that way. I don't know, maybe it comes down to money problems. We don't really have money problems. But to him it's a mighty big thing. At times I just like to go out and have a good time, go to a dance. But he doesn't dance. If I want to take the girls to a show, I do it myself. He'd rather sit home and watch those damn ball games. (Cries bitterly.) It seems that I can't say anything. I can't express my point of view. Because I'm never right. I mean, when it comes down to politics, well, he'll say, "Vote this way. There is no sense in voting against me. That will only cancel both our votes." I just don't know what it is. Like, coming here today, he says the only thing my doctor sent me over for was to see whether there was something wrong with my throat. He says, "How many times are you going to come back here, run up a big bill?" He says, "This is it, this is the last time. You can't be chasing back and forth." There he's . . . telling me again (extremely angry) . . . and as far as I'm concerned I want to get down to the bottom of it, to find out why I'm losing my voice. (Breaks down again.) And I don't care how much money it costs! (Long pause while patient composes herself.)

C: How long have you been married?

P: Oh, a little over 11 years.

C: How do you basically feel about your husband?

P: Oh, I love him. He is a good man . . . I don't know, maybe the thing that bothers me the most is he's too much of a perfectionist on how the house should be run. I know his own mother told me she was glad to get rid of him, because she could sweep the floor and he'd go right after her and sweep it again. This thing about having the house being just so, so often he'll refer to back to being in the Army . . . I have to hang the shirts on the hangers all one way, all facing one way . . . The roll of toilet paper even has to be on one way . . . Even with the girls, if they don't make their beds just right, he threatens them. He says that he'll come up there and rip them all apart and start 'em all over. He says, "That's what they do to you in the Army." So, I don't know if it's got to do with that or what. (Long pause.)

But, I didn't think it was any of this that was causing my trouble, I figured I was . . . working too many hours trying to be a good guy, trying to fill in until they got somebody hired . . . I just keep getting further and further behind in my housework, and this bothers me, too.

* * *

Patients with psychogenic voice disorders are referred to speech pathologists who practice in hospitals as well as in clinics. The following experience concerns a young woman from a South American country who came to the United States for surgery unrelated to the larynx. She had had endotracheal anesthesia and awoke with a severely breathy dysphonia. The laryngologist wrote:

"She gets a good glottic closure and has a normal voice at times. Should be a functional dysphonia. Get speech pathology to see her."

The door to the hospital examination room opened, and a nurse escorted the patient into the room and then disappeared.

* * *

The patient collapsed into the chair opposite mine and then jackknifed forward, her head falling into my lap. She burst into great sobs, through which she managed to blurt out, "Oh, doctor, doctor, my family, they are driving me crazy!" Her sobbing subsided, replaced by great sniffling noises. Then she was quiet and finally sat up in her chair. I withdrew a clean handkerchief into which she noisily blew her nose, then smiled. Her eyes, although wet and red, were large and dark, and her skin had a reddish hue. Her lips were full, red, and etched in a cupid's bow. When she smiled, her teeth shone in white contrast against her dark skin. She spoke again, "I'm sorry, doctor, for having troubled you like this." Her English was excellent, delicately graced with a Portuguese accent. Her voice was severely breathy bordering on aphonia, but it retained the faint outlines of pitch and inflectional changes, which gave her voice expression. Her cough was sharp, giving evidence of her fundamentally sound larynx. What did she mean, I asked, that her family was driving her crazy. Angrily, she told of how, just before I had arrived, she had a telephone call from her mother, who had reprimanded her for not telling her she was going to leave the country for surgery.

Born in Brazil, the daughter of a coffee plantation owner, the patient had been educated in a Catholic girl's school in the United States where she had met her husband, aged 38 years, 6 years older, who was also a student in the United States studying chemistry. She withdrew from her wallet a color photograph of her husband perched high upon a chestnut brown horse. He wore a red beret and an ascot and was, she said, an excellent polo player. She also showed me photographs of her two sons, 10 and 12 years old, both blond and handsome.

Then she lowered her head, and when she looked up again, tears were in her eyes. Her jaw was clenched, and her eyes were wide, and, in what seemed like mock anger, she rasped, "But, he is like so many Latin men. He makes me so angry." Then she stopped and smiled at me through her tears, her head cocked to one side, waiting for me to respond. "What do you mean?" "He treats me like a child, and he doesn't pay enough attention to me. When he comes home at night, he sits and reads the newspaper or a book and doesn't speak a word." Her lower lip bulged and set. "What else?" I asked. She paused. Her eyelids fluttered three times. She smiled sheepishly. "You'll think I'm silly." "No I won't," I insisted. A long pause. "Well, I don't like him to look at other women. You are surprised?" She smiled, and proudly flicked her head obliquely upward. "You don't understand Latin men. They all think they are great lovers and spend every minute trying to prove it. We were at this big banquet and he was sitting next to me and across from us was a girlfriend of mine, and he kept staring at her decolletage all evening!" We both laughed.

Then we talked more seriously, and she told me she had, a year ago, lost a child at birth. Then two weeks before her surgery, she received a phone call from her cousin that she too had lost her baby during childbirth. I tried symptomatic voice therapy but was unsuccessful. I saw her the day before she left the hospital, and except for her voice, she looked and felt well. I apologized for being unable to help her toward a more normal voice, but she reassured me that my visits, she called them "moral support," were more helpful than I could realize.

Three months later she wrote:

The first time I had a real voice was in New York, three days before coming home. I had a dream that night. I dreamed that I was sitting down in a drawing room with my cousin and his wife, the ones I told you had lost their second baby. I was doing all the talking, and I could listen to my own voice. I was cheerful and happy, telling them all about my visit to the United States. Suddenly I told them: "How funny. Do you know what happened to me when I heard of your baby's death? I lost my voice." As soon as I said this I woke up and knew I could speak again. I screamed, and my own voice came out! You cannot imagine how happy and delighted I was. I could not believe it. It was 7 o'clock in the morning. Since then, my voice began to come back for moments: 15 minutes, 10 minutes, half an hour. The day after the trip, which I made all by myself, I had no voice whatsoever. I felt depressed, sad, and very ill. I arrived at my home after a long flight and was excited to see my husband, children, parents; happy to be back home and to think that all I had gone through was over. After my arrival, my voice improved gradually, over a period of days. It has been three months since I had my operation, and sometimes when I get upset I notice a slight sore throat and I feel that my voice begins to change. But that is all. Luckily I feel very well; strong, happy, and so mentally different from what I felt last year.

* * *

SUMMARY

1. Knowledge of the principles and possession of the skills of psychologic interviewing and counseling are indispensable in the diagnosis of and therapy for voice disorders.

2. Virtually all patients with voice disorders, whether organic or psychogenic, have some degree of emotional disequilibrium, either as a cause or as an effect of the voice disorder.

3. Many nonorganic voice disorders diminish or disappear during discussion of life stresses responsible for those disorders.

4. Sensitivity to more serious emotional illness in patients who have voice disorders can facilitate referral to proper mental health specialists.

5. The speech pathologist who is most likely to succeed in providing psychologic support of the patient with a voice disorder is one who has a high degree of acceptance of self and others, is understanding, is skillful in asking questions, knows how to listen, is sympathetic and trustworthy, and is persistent.

SUGGESTIONS FOR ADDITIONAL READING

Butcher, P., Elias, A., Raven, R., and Yeatman, J.: Psychogenic voice disorders unresponsive to speech therapy. Br. J. Disord. Commun., 22:81–92, 1987.
  This interesting article on the feasibility of speech clinicians administering counseling and psychotherapy to patients with psychogenic voice disorders conjointly with psychologists is an innovative and forward-looking approach to the treatment of psychogenic voice disorders.
Hejna, R.F.: Speech Disorders and Nondirective Therapy. New York, Ronald Press, 1960.
  Deals exclusively with the issue of counseling and psychotherapy for all communicative disorders. See especially pp. 22–25 on voice problems.
MacKinnon, R.A., and Michels, R.: The Psychiatric Interview in Clinical Practice. Philadelphia, W.B. Saunders Co., 1971.
  A practical, basic, and eminently readable textbook on the technique of the interview. Introduces the student to psychologic interviewing and lucidly distinguishes among different psychoneurotic and personality disorders.
Rogers, C.R.: On Becoming a Person. Boston, Houghton Mifflin Co., 1961.
  This collection of the best articles and lectures by the well-known clinical psychologist provides a deeper understanding of the objectives of clinician and client in interviewing and psychotherapy.

REFERENCES

Butcher, P., Elias, A., Raven, R., and Yeatman, J.: Psychogenic voice disorders unresponsive to speech therapy. Br. J. Disord. Commun., 22:81–92, 1987.
Kolb, L.C.: Section one: Major clinical syndromes, *In* MacKinnon, R.A., and Michels, R.: The Psychiatric Interview in Clinical Practice. Philadelphia, W.B. Saunders Co., 1971.
MacKinnon, R.A., and Michels, R.: The Psychiatric Interview in Clinical Practice. Philadelphia, W.B. Saunders, Co., 1971.
Rogers, C.R.: On Becoming a Person. Boston, Houghton Mifflin Co., 1961.
Elias, A., Raven, R., Butcher, P., and Littlejohns, D.W.: Speech therapy for psychogenic voice disorder: A survey of current practice and training. Br. J. Disord. Commun., 24:61–76, 1989.
Green, M.C.L.: The Voice and Its Disorders, 3rd ed. London: Pitman Medical, 1972.

Chapter Twelve

STUDIES IN CLINICAL DIAGNOSIS

The first principle is that you must not fool yourself—and you are the easiest person to fool.

—Richard Feynman, physicist

INTRODUCTION

The purpose of this chapter is to help the student develop a comprehensive grasp of the clinician-patient relationship in voice diagnosis and treatment. The clinician needs to know much more than "techniques" in order to treat successfully patients who have voice disorders. An understanding of the overall picture is indispensable because, although the range of voice disorder types in the human population is limited, no two individuals *present* their voice disorders in the same manner owing to the following variables: age and sex; duration, etiology and severity of the voice disorder; concurrent physical illnesses; personality; premorbid and concurrent psychiatric predisposition; nationality and cultural background; education; socioeconomic level; motivation; verbal ability; and insight.

Inherent, and necessary, in the traditional textbook format is that material be presented in a logical, orderly manner. Textbook knowledge is one thing, clinical thinking and action are another. In practice, the clinician is required to work backward from fragments of data, in this case the abnormal voice, and must use surface auditory-perceptual and visual-perceptual signs as means of reasoning toward probable abnormal laryngeal physiology and, even further remotely, to the underlying etiology behind that physiology.

VOICE CLUSTERS

Recognizing this practical necessity, the *voice cluster concept* was devised to help organize our thinking about abnormal voice unknowns. The concept is based on the fact that abnormal voices have a tendency to group themselves into perceptually distinctive colonies. A voice *cluster* is an abstraction, or prototype—it is no single patient's voice. For example, one cluster is the *husky breathy whispered-continuous group* under which all breathy voices are gathered. The common anatomic denominator is that the vocal folds do not meet firmly to form a tight seal. The specific anatomic, physiologic, and etiologic reasons can be very different from patient to patient, however, and finding out the reasons will require further investigation. The point to be made is that we have to begin somewhere to categorize the sound of the voice in order to further our logical thinking about its cause. Following are eight distinctive voice clusters. After listing them, each will be discussed in detail. The clusters are:

    I. *The husky breathy whispered-continuous group*

    II. *The strained hoarse-continuous group*

    III. *The strained hoarse voice arrest-intermittent arrhythmic group*

    IV. *The strained hoarse voice arrest-intermittent rhythmic group*

V. *The voice tremor group*

VI. *The breathy whispered-intermittent group*

VII. *The low-pitch hoarse group*

VIII. *The high-pitch group*

Clinical case studies for the purpose of enabling the student to apply the cluster concept will be presented. These studies have been selected as much for their unusual as for their ordinary occurrence in clinical practice. A prevalent misconception abounds that the atypical case is not worthy of attention for the very reason of its rarity; specifically that time should be spent on the more commonly occurring voice disorders. Experienced clinicians, particularly those who have medical differential diagnostic experience, will testify as to the danger of that idea. The reason is that the least frequently seen voice problem almost always provides the clinician with the greatest chance of making a mistake. It is important to emphasize that the case studies selected here are not intended to be all-inclusive or systematic accounts of every kind of voice sign or disorder that could occur in clinical practice. Rather, the objective is to give the student a sense of the often convoluted nature of the diagnostic and decision-making process. While reading these studies, the student should keep in mind that matters are not always as they appear to be and should look for alternative, and sometimes surprising, explanations to what might have begun as a simple, straightforward diagnostic unknown. These studies can be somewhat confusing and frustrating, and this is intentional, to reflect actual practice. At selected points during each presentation, questions are asked that will encourage the student to consider alternatives in problem solving. Following each case study is a discussion that contains the answers to most of the questions raised during the narrative. They can be used as bases for class discussion. Answers also can be found in other chapters of the book.

I. THE HUSKY BREATHY WHISPERED - CONTINUOUS GROUP

When we hear a voice that is continuously or steadily husky, breathy, or whispered the first question asked should be: *"What might be happening at the vocal fold level to produce this kind of voice?"* The answer is "incomplete glottic closure."

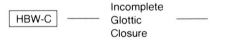

"What are the possible reasons for such incomplete approximation of the vocal folds?" One major cause is a *mass lesion* that produces a rough or irregular surface on one or both vocal folds preventing them from forming a smooth seal in the midline.

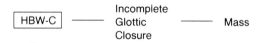

"What specific kinds of lesions are capable of producing such interference?" The most common are polyps, nodules, webs, and carcinomas. Glottic insufficiency from postsurgical loss of tissue, such as after cordectomy, can produce similar results, and so can loss of mass from senile bowing of the vocal folds.

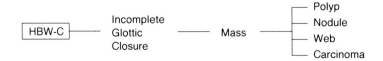

Whether any of these lesions is responsible for the breathy type of voice found within this cluster will be determined by laryngoscopic examination.

Assume that such examination has taken place and has failed to identify any of the lesions just described. The next question should be, *"What other causes could produce a voice that falls within this cluster?"* The answer is neurologic disease, which is the next major cause within the HBW-C cluster group.

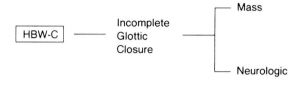

"What is the reason that a neurologic lesion could produce a voice of this cluster description? Where could such lesions in the nervous system take place to produce such a voice? With which neurologic syndromes could such voice be associated?"

Neurologic lesions can prevent adduction of the vocal folds. Any interference with functioning of the Xth cranial nerve will produce unilateral or bilateral vocal fold paralysis preventing their approximation.

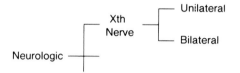

Careful laryngologic examination will probably establish whether or not such paralysis has taken place.

Assume that such examination has failed to disclose paralysis. We must then entertain another possibility, that of myoneural junction disease, or myasthenia gravis, having a prominent laryngeal representation.

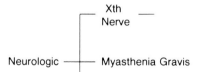

Further neurologic examination, including motor speech examination, would be necessary to confirm or rule out this disease.

A third possibility is early parkinsonism, since breathy voice is one of its first indications. The location of the lesion is within the basal ganglia.

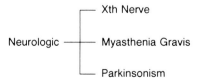

Further possibilities are apraxia of phonation producing loss of recall for phonatory movements and frontal lobe disease producing defects of personality, motivation, and insight.

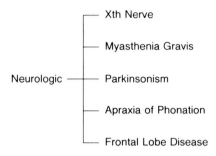

The importance of a complete neurologic examination to clarify the differential diagnosis among these various possibilities is obvious. It should also be apparent that these dysphonias are classifiable under such larger categories as dysarthria, apraxia, and dementia.

The sequence of clinical diagnostic screening from *organic to psychogenic* causes follows a practical rationale and for three important reasons: (1) It is mentally difficult to think about organic and nonorganic causes together without becoming disorganized and even confused. So, taking these two major categories one at a time will keep us from becoming entangled in a morass of conflicting clinical signs and symptoms. (2) The reason that organic causes are examined first is because they are potentially life-threatening. (3) It is easier to communicate with patients and inform them of nonorganic causes once we are convinced no such organic causes are present.

At this point in our schema, let us say we have satisfied ourselves that the patient who presents with a voice of this cluster does not have any of the mass lesions or neurologic diseases suspected. *"Where do we go from here in our thoughts and procedures to help explain this type of abnormal voice?"* We must seriously consider that the abnormal voice is not caused by organic disease and begin to look for psychogenic causes.

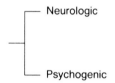

In order to find out if such psychogenic causes exist, it is mandatory that a serious, probing psychosocial history be administered. In the broadest general terms we are looking for evidence of acute situational conflicts or chronic life stress, time-related to onset and development of the abnormal voice. Depression, anxiety, and conversion reaction are the most common effects of such stresses. They produce laryngeal musculoskeletal tension, laryngeal elevation and muscle tension pain, and "globus."

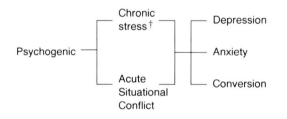

To summarize, the majority of voices that fall within the cluster under discussion can be analyzed according to the following composite schema:

---

†Important to note that chronic stress is a causative factor in the development of vocal nodule.

HUSKY BREATHY WHISPERED-CONTINUOUS GROUP

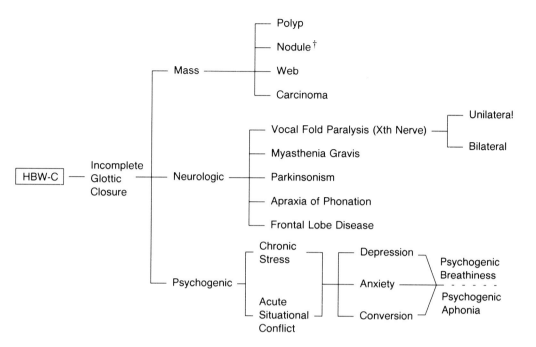

The following specific case studies illustrate in detail the evolution of voice disorders requiring the kinds of procedures and reasoning heretofore discussed. After this first series of case presentations, schematic flow diagrams will be presented for the remainder of the cluster groups, however, without detailed commentary as in this one, allowing the student to work out the meaning of the charts independently.

Case Study Number 1

A 40-year-old female unemployed high school science teacher who is married with three children had a normal voice until two years ago when she underwent thyroid surgery. Upon recovering from the anesthesia, she was alarmed to discover that her voice was almost a whisper. She would choke on liquids unless she swallowed small amounts at a time.

   Q1: What do you suspect is the etiology of her dysphonia?

   Her nurse had written that her cough sounded "mushy and weak." On laryngoscopic examination, the surgeon found a right unilateral vocal fold paralysis. He told her that it would be wise if she used her voice very carefully, whereupon he prescribed voice rest for one week. When she resumed talking, she found that her breathiness was as bad or worse than before. The surgeon referred her for voice therapy. She was treated twice a week for two months, and showed "considerable improvement," but she retained a degree of breathiness that left her dissatisfied. She returned to her otolaryngologist, who recommended Teflon injection, but the patient, wary of further surgery, declined.

---

†Important to note that chronic stress is a causative factor in the development of vocal nodule.

Q2:   What is the rationale for recommending Teflon injection?

The psychosocial history is normal. She describes her relationships with her husband and children as happy, and she expresses much optimism about her life, but she does become upset by her voice, particularly under noisy conditions. She wants to return to classroom teaching and knows she will not be able to do so as long as her voice is abnormal. She is dismayed that her poor voice deprives her of pleasurable social conversation. She cries frequently during the examination.

Her voice quality is moderately breathy, loudness level is reduced, and mild friction noise is heard during inhalation. She sustains the vowel /a/ with a remarkably low volume. You are startled by her ability to triple her volume on demand, during which she produces nearly normal voice. Her cough and glottal coup are normal. A repeat laryngoscopic examination shows that the right vocal fold is still paralyzed.

Q3:   Explain, anatomically, why thyroid surgery should have produced a unilateral vocal fold paralysis in this patient.

Q4:   Draw a superior view of the patient's vocal folds during phonation immediately after surgery.

Q5:   How does your drawing explain the patient's voice signs and symptoms immediately after surgery?

Q6:   Why was she having trouble swallowing liquids?

Q7:   What is the explanation for the nurse's note that, immediately after surgery, her cough sounded "mushy and weak"?

Q8:   How might you explain the fact that, on your examination, even though the right vocal fold was still paralyzed, her cough and glottal coup were normally sharp?

Q9:   How might you explain the fact that when the patient was asked to sustain vowels loudly that her volume tripled and her voice quality became nearly normal despite the persistence of her vocal fold paralysis?

Q10:   What information in the history gives a clue to the etiology of her persistent dysphonia?

Q11:   From the data given, how would you proceed with therapy?

DISCUSSION

This patient's voice disorder teaches an important lesson about the psychologic repercussions of organic voice disorders. Here is a woman who obviously had a unilateral vocal fold paralysis after thyroidectomy, a relatively common occurrence owing to the proximity of the thyroid gland and the recurrent laryngeal nerve. She was frightened when she awoke from the anesthesia to discover that, in effect, she could not talk. The emotional trauma of sudden voice deprivation in a basically healthy woman who has the responsibilities of a family and a career, both of which place a high demand on the ability to speak, may not be as well appreciated as it ought to be. Such anxiety is further heightened by the fact that no one can give her a satisfactory answer to her question as to when, or even whether, her voice will return to normal. The surgeon then places her on voice rest, which communicates to her that not using her voice is good, which must mean then that to use it is bad. The speech clinician who subsequently sees her for therapy and brings about voice improvement fails to reverse the patient's concept of guarded voice use, and she reaches a plateau in therapy that she never surmounts.

The clue to her potential for better voice should have been the discovery that the patient's cough was disproportionately sharp in contrast to her breathiness and reduced loudness. Moreover, despite the persistence of her unilateral vocal fold paralysis, examination showed good compensatory approximation of the normal vocal fold against the paralyzed one. The final proof of her untapped capacity for a nearly normal voice was when she produced a loud, clear voice on demand. Her discovery that she could do this provoked in her genuine surprise; she had not been aware of her potential. What she had done, quite unconsciously, was to partially shut down her depth of respiration and force of vocal fold adduction in a misguided attempt to avoid damaging her vocal folds.

Therapy consisted of helping the patient to divest herself of the notion that vigorous use of her voice was bad. On the contrary, the more she used it the better her voice would become. She was given supervised practice using a much louder, clearer voice. She wrote one month later saying that her voice was nearly normal under most speaking conditions. She still has a unilateral vocal fold paralysis.

Case Study Number 2

The 47-year-old wife of an American industrialist living in London, England, came to the Clinic because she has been unable to find a satisfactory explanation or help for the following complaint: During the past six months her voice has been getting softer. It has reached the point where people have to ask her to repeat what she is saying. She was examined by two laryngologists before coming to the Clinic. One said her vocal cords were normal, the other said that the posterior region of the cords were not closing completely but could make nothing of this finding. He described her voice complaint as "functional."

She has just been re-examined by a laryngologist and, for the first time, a neurologist. Neither was able to diagnose her problem. The laryngologist wrote, "Her voice sounds pretty normal to me." The neurologist, having just completed her residency, was perplexed by the case because the complaint was confined to the patient's voice and she "didn't have much else to go on." She eventually decided that the voice complaint was "non-organic." The referral note says, "Evaluation and therapy for functional voice disorder."

The patient is a tall, exceptionally well-groomed woman whose manner and language reveal a keen intelligence and capacity for detailed recall. She was at a cocktail party for her husband's executive friends when she first noticed she could not speak loudly enough to make herself heard over the noise. Since that occasion, over six months ago, she has had several similar episodes, except that within the past three months she's noticed it even when there is little or no extraneous noise. Also, it is no longer just occasional but is "present more and more of the time."

The psychosocial history is completely unremarkable; the patient and her husband are well suited to one another. Their children are grown and successfully on their own; their daughter is an attorney for a utilities company, and their son is finishing a surgical residency. The patient does admit that when she is under the stresses of everyday life her voice is noticeably worse.

Speech evaluation reveals that her conversational loudness level is, in fact, reduced and her voice is mildly breathy or husky. Her cough is so near normal that you are unable to consider it anything but that or, at most, a mild variant of normal. One thing you note is that she does not use much pitch or loudness variation. When you point this out to her she quickly agrees, because a close friend had told her just the other day that, on the phone, she sounded "flat and depressed" and had expressed concern about the patient.

Q1: *What might be the diagnostic possibilities of the voice findings obtained up to this point?*

Q2: *What is the diagnostic significance of the finding that the patient's voice is worse when she is under stress?*

You ask her to sustain the vowel /a/ as long and steadily as she can. The first time she does this you note that her voice definitely is breathy, but you think you hear something else, a faint irregularity of some kind. On the second and third trials, you are certain that, buried within the breathy quality is a rapid tremor, so subtle as to escape any but the most discriminating ear.

Q3: *What conclusions might you draw about the breathy voice quality?*

Q4: *What are the possible interpretations of the rapid tremor?*

Q5: *Why was the tremor heard only on vowel prolongation?*

On routine motor speech examination you find that her alternate motion rate and regularity on /pʌ/, /tʌ/, /kʌ/ repetitions are normal, but here, again, you find yourself further perplexed that she does not open her lips very widely as she repeats the syllables.

Q6: *Comment on the possible significance of the lip movements just described.*

Q7: *How might this finding relate to those accumulated thus far?*

Finally, because you have been taking special note of the patient's facial expression during the latter part of the examination, you remark to yourself that it is not expressive, except when she speaks with emotional emphasis or smiles. Toward the end of the examination she volunteers, "for whatever help it might be," that her golf game has deteriorated during the same period as her voice complaint.

Q8: *What do you think are the possible causes of the patient's voice disorder?*

Q9: *What steps would you take at this point in the examination?*

DISCUSSION

This study illustrates the importance of being sensitive to the fact that signs of neurologic syndromes in the very early stages of their evolution often appear to others as "functional," and that we are not often blessed with their full, classic clinical characteristics. Here is a diagnosis that was missed by four physicians, primarily because the patient's signs and symptoms were limited to her speech. This is common in early voice signs of neurologic disease; after all, breathiness and reduced loudness are also signs of psychogenicity. That is why we must look for any additional signs, which, when assembled may form a pattern that might explain the patient's dysphonia or other chief speech complaint. The first clue we get about this patient is that her demeanor does not fit with the typical patient with psychogenic or "functional" dysphonia. We then learn that, in addition to her breathiness, one laryngoscopic examination showed that the interarytenoid portions of the vocal folds were not approximating completely. In addition to the breathiness we have evidence of a loss of pitch and loudness variations. During the speech examination, she had a barely detectable, rapid voice tremor on vowel prolongation that could never have been detected during ordinary speech owing to its mildness. The failure of her lips to make normally wide excursions on alternate motion rate for /pʌ/ for the first time became an important finding. The information that her voice was worse under stress proved nothing either way; patients with both organic and psychogenic voice disorders report these variations. Only after putting these findings together did her lack of facial mobility take on importance.

By now it should be apparent that the suspicion of early parkinsonism has been raised. You telephone the neurologist who had last examined her and ask if you might speak with her about your findings. You tell her that the patient's voice and associated speech findings may be suggestive of early parkinsonian dysarthria, which might be revealing itself primarily via her larynx. After expressing ill-disguised surprise, she thanks you and suggests that another neurologist who specializes in Parkinson's disease examine the patient. He does. His note reads: "This patient has mild masking of facies, mild rigidity of her upper extremities to passive movement, and mild reduction in arm swing and distance between her steps as she walks. This, in all probability, is early Parkinson's disease. The mildness of her signs does not warrant any treatment at this time. The patient should be scheduled for re-examination in six months."

Case Study Number 3

A 24-year-old airline stewardess comes to you for advice concerning vocal nodules. The referring laryngologist describes "well-developed, probably encapsulated, nodules in the middle of the vocal cords, bilaterally." The patient went to the laryngologist after a friend had advised her that she ought to have an examination because someone else she knew had a similar voice and she was found to have serious organic disease.

The patient says that her voice has been "kind of husky" for as long as she can remember. She was a cheerleader in high school and describes herself as one who talks incessantly; even when she is alone, she talks to her dog. She does not smoke and drinks only socially with moderation. On examination, her voice has a noticeably breathy-husky quality.

Q1:   *What is the physical explanation for the patient's "breathy-husky" voice quality?*

Q2:   *What is the most likely etiology of her vocal nodules?*

Q3:   *Do you feel comfortable making a therapy decision at this point? If so, what do you think ought to be done? If not, what further information do you think you need?*

The psychosocial history is as follows. After high school graduation and two years of college, she was accepted for airline stewardess training. One year later, she married an accountant and continued to work at her airline job. She says her marriage is "quite satisfactory," although recently she has been unhappy about her husband having to work long hours because of increased responsibilities. She wishes she could see more of him. She conveys the impression that there are no deeper problems.

As far as she is concerned, her voice has never been a problem. Many people even tell her they like the quality of her voice. Actually, her main reason for coming to the Clinic was that she feared a disease of her larynx, not because she wanted help for her voice.

Q4:   *Do you think this patient is a candidate for voice therapy? Why?*

Q5:   *Should this patient's vocal nodules be removed surgically? Why?*

Q6:   *What would you have done if the laryngologist had recommended surgical removal?*

DISCUSSION

The "breathy-husky" voice quality in this patient is typical of those who have vocal nodules. The voice quality is the effect of the nodules projecting medially from the vocal folds so that when they approximate during phonation the vocal edges do not form a complete seal; instead, spaces are left in the region of the nodules allowing air to escape during phonation, hence the breathy quality.

From the history provided, and the laryngologist's description of probable encapsulation, it would appear that these nodules have been present for a long time. Quite likely, they were formed when the patient was a cheerleader, or before, and that her greater-than-average voice use has caused them to persist.

There is serious doubt that voice therapy is necessary or even desirable. The patient is satisfied with her voice even though most clinicians would agree it was defective. In many vocal abusers excessive voice use is inseparable from their basically extroverted personalities, making voice modification difficult to achieve. Even if she were motivated, reducing vocal abuse probably would not diminish the size of the nodules owing to their encapsulation. In view of the poor prognosis for reducing encapsulated vocal nodules by means of voice re-education, there is a strong tendency to advocate surgical removal. Although in some instances this might be advisable, there are risks associated with surgery; often the dysphonia remains or even becomes worse.

Case Study Number 4

A patient is sent to you with the following history. She is a 52-year-old woman who complains of general fatigue and episodes of voice loss for about two years. Twenty years ago she had an episode of anxiety, hyperventilation, and a sense of impending doom. She was helped with psychologic counseling and has had only rare occurrences of these complaints ever since. Three years ago she choked on a carrot; said it stuck in her windpipe and that she nearly died. Two years ago she began to have what she describes as "severe fatigue, no stamina, generalized weakness, a need to walk slowly—like I'm 90 years old." She says her symptoms are getting progressively worse.

When she talks on the telephone for long periods, her "voice loses volume and becomes a whisper" accompanied by chest discomfort and a pulling sensation in her epigastrium. She feels more fatigued and weak during these spells, and three or four times she felt light-headed when she had them. At first these episodes occurred only once or twice a week, but now they occur daily "anytime I talk." All of her symptoms are now worse.

The neurologist, who wrote these findings also noted that when he asked her to count to 100 her "voice deteriorated to a whisper."

Q1:   At this point, what causes of her voice disorder might you consider?

During your examination, you discover that her voice is intermittently breathy during contextual speech. Her cough is normally sharp. She complains of pain in the region of her larynx. She gives no evidence of hypernasality or nasal emission, and her articulation is normal. You ask her to count vigorously from one to 150. She becomes nearly aphonic by the time she reaches 60, but with no signs of hypernasality or articulatory disturbance accompanying the voice change. Her cough during her aphonia retains its sharpness.

Q2:   Does this patient show the classic signs of the dysarthria of myasthenia gravis?

Q3:   What is the neuroanatomic type of dysarthria that can accompany myasthenia gravis and what are its classical signs?

Q4:   Is it possible for someone to have myasthenia gravis localized to the larynx only?

Q5:   If the voice had deteriorated to aphonia for reasons of muscular weakness after the stress test of counting, what do you think the quality of her cough should be?

You discuss your findings with the neurologist, who suggests that Tensilon be administered after voice deterioration but, in this case, he suggests injecting sterile water prior to the Tensilon test.

Q6:   Why do you think the neurologist wanted to inject sterile water before Tensilon?

The neurologist inserts the needle of a syringe filled with sterile water into the patient's arm, but she has not been informed that water is the substance being injected. Her voice, which begins as a whisper after having been first fatigued, becomes steadily louder and clearer as she counts, even before the neurologist has injected the water. The patient complains of "feeling funny." The water is then injected with no further effect.

Q7:   What do you conclude from the events just described?

Q8:   How do you think the speech pathologist and the neurologist should proceed with the patient from this point?

Further discussion with the patient reveals, for the first time, that ever since she had been placed in a cardiac intensive care unit two years ago for cardiac arrhythmia she has been chronically anxious about her heart. Even though the cardiac findings were diagnosed as benign, she still becomes extremely anxious whenever her heartbeat is irregular.

Q9:   Discuss the relevance of this latest information to the patient's total neurologic and speech signs and symptoms.

Q10:   What further action do you think should be taken?

DISCUSSION

On the face of it, any speech deterioration during prolonged or effortful speaking should bring to mind myasthenia gravis. The question that often confronts us is whether a given patient with myasthenia gravis needs to show all of the classic signs of flaccid dysarthria, i.e., whether all speech systems—respiratory, phonatory, resonatory, and articulatory—need to be implicated before we can reasonably suspect this type of dysarthria. The answer is "no." Although rare, bulbar myasthenia gravis can become manifested at the laryngeal level only, so it is reasonable that this patient was suspected of having the disease, especially when her voice had deteriorated during stressful counting. But, all findings did not fit with the idea of progressive muscular weakness as the underlying cause of her bouts with dysphonia. Rarely, if ever, does the myasthenic patient's voice deteriorate into a complete whisper, as this patient's had. However, most telling was the preservation of her sharp cough during the time she was aphonic. The typical patient with flaccid dysphonia from true muscular weakness of the laryngeal adductors will produce a weak or "mushy" cough proportional to the degree of dysphonia present. The neurologist suspected that something about his entire examination did not fit with organic disease, and when presented with evidence of the sharp cough decided to do a placebo test—sterile water instead of Tensilon—first to see if the patient would respond as if she had been given the drug. Our suspicions were confirmed when the needle had been inserted into the vein and her voice began to improve *as if* she had been given Tensilon, even before the water had been injected. The test was discontinued with confirmation of psychogenic dysphonia.

It is curious that a small percentage of patients will develop nonorganic musculoskeletal reactions, which in some cases are conversion reactions, that simulate neurologic syndromes relatively well-known to the general public, such as myasthenia gravis or multiple sclerosis. Often the idea is inadvertently suggested by prior medical consultations or by the patient's experience with a relative or friend who had the disease.

In our patient, the reason was never found as to why she happened to acquire a nonorganic dysphonia that resembled myasthenia gravis, but the neurologist strongly suspected that it had something to do with her anxiety about her heart. His course of action from that point was to schedule a complete examination by a cardiologist for a new opinion, with the intent of educating the patient as to her true cardiac status. Held in reserve was a psychiatric consultation should the cardiologist's counseling prove ineffective.

II. STRAINED HOARSE - CONTINUOUS GROUP

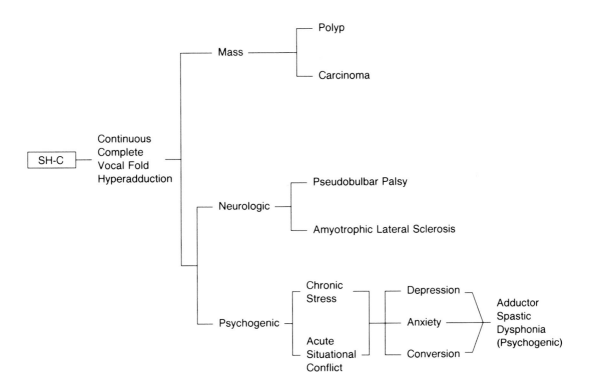

Case Study Number 5

A 47-year-old male instructor in economics at a community college comes to you with the complaint of hoarseness that seems to have developed during the Fall semester. Now Christmastime, his voice is worse than it has ever been. He thinks he has been under stress because of a change in his teaching duties, having been given increasing responsibilities owing to the loss of a faculty member. He finds that about halfway through a lecture his hoarseness increases and he feels pain in his throat. He recently visited an otolaryngologist who said that his vocal cords looked nearly normal except for some slight reddening. Until his voice disorder began four months previously, he had been in excellent health and had had no previous trouble with his voice in spite of an active teaching career spanning 20 years. On voice evaluation you hear a continuously strained-hoarse voice quality. On vowel prolongation there is a "wet" sounding noise superimposed on the hoarseness, and, at times, it sounds as if there is a very subtle, rapid tremor or "flutter" in the patient's voice. The psychosocial history reveals that he is happily married with two teenage children, both of whom are doing well in school. His wife is a social worker employed part-time. The patient admits that he has always been high-strung, that lecturing has always been extremely important to him, and that he derives most of his work satisfaction from that activity, finding students stimulating and challenging. This past semester has been more upsetting than previous years owing to having to teach two additional courses, which interferes with preparation for his lectures. Being compulsive and meticulous, he becomes anxious if he has not prepared adequately for every lecture.

Q1: *What possible etiologies of this patient's dysphonia do you entertain?*

Q2: *What evidence can you muster to support your position?*

Q3: *What is the significance of the specialist's observation of erythema of the vocal folds?*

Q4: *What significance do you give to the observation that his voice sounded "wet" on vowel prolongation?*

Q5: *What interpretation do you give to the observation of a rapid tremor or "flutter" during vowel prolongation?*

Q6: *How would you progress with the examination and the management of this patient from this point?*

The patient's cough sounded reasonably normal. However, his glottal attack on a vowel seemed to be produced with less than normal percussion.

Q7: *If valid, what interpretation would be given to a less than normal glottal attack on a vowel?*

Q8: *Why would the cough be sharper than the glottal attack on a vowel?*

You decide to perform an oral-physical examination. With a tongue depressor, you stroke the patient's lips from the angles of the mouth toward the center and think you see a slight pursing of the patient's lips. Upon opening his mouth, you find that his mouth glistens with a coating of saliva, and you ask if he has noticed any wetness of his pillow upon arising in the morning. Upon protruding his tongue approximately 0.5 inch beyond his incisor teeth and resting it there, you think you see an irregular surface of his tongue along both sides. Every now and then you see dimpling movements in different areas of the surface of the tongue along the sides.

Q9: *What interpretation do you give to the wetness on the surface of the mouth and tongue?*

Q10: *What is the significance of the question about the wet pillow in the morning?*

Q11: *What is the meaning of the irregular tongue surface along the sides?*

Q12: *What relevance are the dimpling movements scattered over the edges of the tongue?*

During the interview you note further that two or three times when you touched on personal issues, the patient seemed to be on the verge of crying. When asked about it he said, almost puzzled by his own loss of control, that he had been doing that quite often during the past two months, sometimes with only the slightest provocation. You note also, as he speaks, that in addition to the hoarseness his prosody is somewhat lacking in pitch variations.

Q13: *What thoughts come to mind about the patient's tendency to cry easily?*

Q14: *Does the observation of a tendency toward monopitch contribute anything to your differential diagnostic thinking?*

Continuing with a routine motor-speech examination, you are further alerted to the possibility that on testing alternate motion rate for /p ʌ /, /t ʌ /, and /k ʌ /, his ability to repeat these syllables may not be quite within the normal speed range, something that did not appear abnormal during contextual speech. You decide to measure his rate and discover that for the /p ʌ / his maximum rate is 5 Hz, for /t ʌ /, 4 Hz, and for /k ʌ /, his rate fluctuates between 3 and 4 Hz.

> **Q15:** *What significance do you give to the alternate motion rates obtained?*

Further background information reveals that the patient has been having difficulty lately swallowing liquids, tending to choke occasionally unless he drinks slowly. His gag reflex, on your continued motor-speech examination, is quite active and yet, even though you do not hear any hypernasality, he seems to have mild nasal emission producing moisture on a mirrored surface.

> **Q16:** *What is the potential significance of the patient's occasional tendency to choke on fluids?*
>
> **Q17:** *In view of the active gag reflex, what significance, if any, is the mild degree of nasal emission observed during mirror testing?*
>
> **Q18:** *What diagnostic possibilities are you entertaining concerning this patient's voice disorder?*
>
> **Q19:** *What decisions would you make concerning further procedures to be taken with this patient?*

DISCUSSION

The case depicted here is not unusual. A patient comes with a focal voice disorder in which most or all attention by various clinicians has been directed toward the larynx, obscuring other deviations of speech, which admittedly can be borderline and appear normal until scrutinized carefully. Such was the situation with this patient who, because of no mass lesions and because of symmetric movements of the vocal folds, was considered to be free of organic disease. The inflammation noted by the otolaryngologist is so common in patients, and especially in those who have a tendency toward vocal misuse, it is considered to be insignificant. It would have been reasonable for the average clinician to attribute the strained-hoarse dysphonia to vocal misuse in a teacher under stress in his job, but concurrent events are not necessarily causally related.

Piecing the evolving historical and examination findings together, the clinician should have become increasingly suspicious that there was more going on with this patient's speech mechanism than a phonatory disorder. In retrospect, we see a picture forming of a man developing emotional lability, dysphagia, reduced ability to swallow accumulating saliva, possible tongue atrophy and fasciculations, velopharyngeal insufficiency (which can occur even in the presence of an active gag reflex), a positive sucking reflex, and borderline slow reciprocating muscle movements as demonstrated on alternate motion rates.

The differential diagnostic choices in this patient are between psychogenic voice disorder with or without vocal abuse and very early spastic (pseudobulbar) dysarthria having a major laryngeal-phonatory expression.

The decision at the termination of the speech pathologist's examination should have been, and was, to refer the patient for a neurologic examination, whereupon signs of spasticity were found elsewhere in the body, as was evidence of muscle denervation on electromyographic examination, implicating the lower motor neuron in addition to the upper motor neuron system. The neurologist's diagnosis was motor neuron disease, probably amyotrophic lateral sclerosis.

III. STRAINED HOARSE VOICE ARREST - INTERMITTENT ARRHYTHMIC GROUP

Case Study Number 6

A 32-year-old woman enters your office. Three chairs line the wall, each extending further from your desk. She sits on the one farthest from you, piling her coat, purse, and paperback book on her lap. She smiles, sits erectly, and leans away from you.

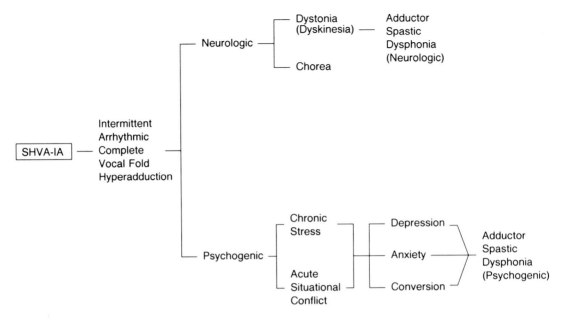

Q1: What early inferences might be made about this person based on the information given?

Q2: Which statement to the patient do you think would be the most appropriate to make at this juncture in the examination?:

   a. *"I see you've been reading the latest best seller. I've been wanting to get it myself. What do you think of it?"*

   b. *"Your doctor sent me a report about your voice disorder. From his letter, it looks as if you've been abusing your voice quite a bit lately."*

   c. *"You might be more comfortable if you put your belongings on that chair and sat next to my desk. I think we'll be able to converse more easily that way."*

*   *   *

C: What brings you to the Clinic?

P: My voice. It's been like this for three months, and it's like about to drive me up the wall.

C: Could you describe it? What's different about it now, compared with the way it used to be?

P: Gee, that's going to be hard . . . Well, I guess it's kind of hoarse. Well, not exactly hoarse; it's different from the hoarseness I usually get from laryngitis. It's, uh, kind of strained or rhaspy; like I'm pushing or pulling everything from way down here. (She lays the flat of her hand on her abdomen.) It's very tiring. Sometimes it gets so bad I just don't talk.

C: How did this voice trouble start?

P: It actually began with a cold and sore throat. (Laughs wryly.) Then, the cold went away, but the hoarseness didn't. My neck feels sore, too. (She runs her hand from her chest to under her chin.) And, I get this pain in my ears. The doctor looked but he couldn't find anything wrong with my ears or my lymph nodes.

*   *   *

Q3: Why didn't the clinician launch directly into a voice evaluation instead of conducting a preliminary discussion?

Q4: Even though you have not performed a formal voice evaluation, what might you deduce about your patient's vocal fold activity from her description of her voice?

Q5: What do you think is the physical basis for her complaints about increased efforts to talk?

Q6: What do you make of her statement that her voice trouble persisted?

Q7: What might be the significance of her complaints of neck and ear pain?

* * *

C: So, if I have this correctly, your voice trouble began about three months ago with a cold and persisted after the cold cleared. I want to go into the history of the voice disorder in greater detail, but before we do, I want to examine thoroughly your speech mechanism and voice.

C: First, read this paragraph aloud while I tape record your speech.

P: (She reads the "Grandfather Passage" aloud.)

C: Now I want you to sustain the vowel /a/ as long and steadily as you can. Do that three times.

P: (As she reads the passage you hear irregular, fluctuating moments of strained hoarseness. On vowel prolongation, her voice is also strained but not as much as during oral reading. You hear moments of clearer voice which is even more apparent at higher pitch levels.)

C: Allright, now will you cough as sharply as you can?

P: (She does so with a sharp, well-defined glottal attack.)

C: What we want to do now is to examine your speech mechanism. I'd like you to sit up straight and rest your hands in your lap. Look straight ahead.

P: (The clinician observes her during complete rest for several seconds.)

C: Now, open your mouth, but keep your tongue at rest on the floor of the mouth.

P: (The tongue is of normal size and shape and is symmetric.)

C: Now, gently rest the tip of your tongue over your lower teeth.

P: (The tongue surface remains quiescent.)

C: Stick your tongue straight out of your mouth.

P: (She does so symmetrically.)

C: Wiggle it from side to side as fast as you can.

P: (These movements are performed rapidly with good range of motion.)

C: Put your tongue in your left cheek and don't let my finger press it in.

P: (This is done in the right cheek as well. Her tongue resists pressure well.)

C: Press your tongue forward against the tongue depressor as I push in.

P: (She does this with good strength.)

C: Lift the tip of your tongue and touch your upper lip.

P: (This is performed normally.)

C: Hold your mouth open quietly again while I look at your soft palate.

P: (It hangs quietly and symmetrically.)

C: I'm going to take this tongue depressor and stroke the sides of your soft palate and pharynx.

P: (She gags easily and both sides of the soft palate rise symmetrically and with good medial pharyngeal wall movement.)

C: Open and close your mouth.

P: (She does so without any deviation of the mandible.)

* * *

Q8: *What words might you use to describe the patient's voice signs?*

Q9: *What kinds of information did you expect to obtain from asking her to read a standard paragraph aloud?*

Q10: *What kinds of information did you expect to obtain from asking her to sustain a vowel sound as long as she could?*

Q11: *What is the significance of her clearer voice at a higher pitch level?*

Q12: *What is the purpose of asking her to cough as sharply as possible?*

Q13: *In light of the fact that she has been referred to you with a voice disorder, for what specific reasons did you perform a complete oral-physical examination?*

Q14: *What was the purpose of asking her to sit as quietly as possible while you observed her head, neck, and other bodily structures?*

* * *

C: If you will look straight ahead, now, I'm going to feel your neck.

P: (Her larynx is rigid; it is difficult to move from side to side. Her thyroid cartilage is pulled up high in her neck, and her thyrohyoid space is narrow. You encircle the hyoid bone with the thumb of your left hand over the tip of the left major horn of her hyoid bone and the middle finger over the right, and pressing inward, rotate your fingers over this area.) "Ow. Do you have to do that? (Then, with the thumb and middle finger over the superior borders of the alae of the thyroid cartilage and your index finger in the thyroid notch, you try to maneuver the larynx downward, away from the hyoid bone. As you are doing this, you ask.)

C: How does that feel?

P: Oh, it hurts. It really does. (*As she says this, you hear a sudden clearing of her voice.* She looks at you with surprise.) Say. That sounded different, (her voice returning to its strained-hoarseness).

* * *

Q15: *What is your interpretation of the elevated larynx, laryngeal rigidity, and diminished thyrohyoid space?*

Q16: *Name the muscles most likely to be involved in these physical findings.*

Q17: *Why did she respond with pain when you pressed your fingers and rotated them in the hyoid region?*

Q18: *How does this information contribute to your understanding of the etiologic diagnosis of her voice disorder?*

Q19: *What is the significance of the momentary clearing of her voice as you pulled downward on her larynx?*

* * *

C: Let's continue with the history of your voice trouble. Tell me, from the time it began, is it getting better, worse, or staying the same?

P: It fluctuates. Sometimes it's better, sometimes worse.

C: How about time of day; does that affect it?

P: Yes. It's usually better in the morning. In fact, there are times when I first get up in the morning it's normal, and that may last for 15 to 20 minutes.

C: Have there been other times that the voice has returned to normal?

P: Yes. About a month ago it was normal almost the whole time I was on a trip alone to San Francisco, but it got worse again after I came home.

C: So, your voice disorder is not a steady thing; it fluctuates with time of day and where you are. Your doctor wrote in his referral letter that you are in TV production. Tell me about that.

P: I'm an assistant manager.

C: How long have you been in that kind of work?

P: About 10 years. I joined the station right out of college.

C: Do you use your voice much in your work?

P: (She smiles and angles her head toward you for emphasis.) You bet I do. I'm on the phone all day talking to salesmen, technicians, personnel. Some days by late afternoon I can barely talk.

C: And, have you always had to use your voice a lot in your work?

P: Yes. It's been that way from the beginning when I took the job.

* * *

Q20: *What is your reaction to the information that the patient's voice fluctuates depending upon situations and time of day?*

Q21: *What is your reaction to the information that at times the voice has returned to normal for several minutes to several days?*

Q22: *What conclusions do you draw about the possible etiology of her voice disorder from the information that she uses her voice far more than the average person in her daily work?*

Q23: *With the information you have at this point, are you satisfied that you understand the etiology of her voice disorder and are ready to begin therapy? If so, what procedures would you next initiate?*

Q24: *If you are not satisfied that you have the entire picture of her voice problem, what further information would you wish to obtain?*

* * *

C: Let's stop at this point and review what we have so far. Did your doctor explain the results of his laryngologic examination?

P: Yes. He said my vocal cords were normal except for some slight reddening that couldn't account for my abnormal voice. He said the redness could have come from a cold or it could be due to irritation from abusing my voice.

C: Good. Because I want you to understand that basically there is nothing physically wrong with your vocal cords. There are no growths, infections, or paralyses that might account for your voice trouble.

P: Well, I'm certainly glad to hear that. You hear so much about cancer and things like that. I was really worried. . . . But, then why does my voice sound this way? Are you going to tell me this is all in my head?

C: That's a good question, because, here you have this very abnormal sounding voice and we're telling you there's nothing physically wrong with the voice mechanism.

P: Yes. And, that feeling of stiffness and pain—if that's not physical, what could it be?

C: I appreciate how confusing this must be, so, I want to introduce an idea to you that, for the time being, might help to explain your complaints. A person can have considerable changes in voice along with real feelings of stiffness and pain because of excess contraction of the throat muscles. Most people have had similar tension and pain in other parts of the body. When such tensions occur in the throat muscles, they can cause changes in the voice along with these abnormal feelings.

P: All right. So, what causes the tensions? I think I'm pretty well adjusted. (Slight note of irritation in her manner at this point.)

C: Let's talk about that, if we may. Specifically, was there anything unusual in the way of personal problems when you started having trouble with your voice?

P: Not that I can think of. I was working as usual. Everything is going real well at the job. In fact, I just got a promotion and a raise. No, there's nothing. (As the patient tells you this, she averts her gaze and frowns, looking down at her lap. There is a long pause.)

* * *

Q25: *Which of the following steps would you take at this point?*
  a. Accept her denial of problems and continue on another subject.
  b. Point out to her that she seems upset by something.
  c. Discontinue the examination and make another appointment.
  d. Wait and say nothing.

* * *

(She looks up at you, smiles and shrugs her shoulders as if to say: "That's it; nothing else comes to mind".)

C: This is a difficult question for most people. Sometimes we are unaware that certain things are bothering us.

P: Well, like what kinds of problems are you referring to? I mean, uh, I guess maybe there has been something bothering me, but I didn't think it would have anything to do with my voice. (Pauses) Now that you mention it, I have been unhappy in a situation that I haven't done anything about. Normally, when I'm unhappy in a situation, I change it. (Pause) The marriage.

C: Would you mind telling me more about that?

P: Well, he is very . . . he doesn't want to accept the fact that we don't have a marriage, and it's very difficult for him. He doesn't understand a lot of things about it which I understand. I've never been a nervous person or shaky, you know, about anything, and just since we've been married, I've been fighting the divorce or separation. For my husband's sake, I want to stay married.

C: What, in your opinion, is wrong with the marriage?

P: I guess the fact that I don't like closeness. I loved being single. My favorite things are to ride my horse out in the woods for days or read books. Of course, I love being with people also. I am an executive, so I have to be with people. But, marriage isn't anything like I thought it would be.

C: What did you think it was going to be like?

P: Well, I thought it would be a great deal of sharing emotionally and materialistically—all the things that you share—but I didn't think it would be sharing *everything,* meaning the husband; he doesn't want to do anything unless I do it with him. To me, it has been very draining, because I never in my life, even when I lived with a big family, had all that closeness. I've never had that much closeness in that way; to me, it's like 24 hours of . . . (pauses, searches for the right word).

C: Being stifled?

P: Yes. And I've told him that and explained it to him and he doesn't do it purposely. I think it's the first time he's ever been in love, and he's gotten carried away with it. And the difference being he's a person that needs me and I don't need him. I don't need him in the way, I mean, to fulfill my life, and that is a big difference in our relationship.

C: Did you have trouble confronting your husband with your feelings about the marriage?

P: Not at all. In fact, before we got married, I was really fighting getting married.

C: Why did you?

P: I wish I knew, because it just happened real suddenly, and my husband is very persuasive, and I've always really cared for him, too. (Long pause)

C: How and when did you meet him?

P: We were attending the same advertising convention. That was about nine months ago. He's older, 52, and has made a lot of money and had been recently divorced. It was a sort of a whirlwind courtship, at least for me. He sort of pursued me during the whole convention. We started going out together. After that, he was very insistent; said he needed me desperately. We were married after three months.

C: So, that was about six months ago, and your voice trouble started three months ago. But, in spite of your feelings about wanting to remain single, you went ahead with the marriage anyway. Did you express your misgivings to your husband before you were married?

P: Very much. I told him I was not a touchy-feely person. I mean, I'm loving, and I have a lot of love to give, and I can accept love, but he is starved for love in the way that he really needs constant patting on the head and a lot of attention, and a lot of what I can't, I guess, give. And, I don't know if there is any reason for him to lack that just because of me.

C: Do you and your husband have much in common?

P: Oh gosh! We have everything in common. We are both very adventuresome; we love to travel, camp, ski.

C: Do you think your voice is better right now than when we started?

P: Much better.

C: I'm glad you recognize that. It's 50 to 75 percent improved since we began discussing this marital situation. Do you feel better about having talked about that?

P: Yes. Much better. Up until now, I kept rejecting talking to anybody professional about it. I kept thinking, well, whatever it is it will go away tomorrow, because tomorrow would be fine. I got to the point where it was so frustrating not being able to converse and express or even go to a counter and order a bottle of perfume without somebody asking: "What are you saying?" This confirms my feeling that my voice has something to do with keeping things in. In other words, I've always been a happy person, and I'm always jovial and never depressed, and just lately I've been in a state of depression.

C: Can you estimate for how long?

P: Well, I'd say about three or four months.

C: That's about the time you've had your voice problem.

P: I feel like it has. Because I feel like it, in other words, as I said earlier, I've never been a nervous person. Well, lately I've been very, very tense. I lay down to go to sleep and try to sleep and then just start thinking.

C: Do you think our discussion has been helpful?

P: I'm sure it has. Before, I thought this voice thing was physical, but I realize now I don't have something physical. I feel more comfortable about that. I also feel more comfortable because until now, I hadn't talked to anybody at length about this.

* * *

Q26: *What would you say next to the patient? Why?*

* * *

C: How do you think we should proceed from here?

P: (She becomes silent for almost a minute, thinking deeply.) Obviously, my voice is better. Sounds almost normal, now. I came to have my voice helped, but here I am with an entirely different problem. That I didn't expect.

C: That's something you're going to have to deal with, isn't it? What do you want to do?

P: I think a separation is worth a try; be away from each other for six months or so and for me to seek whatever therapy I need during that six months.

C: Therapy? What did you have in mind?

P: Counseling, marital counseling I suppose.

C: Do you know of anyone locally who could help? Or, would you prefer that we arrange for you to see someone?

P: No, I know someone who's really good, has a good reputation. May I ask that you send a report of your examination to her?

C: Of course. And, I'll send a full report to your laryngologist within the next few days.

P: But, do you really think all this has caused my voice trouble?

C: What do you think?

P: (She smiles.) I think it has.

C: I'll say goodbye, then. Please keep in touch and let me know how things turn out?

P: I will. I promise.

* * *

Q27: Is there a relationship between her marital problem and her voice disorder? Or, are they just coincidental?

Q28: How do you think the clinician in this case handled the situation?

Q29: Do you think the patient was in need of psychiatric help? Explain.

Q30: What formal diagnosis would you give to her voice disorder? Why?

Q31: What do you think is the prognosis for her voice disorder and her relationship with her husband? Why?

Q32: Should the patient have been given conventional voice therapy?

The patient wrote the following letter to the speech pathologist:

It has been two months since I came to see you about my voice disorder, and I hope you will recall the circumstances surrounding the disorder. As we had decided then, I went to see a psychiatrist in my hometown who specializes in marital problems. Both my husband and myself had several sessions with her, and after getting our differences into the open, which took several consultations, we decided, with the approval of the psychiatrist, to separate. This happened three weeks ago, and while my voice had remained improved after having seen you, it continued to do so after our separation and as I write my voice is completely normal.

I would like to thank you for all your help and for enabling me to see what was bothering me.

INSTRUCTIONS

1. Write a clinical report of your examination of this patient.
2. Write a letter to the referring otolaryngologist.

SAMPLE REPORT OF CLINICAL VOICE EXAMINATION

Mrs. _____ is a 32-year-old television station assistant manager who was referred by Dr. _____, laryngologist, with a diagnosis of a "voice disorder secondary to vocal abuse." Based on his laryngoscopic examination, except for some evidence of vocal fold irritation, the vocal folds were essentially normal in structure and movement.

The patient began noticing signs of strained voice quality approximately three months following her marriage. It has persisted since then, although it fluctuates, depending upon time of day, fatigue, and whether or not she happens to be experiencing an optimistic or pessimistic outlook. On one occasion the voice was completely normal while she was alone on vacation.

Oral-physical examination failed to disclose any evidence of facial, lingual, velar, or mandibular weakness or asymmetry. She gave no evidence of unusual movements about her face or other parts of her head, neck, or extremities. Articulation, both during contextual speech and on alternate motion rate, failed to disclose any evidence of a motor speech disorder.

The physical history indicates that although Mrs. _____ has been under considerable pressure at work using her voice a great deal, this situation has existed for many more years than the short duration of her current voice disorder. After initial reluctance, she disclosed that she was dissatisfied with her marriage owing to its confining nature. As the patient disclosed this information her voice gradually improved. She recognized the improvement and understood the relationship between her voice disorder and her martial dissatisfaction.

We discussed the advisability of her obtaining counseling in order to help her resolve her marital problem. Symptomatic therapy of the voice disorder would be ill-timed in view of her emotional conflict and its priority over her abnormal voice.

We decided that the patient would seek professional help for her marital problem. She will keep us informed as to her progress.

SAMPLE LETTER TO THE OTOLARYNGOLOGIST

Thank you for your kind referral of Mrs. _____. I have enclosed the report of my clinical speech evaluation. While I think that vocal abuse might have exacerbated her voice disorder, it was my impression, as noted in the enclosed report of clinical examination, that the fundamental cause of her dysphonia has been psychologic and related to an unresolved marital problem. I think you would be gratified to learn that her dysphonia improved significantly during her disclosure of her dissatisfactions, and that she recognized the relationship between her voice disorder and these tensions. My impression was that symptomatic voice therapy would have been premature at this point inasmuch as her entire attitude shifted from attention to her voice to that of her martial dissatisfaction.

I offered the patient the names of psychiatrists and clinical psychologists in her local area, but she elected to see someone of her acquaintance with an excellent reputation. I will keep you informed as to her progress. I suggested that she contact you at some date in the future to let you know how she is doing.

If there is any further information that you would like to have, please do not hesitate to call or write.

DISCUSSION

It is usually a good idea to begin with general conversation rather than going directly into the mechanics of the voice examination. To do so is not only a sign of personal interest in the patient but also gives the clinician an impression of the patient's total communication in addition to the voice, i.e., resonation, articulation, language, ideation, and affect.

From the transcript, we read the description "strained or effortful." Although it is difficult to know what the voice was like without hearing it, the term "strained" ought to have conjured up hyperadduction of either the true vocal folds, false vocal folds, or both. Complaints about increased effort to talk along with strained hoarseness is also evidence of vocal fold hyperadduction. The increased physical effort indicates that the patient was having to exert abnormally intense thoracic and abdominal muscle contraction in order to force air through the hyperadducted vocal folds. The patient's complaint of neck and ear pain are usually signs of chronic excess intrinsic and extrinsic laryngeal muscle contraction.

The statement that the voice disorder began with an upper respiratory infection that disappeared whereas the voice disorder persisted, usually indicates psychogenic dysphonia, since a high percentage of psychogenic voice disorders begin in this way.

Laryngeal elevation, rigidity, and diminished thyrohyoid space are usually signs of chronic hypercontraction of the extrinsic, and probably the intrinsic, laryngeal muscles and are associated with musculoskeletal tension disorders. The muscle groups most likely involved in such laryngeal malpositioning are the suprahyoids and infrahyoids. Pain when the tissues around the hyoid bone and thyroid cartilage are kneaded supports the inference of excess musculoskeletal tension. (*Many clinicians are reluctant to touch the patient, let alone cause pain. Yet, it is essential to determine if, in fact, pain and tension exist if a proper etiologic diagnosis is to be made.*)

Momentary clearing of the voice as the larynx was pulled downward reinforces the suspicion of a musculoskeletal tension voice disorder. That the patient's voice fluctuated depending upon situation and time of day further supports psychogenicity; however, it must be strongly emphasized that organic voice disorders also vary in this manner, although they rarely return to normal. That her voice returned to normal, not just improved, from several minutes to several days, almost certainly indicates that the entire voice disorder is psychogenic.

From the written descriptions of the voice, such words as spastic, spasmodic, hyperfunctional, or strained-hoarseness come to mind. Asking the patient to read a standard paragraph aloud not only provides information about how the dysphonia fluctuates with the production of phonemes in different contexts, but it also reveals other aspects of motor speech. Asking the patient to sustain a vowel provides information about the quality, pitch level, and steadiness of the voice. During such steady-state activity, the clinician can listen carefully for subtle voice aberrations and for fluctuations in laryngeal-respiratory control. Also, in certain voice disorders, vowel prolongation can produce a very different voice than during contextual speech, which may have important differential diagnostic significance.

The fact that the patient's voice was clearer at higher pitch levels should have led the clinician in the direction of considering the voice disorder to be one type of adductor spastic dysphonia, in which there is strained voice at conversational pitch levels but clear voice at higher ones.

Asking the patient to cough or produce a sharp glottal attack provides important information about her ability to adduct her vocal folds adequately. In patients who have organic weakness, the cough and glottal coup lack sharpness. A complete oral-physical examination is always important, even when the clinician suspects that the disorder is confined to the larynx, because motor-speech disorders can begin with a dysphonia, *predominantly*, while very careful examination of remaining motor-speech structures may disclose the beginnings of a dysarthria in other regions of the speech musculature.

Asking the patient to keep her mouth, tongue, and jaw at rest while the clinician observes her head and neck structures is important to determine the presence of subtle neurologic movement disorders that have a tendency to show themselves only when the patient is quiescent.

There was a definite link between the patient's marital problem and her voice disorder. Only during her marriage did she develop the voice disorder for the first time in her life. Her voice became normal while she was away from her husband. Her dysphonia improved during the interviews as she described the conflicts created by her marriage. There was little question that the patient needed counseling. She was in a serious conflictual situation that was already having somatic repercussions, and it was apparent that she was unable to manage this situation on her own.

Based on the intermittent strained voice quality and associated laryngospasm, the history, and the changes in voice, it would be appropriate to conclude that this patient had *adductor spastic dysphonia, psychogenic, probably of the conversion-reaction type*.

Case Study Number 7

A 43-year-old married woman with grown children who works for a real estate firm came to the Clinic for help with a voice problem of one year's duration. She describes her voice as "tense, strained, and high in pitch, and some words won't come out at all." Her disorder began gradually with a nondescript hoarseness that continued to deteriorate to its current strained quality. It had improved on occasion; she had been receiving voice therapy "to produce a more relaxed and clearer voice." While she found that she could, in fact, produce a clearer voice with concentration, these techniques did not hold up in most speaking situations outside of the Clinic. She volunteers that her voice disorder has interfered with her supervisory responsibilities at work and has been equally damaging to her social life. The most important ability had gone out of her life, she said, and at fleeting moments during the past few months, she has had suicidal thoughts.

Lately, she has been complaining of "a tight neck and shoulder" and that especially when driving, she has noticed a tremor of her head. At about the same time she began to notice a tremor in her voice, but this was prior to its worsening.

Voice examination revealed a pronounced strained-strangled voice, but vowel prolongation was clear and steady, except at a higher pitch level where mild tremor was detected. During the oral-physical examination, she had intermittent head tremor and a tendency for her head to turn to her right side.

The psychosocial history was nonproductive. She was not under any particular stress or anxiety at work, and her marital and other domestic relationships, including those with her children, were pleasant and free of all but the usual day-to-day variations.

The ear, nose, and throat examination report came back with the notation, "normal laryngoscopic examination; functional dysphonia."

> *Q1:   From this description of the patient's voice, what terminology would you use to describe the voice signs and symptoms?*

Q2:   *What muscular actions within the larynx and surrounding structures could be producing this kind of voice?*

Q3:   *What significance, if any, would you give to the patient's complaint of turning of her head and head tremor?*

Q4:   *What are your thoughts, your reactions to the examination report of a normal larynx and that the disorder was "functional"?*

Q5:   *With the information that you have in hand, what next steps would you take in the management of this patient?*

Because of her complaint of mild turning of her head and head tremor, a neurologic examination was scheduled. After a complete examination, the neurologist summarized his findings as follows: "For the past two years, the patient has been aware of a sense of aching in the back of her neck in the region of the left trapezius muscle. A few months later she began to be aware of a tendency for her face to turn to the left and the vertex of her head to the right, which she can voluntarily straighten with her left hand. No one else observed these movements owing to their mildness. She is most aware of this movement while driving a car and watching television or a movie. Also a few months after the onset of aching in her neck, she became aware of a horizontal head tremor, intermittently, most noticeable when she was in a motor vehicle. A few months after that she began to detect a tremor in her voice. Laughing or yawning transiently corrected the aberrant head posturing. Because of her voice disorder, her future career is at stake, and if something is not done about her voice she may lose her position in her firm. She admits to a reactive depression to her voice that has also caused her to become withdrawn. In addition to the voice and head and neck findings, it is also important to note that she holds a writing instrument tightly and comments that, within the past year, her penmanship has declined. The remainder of the examination is normal. *Impression:* The neurologic examination gives evidence of extremely mild, but observable, spasmodic torticollis and associated head tremor."

Q6:   *What is spasmodic torticollis?*

Q7:   *What is the significance of the head tremor in association with spasmodic torticollis?*

Q8:   *What is the connection, if any, between the spasmodic torticollis, head tremor, and the patient's voice disorder?*

Q9:   *What is the significance of the change in her writing?*

Conference with both the laryngologist and the neurologist discloses that there is no therapy that could be suggested from the standpoint of their specialties; that there were some drugs that have been used to treat a variety of movement disorders but that none had shown any promise.

Q10: *What steps would you now initiate with this patient in order to help her with her voice disorder?*

Q11: *The patient is now back in your office and it is your responsibility to summarize the results of everyone's examinations and to counsel the patient further pertaining to future therapy, if any. What would you tell the patient as to the nature of her voice disorder, its cause, and the options for treatment?*

The patient was told that she had a disorder that has gone by the name of adductor spastic dysphonia, and that in some cases the disorder is psychologic and in some cases it is neurologic. In her case—in addition to the fact that previous psychiatric and psychologic studies had failed to show any significant psychopathology, and that the neurologic examination had disclosed mild but positive signs of a movement disorder—in all probability (although no one can say with complete certainty), this was an adductor spastic dysphonia of the dystonic type involving both torticollis and tremor. Because previous therapy performed by a competent speech pathologist had failed to produce an enduring improvement in her voice, the patient was told the only remaining therapy option available at that time was the recurrent laryngeal nerve resection procedure.

The patient, it turned out, had studied this disorder and its causes and she knew about the surgery for it. She expressed skepticism owing to the conflicting reports about its effectiveness, especially in the long term, and was concerned about the kind of voice quality that would result from the surgery. On the other hand, she said that she was thoroughly "fed up" with the voice, that she had to do something, and that she was willing to risk failure if there was any chance the surgery might prove to be of benefit for her.

After evaluating videotapes of previous patients who had undergone the surgery, the patient decided to proceed with the lidocaine injection procedure.

> *Q12:* *What is the purpose of the lidocaine injection? Explain, physiologically, its effects on the patient's vocal folds, the kind of voice that will result from the injection, what it can predict about the effects of surgery, and indications and contraindications to surgery based on the injection procedure.*

Sitting upright in the laryngologist's examining chair, a needle filled with 1 percent lidocaine was injected in the region of the cricothyroid space on the right side of the neck.

> *Q13:* *Why was the injection made at this particular anatomic site?*
> *Q14:* *How soon after the injection should the voice change?*
> *Q15:* *How long should the effects of the injection last?*
> *Q16:* *How can you tell if the injection has paralyzed the vocal folds?*
> *Q17:* *What kinds of voice testing material should be used to enable patients and clinicians to evaluate the effects of the injection?*

It required four injections before the laryngologist was able to hit the nerve and the voice became smooth, slightly breathy, and completely free of spasm. The patient expressed immediate gratification at these voice and physical changes and said that she wished to proceed with surgery without further need for contemplation. The patient underwent a pre-anesthesia medical examination during the afternoon of that day, entered the hospital at suppertime, and went into surgery at 7:30 the next morning. The patient was anesthetized, a primary, collar incision was made at the base of her neck, and the right recurrent laryngeal nerve was identified. After certainty of identification by mechanical stimulation of the presumed nerve and looking for momentary vocal cord movement via direct laryngoscopy, a section of the nerve was taken and the neck was closed. The pathologist's report identified the specimen as nerve tissue.

During the next few hours, the patient became increasingly alert, remained in her hospital room that night and was wheeled to the speech pathologist's office the next morning for a 24-hour postsurgery evaluation.

> *Q18:* *What would you expect the patient's voice to sound like at this postsurgical period?*
> *Q19:* *What would you tell the patient when she asks whether this is the way the voice is going to be or whether it will change?*
> *Q20:* *What advice should be given to the patient at this point as to how to use the voice?*

The 24-hour postsurgical voice was breathy and each time the patient increased the intensity of her voice, it became rhaspy and contained falsetto pitch breaks. She expressed satisfaction, at this point, mostly with the increased ease of voice production. She looked calm, her facial expression having changed from one of strain to one of relaxation. Her voice was recorded.

The next morning, 48 hours after surgery, her voice had lost some of the breathiness and was louder. She looked less groggy and continued to express approval of the sound and feel of the voice. Her voice was recorded again and she returned to her hospital room.

On the third morning, 72 hours after surgery, her voice had continued to improve in clarity and loudness. She had just been discharged from the hospital and was going home. She was advised to use her voice fully and not to be afraid of using it, although loud abusive talking would obviously be ill-advised. One week later the patient wrote:

It is still difficult for me to believe this "miracle" has really happened. Each day is a gift from God. The most wonderful change is that I can again enjoy being with people I love rather than wishing they would go away and let me have some peace.

I am still a little hesitant to talk too much; I don't want to "wear it out."

I can barely remember the constant fatigue and depression I felt only a week ago. The future looks bright and sunny. I believe faith and a realistic expectation of success will keep this "miracle" working.

There are no words adequate to express our gratitude. You have touched our lives in a very special way.

One year after surgery, her voice could be described as nearly normal. It is smooth, melodious, free of any hint of spasm, and, most importantly, has remained consistently so without any sign of deterioration.

Q21:   *What accounts for the voice improvement as time passes following surgery?*

Q22:   *Can all patients who have recurrent laryngeal nerve surgery expect the degree of improvement experienced by this patient? What would you say to a patient who asked about the probabilities of improvement as a result of surgery?*

DISCUSSION

This patient had the neurologic adductor spastic dysphonia of the dystonic variety with associated tremor. The strained-hoarse arrests of the voice arose from intermittent hyperadduction of the true and false vocal folds. The first clue to the neurologic nature of her spastic dysphonia was the tremor in her voice and head, and the complaint of turning of the head. Tremor and spasmodic torticollis commonly occur in association with each other, and adductor laryngeal spasms can often be a sign of either disorder. The patient's complaint of difficulty grasping a writing instrument may have indicated some dystonic involvement of her hand. After ruling out primary psychogenic factors and obtaining a neurologic examination, and knowing that previous efforts toward voice therapy were unsuccessful and that the patient was approaching the desperate stage of her experience with disorder, it was obvious that something more drastic needed to be done. Informing the patient as much as possible was necessary. The advantages and disadvantages of surgery needed to be presented, preferably with actual case demonstrations to show the patient what might be expected from the surgery.

The purpose of the lidocaine injection is temporarily to paralyze one vocal fold, simulating the surgery. The kind of voice that results from the injection is not exactly like that from the surgery owing to the frequent involvement of the superior laryngeal nerve affecting the cricothyroid muscle. The patient has to be informed of this fact, and the rule of thumb is that if the patient can accept the lidocaine voice, acceptance of the postsurgical voice will certainly be as good or better. The injection is made in the cricothyroid space because that is the entrance site of the nerve into the larynx. The injection lasts anywhere from 10 to 45 minutes, depending upon how much of the anesthetic infiltrates the nerve. The laryngologist can tell if the injection has paralyzed the vocal fold by performing a laryngoscopic examination after injecting the anesthetic. The speech pathologist can hear the loss of sharpness of the cough, and the voice changes—sometimes rather suddenly—to a husky smoothness, and strained voice arrests suddenly disappear. The voice should be recorded during this period for a further evaluation using the same test materials as those used prior to evaluation—usually a standard paragraph, vowel prolongation, and production of coughing and the glottal coup.

The immediately postsurgical voice is usually breathier and weaker than after the passage of several days owing to the fact that the glottis is widest at this time and that the intact vocal fold has not yet learned to compensate. The patient needs to be reassured that this immediately postsurgical voice will not be permanent and that improvement can be expected within a matter of days. Because there is some evidence to indicate that maintenance of a higher, smoother voice may help to avert spasm in the future, the patient is advised to phonate in a slightly higher pitch than usual and that this be felt in the "mask" region of the face. Finally, it is always wise to maintain contact with the patient and request follow-up recordings or return visits to monitor the progress of the voice and to provide counsel, if necessary.

IV. STRAINED HOARSE VOICE
ARREST - INTERMITTENT RHYTHMIC GROUP

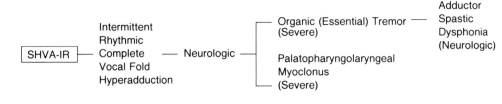

Case Study Number 8

A 47-year-old married woman, referred by her family practitioner, complains of a voice disorder that she has had since age 25 years. Until five years ago, it was intermittent, but since then it has been persistent. She describes her voice as tremulous. One doctor years ago said she probably had parkinsonism.

The internist's note states that her voice symptoms occurred at first only when she was excited or under stress, but over the years they have become persistent. Tension or stress aggravate her voice disorder. Although not disabling, it is embarrassing.

The patient has had hypertension for four years, which is controlled by medication. Her dentition is in poor repair with numerous caries, and she has gingivitis. There is no history of diabetes, hypothyroidism, or any other metabolic disease. Her cardiovascular status is normal. She complains of heartburn once or twice a week. She had a hysterectomy 10 years ago when she was five months pregnant. She has had hot flashes for two to three years, which are not troublesome. She does not take estrogens. She has a mild suprapatellar aching arthralgia when she sits for long periods of time.

The patient divorced her first husband 15 years ago because of physical abuse. Her present marriage is satisfactory. She is employed full time as an office administrator. She and her husband have four children.

Laryngologic examination fails to disclose laryngeal disease, and the laryngologist thinks her tremulous voice may be "functional." During speech examination, you find a pleasant, mildly obese woman who says her voice disorder was intermittent when it started, but she has become concerned about her voice recently because it has grown worse over the past three years. It is now a definite communication problem and interferes with her work as an administrator.

During conversational speech, she has staccato voice arrests. When she sustains the vowel /a/, you hear rhythmic voice arrests of the type heard during contextual speech. You record the vowel prolongation on audiotape and obtain an oscillographic tracing (Fig. 12-1). Speech intelligibility is poor owing to the voice arrests. You also notice an almost imperceptible head tremor and possibly tremors around her lips and chin as she speaks, but which are absent when she is silent. Except for her dysphonia motor speech examination is normal. The patient straightforwardly denies any personal problems during the onset or development of her voice disorder.

Q1: From the oscillographic tracing, what is the approximate frequency of the patient's voice arrests?

Q2: What is the significance of the observation that the patient's voice, head, lips, and chin are tremorous during speech but not during silence?

Q3: What could be the connection between the voice arrests and tremor in other parts of her body?

You schedule a neurologic examination for the patient. This examination confirms the history of the voice disorder and adds other important information; that the patient's legs are beginning to shake and she feels as if her body is getting quivery also. Once or twice a week she chokes while

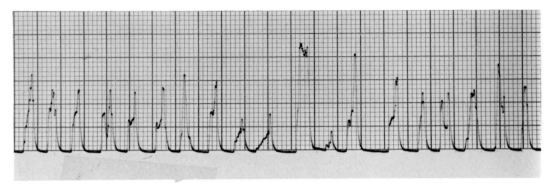

Figure 12-1 Voice arrests produced during vowel /a/ prolongation; 1 sec. equals 25 mm.

eating, and she thinks she has some quivering of her breathing as well. She has previously been told that her symptoms are "all in her head." The neurologic examination discloses a rapid, forward-backward head tremor, voice tremor, and respiratory tremor. Her hands and feet are quite steady. She has a small-fiber peripheral neuropathy in her legs and mildly decreased reflexes. Her blood pressure is elevated.

The neurologist is the first person to ask the patient about any family history of voice or associated tremors; previous examiners had failed to do so. From this single question emerges the most important information of the entire series of examinations—that tremors in different parts of the body are rampant in the patient's family. The Department of Genetics produces the pedigree in Figure 12-2. They reported the following data:

1. The patient's maternal grandmother had tremor of her body and voice.
2. Her maternal-maternal great grandfather had tremors of his voice, arms, legs, and head.
3. Her maternal-maternal great aunt had no outward tremor but is said to have "shook inside."
4. The mother has tremor of her voice and hands, cannot use her hands and has to be dressed and fed.
5. Her maternal aunt has tremor of her voice and arms and cannot use her hands.
6. Her maternal aunt has tremor of her body, voice, and hands but is able to use her hands.
7. Two maternal first cousins are said to have voice and general tremor.
8. Her sister has tremor of her head.
9. Her brother has tremor of his hands.
10. One son has a "halting" speech pattern.

Q4: *What is the etiologic diagnosis of this patient's voice disorder?*

Q5: *With what other voice disorders is this one often confused?*

Q6: *How does the physiology of the voice disorder explain the patient's voice tremor and voice arrests?*

Q7: *What relevance is the history that the voice worsens under stress?*

Q8: *What therapy would you suggest for the voice disorder?*

Q9: *How would you counsel a person with this type of voice disorder as to its prognosis?*

Discussion

This patient's voice arrests are momentary laryngospasms produced by intermittent hyperadduction of the vocal folds. Their regularity or rhythmicity is more apparent during vowel prolongation than contextual speech. Figure 12-1 shows that these arrests occur at a rate of approximately 4 Hz. Rhythmic voice arrests and tremor elsewhere in her body (but only on initiation of movement, not

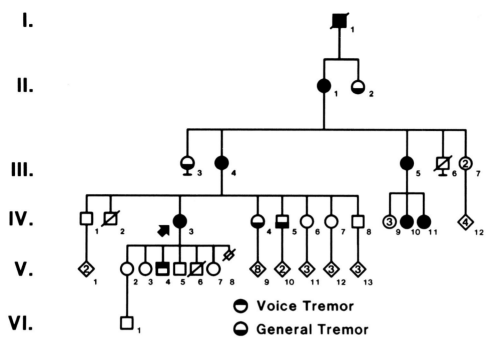

Figure 12–2   Family tree of patient with adductor spastic dysphonia of essential (heredofamilial) tremor. The arrow indicates the patient described in the text.

at rest) mean that she has an *intention* tremor involving her larynx, head, and other body parts. In this particular patient, tremor is present in other members of the patient's family. She qualifies for the diagnosis of essential (heredofamilial) tremor.

Her voice disorder, which some clinicians might have labeled adductor spastic dysphonia without qualifications, needs to be further specified as the *adductor spastic dysphonia of essential tremor,* which is to be distinguished from other forms of adductor spastic dysphonia. The voice disorder is clearly neurologic and highly resistant to voice or drug therapy. At present, the best that can be done for the patient is to educate her as to the etiology of the disorder—many patients are confused about this—and are at least relieved to know that it is a recognized entity and that, although its prognosis is one of continued dysphonia, the disorder is not life-threatening. When the adductor spastic dysphonia of essential tremor becomes severe enough to threaten speech intelligibility, and not all do, consideration of recurrent laryngeal nerve resection should be given with the understanding that its effects may be temporary.

V. VOICE TREMOR GROUP

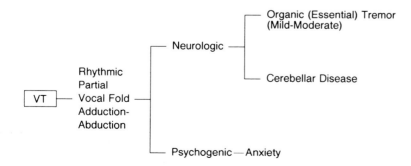

Case Study Number 9

This is a 68-year-old retired female telephone operator referred by a laryngologist who writes that the patient has a tremor of her voice, that it is "functional," and that voice therapy is recommended. The patient is a heavy smoker and has polyps on both vocal folds.

The patient enters your office, and you notice her right hand shakes as she extends her hand in greeting. For a moment, as you look at her sitting in silence, her head seems to be nodding rhythmically, but her hands rest quietly in her lap. Upon responding to your question as to when her voice trouble began, you hear a coarse, low-pitched, quavering voice. The patient says she has been to several doctors about her voice, which is embarrassing to her. She is apologetic about not heeding her local physician's advice to stop smoking. Recently she was told that her voice was a sign of mild Parkinson's disease. Her voice tremor had begun eight years ago, so gradually she was hardly aware of it. However, her head tremor began 30 years ago. Her brother, who is three years younger, has had head and hand tremor for four or five years, but his voice is normal.

The voice tremor came on after the extraction of three teeth for pyorrhea. She was given thiopental sodium anesthesia. All went uneventfully. Two weeks after surgery her teeth were fitted and she had some trouble with her articulation. Six weeks later, a quaver in her voice first appeared. Since then both the voice and head tremor have gradually worsened. Her tremor is worse when she is tired or upset.

> *Q1:* What is meant by voice tremor?
>
> *Q2:* What would you expect to see on laryngoscopic examination during vowel prolongation in a patient with voice tremor?
>
> *Q3:* From the data given, what arguments can you muster in support of the diagnosis of parkinsonism as a cause of the voice tremor?
>
> *Q4:* From the data given, what arguments can be made against parkinsonism as a cause of her dysphonia?
>
> *Q5:* What evidence do we have that the voice tremor is "functional" or psychogenic?
>
> *Q6:* Why does the patient have a low-pitched hoarseness in addition to the tremor?

An oral-physical and motor speech examination revealed the following information:

1. The patient's voice tremor on vowel prolongation averaged 5 Hz. The tremor smoothly varied, but occasionally she would produce a complete voice arrest.
2. Synchronous with the voice tremor were pharyngeal and tongue tremor. Almost unnoticeable were also lip and mandibular tremor.
3. Although no tremor was noticed when the upper extremities were at rest, the patient had fine hand tremor when she extended her arms with fingers spread.
4. The patient casually mentioned during this examination that she has used alcoholic beverages to reduce the severity of her tremors.

> *Q7:* What formal etiologic diagnosis would you postulate for this voice disorder?
>
> *Q8:* How would you proceed from this point on?

Suspecting a neurologic etiology, you arrange for the patient to have a neurologic examination, which showed the following:

1. Terminal tremor of both upper extremities
2. Tremor of her head and mandible
3. Mild reduction in sensitivity to touch over the dorsum of both feet
4. Mild incoordination on finger-to-nose testing, bilaterally
5. Mild incoordination on heel-to-knee testing

The neurologist's conclusion from the history and physical examination: "This seems to be a nonspecific tremor—probably of basal nuclear origin and possibly familial. It falls within the scope of organic (essential) tremor or heredofamilial tremor. I doubt that anything is likely to be helpful."

DISCUSSION

Outside of neurologic circles, tremor of the voice is often misdiagnosed as either "functional" or psychogenic or as associated with parkinsonism. On laryngoscopic examination, during vowel prolongation the vocal folds are easily visualized rhythmically adducting and abducting, the pitch rising during adduction and falling during abduction. When severe, the vocal folds will adduct completely in the midline, producing voice arrests. If these are pervasive the voice disorder takes on the characteristics of adductor spastic dysphonia.

Parkinsonism does not usually produce voice tremor. In some parkinsonian patients one can hear a highly subtle tremorlike "flutter" on vowel prolongation, but it does not possess the coarser type of tremor as in this patient who has organic (essential) tremor, probably familial. Patients with parkinsonism have tremor, but it is a *rest* tremor. Essential tremor is an *action* or *intention* tremor. The patient under discussion was quiescent at rest and exhibited her tremor only during the volitional acts of phonation and extension of her extremities. The student might ask why, then, did she have head tremor at "rest"? The answer is that holding up the head is not actually a resting activity; doing so requires active muscle contraction to overcome the effects of gravity.

Support for psychogenic etiology was unsubstantiated, although, *stressful events can aggravate and even precipitate tremor, as they do in most neurologic diseases.*

The low-pitched hoarseness was consistent with the polypoid changes of the vocal folds secondary to the long history of tobacco abuse and had no relation to the voice tremor.

Alcohol consumption frequently (not always) reduces the amplitude of organic voice tremor and is useful information in diagnostic history-taking.

Management of organic voice tremor is not easy. Symptomatic voice therapy is ineffective. No convincing evidence of the effectiveness of essential tremor medications for voice tremor has been reported, even though such medications are often beneficial for tremors elsewhere in the body. Although many patients spontaneously employ alcohol as a palliative for voice tremor, it is hazardous because of its potential for producing dependency.

Educating the patient about the etiology of the voice tremor is more valuable than clinicians may realize. As with many other disorders about which patients have been given an incorrect diagnosis, or none at all, to learn that essential tremor is organic rather than psychogenic, that it is benign, that it does not necessarily have to worsen, and may even improve, and that the dysphonia is common and is acceptable to many listeners, can be a genuine relief to patients seeking help for this disorder.

VI. BREATHY WHISPERED - INTERMITTENT GROUP

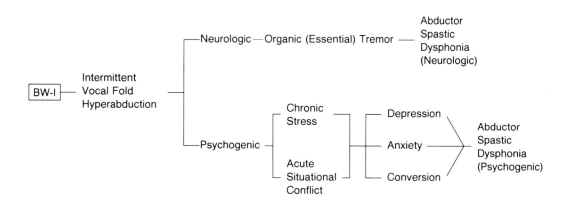

Case Study Number 10

A 39-year-old clergyman is referred to you by a speech pathologist colleague after having had a complete laryngologic examination that failed to disclose any organic laryngeal disease. The referring speech clinician was not experienced in voice disorders and had administered therapy without success. He requests another opinion on diagnosis and treatment of the dysphonia.

The patient, a tall, blond man of striking appearance, has penetrating eye contact and exudes an air of solidity and authority. He is pleasant and straightforward. His language is explicit. He gives the impression of someone who genuinely wants help and will cooperate in any way he can to get it. After completing the preliminaries, he interrupts the examination by asking if his wife could join in the examination, explaining that she has been worried about his voice.

During conversational speech and oral reading of a standard paragraph, you note the following:

1. Every few seconds his normal voice cuts out and becomes breathy or whispered. Then, just as suddenly it returns to normal.
2. These moments of breathiness most often follow unvoiced consonants.
3. They are more often triggered by plosives than by fricatives.
4. These plosives are almost invariably unvoiced.
5. The unvoiced plosives trigger breathiness nearly always when they are in the initial rather than the medial or final positions of words.
6. The patient can produce several sentences without any segments of breathiness.
7. During vowel prolongation, his voice is continuously normal, i.e., free of breathy segments.
8. Each time he produces a moment of breathiness, you notice an abrupt inward movement of his abdomen.

A complete oral-physical and motor-speech examination fails to disclose any evidence of structural or motor disturbances in the remainder of his speech mechanism. The ear, nose, and throat examination is normal. His cough is normally sharp.

You take a careful history. "When and how did his voice disorder begin?" He tells you that it came on five years ago very gradually, increasing to its present level of severity within six months. It has remained this way ever since. He notices that sometimes his voice is better when he is relaxed, and worse when he is under stress, such as while delivering a sermon. He tells you that his voice has never returned to normal for more than a few minutes during the entire history of his voice disorder.

One year after his dysphonia had begun, he sought the help of a speech pathologist who, although not a specialist in voice disorders, agreed to a trial of therapy, because there was no one else available in the patient's locality. For three months, twice a week, the patient was given therapies consisting of grunting, chewing, and relaxation exercises associated with biofeedback sessions during which electrodes were placed over his forehead and jaw muscles. These ministrations were mildly and temporarily helpful, but they benefited his voice least when he needed it most, namely, during the counseling and public speaking demands of his profession. After what he felt was a fair trial of therapy without acceptable results, he broke off further appointments and did nothing about his voice for three years.

"Did the speech clinician ever take a history of any psychologic or emotional problems that you might have had at the time your voice disorder started?" The patient answers that he had asked some general questions but did not go into any depth; he seemed to emphasize voice retraining over other considerations.

You begin to probe the subject of emotional stress. The patient readily accedes to this line of questioning. You ask him about his relationship with his wife and his professional associates and are comfortable with his responses that indicate: (1) He has a stable, amicable relationship with his wife; (2) he is effective and well-respected as a pastor of a small, upper middle-class surburban community.

"Did anything upsetting happen at the time the voice disorder started five years ago?" The following information emerges.

The voice trouble began during a period when their oldest daughter had been arrested for shoplifting. Father and daughter began to have angry "blowups" during which the father was frequently driven to the verge of striking her. The parents tried desperately to help but they had never sought professional assistance.

Commenting on his voice during the height of his conflicts with his daughter, he says: "The more I would yell, the worse my voice would become." During the patient's narrative of this difficult period, his moments of breathy voice are more frequent and of longer duration. Toward the end of his narrative as he brings the history up to the present, he has fewer and briefer moments of breathiness than at the beginning of the interview.

During trial and error therapy, you discover that if the patient makes an effort to sustain voicing during unvoiced consonants, he has fewer and shorter breathy and aphonic breaks.

Q1: Describe the movements of the vocal folds responsible for the voice aberrations during the patient's contextual speech.

Q2: What is the most likely explanation for the fact that the breathy and aphonic periods are more severe following unvoiced plosive consonants?

Q3: Why are the breathy moments less severe or absent in association with unvoiced consonants in medial and final rather than in initial positions of words?

Q4: How do you account for the patient's ability to sustain vowel sounds without breathy or aphonic breaks?

Q5: What is the most plausible explanation for the abrupt inward abdominal movements simultaneous with moments of breathy voice?

Q6: What symptomatic diagnosis would best describe this voice disorder?

Q7: What do you think is the etiology of this patient's voice disorder? Support your interpretation.

Q8: How would you proceed in the treatment of this patient's voice disorder?

Discussion

Patients who have alternately normal voice and breathy or aphonic segments during contextual speech may be described as having abductor spastic dysphonia. This is a descriptive term only; it tells us nothing about its cause, which requires further investigation. A fiberscopic examination of the vocal folds during contextual speech discloses that each time we hear an aphonic break we see the vocal folds abduct, and each time we hear a voiced segment we see them adduct. The sudden inward movement of the patient's abdomen with each aphonic segment occurs because of the sudden drop in vocal fold resistance to the airstream being forced from the lungs by abdominal contractions.

In abductor spastic dysphonia, the abductor laryngospasms seem to be worsened by unvoiced, as opposed to voiced, consonants, especially voiceless plosives. Apparently, these phonemes do not give the vocal folds enough time to inhibit their tendency to abduct, and they overshoot, releasing more than the usual amount of air. Their propensity to do so is greatest when the plosives are in the initial positions of words rather than in medial positions, where they are bounded by voiced phonemes, or the final position of words where they are preceded by voiced phonemes. Presumably, that is why vowel prolongations usually contain few or no aphonic breaks; the vocal folds are adducted and held in a steady state during the entire period of phonation and are not required to shift from voicing to unvoicing and back again.

The psychosocial history strongly points to the probability that this patient's abductor spastic dysphonia is psychogenic, having begun during a period of intense anger and public humiliation brought on by the daughter's antisocial behavior. What is curious is that the dysphonia persists despite resolution of the daughter's difficulties, although the parents still harbor some concern about her. As of this writing, symptomatic voice therapy has not been successful. Deeper psychiatric investigation is probably warranted. However, voice therapy should always be tried. Teaching the patient to voice *all* consonants may help the patient override the breathy or voiceless segments. The etiology of this patient's voice disorder has not been firmly established and, for the present, must be considered idiopathic.

As a final note, we should be aware that, like adductor spastic dysphonia, the abductor type can be of neurologic as well as psychogenic etiology. Two signs of the neurologic type are an absence of a positive psychiatric history and on vowel prolongation instead of steady voice, *there are rhythmic unvoiced interruptions that may indicate abductor spastic dysphonia of essential voice tremor.*

VII. LOW-PITCH HOARSE GROUP

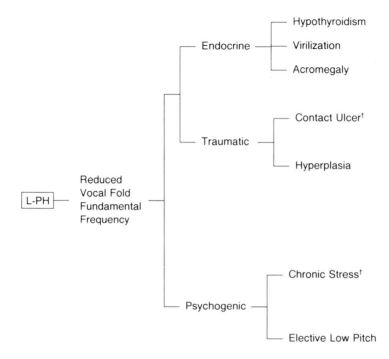

Case Study Number 11

The following case is that of a 41-year-old professor of English literature with a five-year history of episodic hoarseness related to lecturing.* The hoarseness that brought him to the Clinic began 7 months ago and coincided with the beginning of a regular teaching schedule and new duties as a curriculum supervisor. Indirect laryngoscopy shows a contact ulcer granuloma on the posterior third of the left vocal cord.

*   *   *

P: Why, I suspect I've had this kind of voice irritation for several years. The last time I had an examination of the larynx was, I think, about five years ago, and there was some irritation there but no growth. It has just been this fall that I, as I said, had the laryngitis, at least that's what I call it. I was concerned about it and sinus headaches and so forth. But it was the hoarseness and the irritation and the voice loss that concerned me most, and I work hard at teaching. I move around a lot, I push myself. My style is a kind of Socratic, excited, let's-move-ideas-around kind of style, and I work hard at it, and I force, I know I push my voice. I'm pushing it. I don't sit quietly and let my voice assert itself. When I lecture, particularly in a larger group, and I've had classes of 35 and 40 and 50, I tend to really move out, and I do know that I push my voice beyond its, certainly its normal speech level.

C: In terms of loudness?

P: In terms, I think, of volume.

C: Volume. That's what I meant. How about pitch? Do you think you strive for a low-pitched voice, consciously or unconsciously?

P: I don't know. I may do that. I don't know. I may push toward a lower voice range or frequency. I don't know why I might do that. Generally, I'm not conscious of it. I may be doing it and not be conscious of it.

C: Can you think of any ideas as to why you might be pushing for a lower frequency or a lower pitch?

---

†Important to note is the factor of chronic stress as a causative factor in the development of contact ulcer.

*An actual transcription of the following interview can be heard in Aronson, A.E.: Audio Seminars in Speech Pathology, Psychogenic Voice Disorders, Philadelphia, W.B. Saunders Co., 1973. Cassette no. 1, side 1.

P: Oh, I don't know. I suspect it might be more comfortable in a higher range.

C: Any other thoughts come to mind?

P: I don't know whether I feel this is more impressive, if I'm doing this because I think it's more impressive.

C: There's a possibility that that may be true?

P: I can't isolate that.

C: It's a possibility, but not necessarily true.

P: I know that when I can start speaking in Norwegian I can allow a kind of higher range that's easier.

C: It's easier to speak at a higher pitch?

P: Well, it is when I go into a different language.

C: How about in English; think you should go into a higher pitch?

P: I don't know, but it seems to be a little easier and I seem to be pushing it. I seem to be speaking farther forward or getting the vibration farther forward in my head or something. It does hurt more, like when I drop down now, as opposed to speaking maybe up like this.

C: Do you lecture in a large room?

P: Yes, I have.

C: Are the acoustics good or bad?

P: They vary tremendously; generally speaking, they're not very good.

C: Why is that? What is the nature of the acoustics?

P: Just flat. There is a sense that you have to really get up and project. Most of my colleagues have mentioned this, too. I don't think students could really hear you in the back, you know, if I sat and talked as I'm talking now, for example. Even if it were very quiet, some of the students in the back row simply couldn't hear me in those rooms. I have to push more than I'm pushing right now with my voice. I move toward them. I've done everything I can spatially to get close to them, at least in physical proximity. I do think that right now I can feel a little irritation and hoarseness.

C: How about noise levels, background noise levels, as you're trying to lecture?

P: It's very quiet. I've never had a problem with that. I suspect it might be in secondary education, but certainly there's none. I think I am nervous. I'm always overprepared. I'm always very anxious about doing well. I always have, so that I feel very satisfied, and I've always had good responses, but I've had to work hard at it, and I sweat a lot. I know I'm working hard. I'm in there, I get ready for the class, I prepare very carefully, I plan courses very carefully. I work with them very carefully, so I suspect that I am nervous about class.

C: Now, how will your voice fare during the course of, say a 50-minute lecture, when you are in this particular mood and you have this degree of tension or anxiety? Will it last or not?

P: It will last, but I feel the strain will last 10 minutes or so. In fact, there will be a more pronounced hoarseness. I can feel the tightening. On the other hand, well I suspect that no matter whether I'm using the Socratic method or not, or just moving into a kind of casual, easygoing kind of dialogue of some kind, that the differences are a difference of degree, and in those instances I feel the strain and tightening.

C: Will that tightening also be accompanied by, say, a dull aching in your larynx?

P: You're asking me to become conscious of things I haven't really paid much attention to, and I'm always a little suspicious of my own recall and my own awareness of my physiologic processes, but I think that's true. And I think there is even a tendency to bring about some sort of headache, a little bit of a headache from it. That is, I can feel irritation here starting to bring about a headache reaction. . . . But it's never been easy for me to talk. I was always very quiet when I was younger, and through my whole career as a teacher I've worked hard to project, to get away from this. I was fairly introverted and quiet, and I've always had the feeling that other people have had stronger voices, that I have not had a particularly strong voice. But, as I said, I can always remember this kind of, this tendency toward this, this hoarseness, and when I talked for a long time or lectured, I taught high school for 4 years, and I had five hours of class a day, I would be darn sore at the end of the day. I would tend to become very quiet and my wife would say that I would, for the rest of the day, speak very, very quietly if I could.

C: Would you feel sort of worn out in general from talking, sort of fatigued?

P: From that more than anything else. *Just the physical business of talking.* Not the classroom dynamics or anything like that. It was just talking. It has never been particularly easy for me. And I'm in a profession where that's the medium, you see, that's the demand.

* * *

Q1: *What is the physical explanation behind the excessively low pitch of this patient's voice?*

Q2: *What is the reason for the contact ulcer being located at the posterior third of the vocal fold?*

Q3: *What is the contribution of the patient's artificially lowering his pitch to his voice disorder?*

Q4: *What might be the causes of the patient's complaint of tightness and dull aching in his throat?*

Q5: *Comment on the relative contributions of vocal abuse, personality, and emotional stress to the development of this patient's voice disorder.*

VIII. HIGH-PITCH GROUP

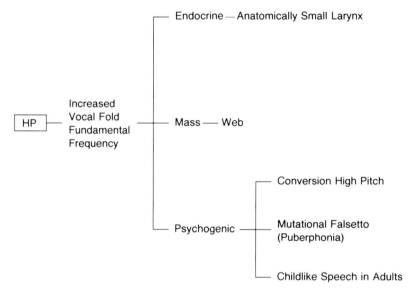

Case Study Number 12

A 23-year-old college student comes to the Clinic complaining of general fatigue. She has a history of mononucleosis. Six months ago she noticed a drooping of her left eyelid that was diagnosed elsewhere as a sign of myasthenia gravis. However, a Tensilon test was negative. During the neurologic history, she does not complain of difficulty chewing or swallowing, double vision, or limb weakness; in fact, she says she runs three miles a day. Her neurologic examination is normal; however, her history of left ptosis leads the neurologist to conclude that she does have ocular myasthenia that is currently asymptomatic. After discussing the pros and cons of continuing her medication, she is referred for evaluation of an accompanying speech disorder.

The patient enters your office casually dressed and looking younger than her 23 years. From the moment she speaks you are startled by her high-pitched, though not falsetto, voice and the way in which she articulates with a slight pursing of her lips and a subtle interdental lisp. Her prosody is that of exaggerated pitch changes. Her speech gives you the uncomfortable feeling that you are talking with a child rather than an adult college student.

She says her speech began to change about four years ago. Two years ago an otolaryngologist said she had a high voice because her larynx was too small. Laryngologic examination here mentions nothing about an abnormally small larynx.

Q1: *How do these speech signs relate to myasthenia gravis?*

Q2: *What further tests would you recommend to determine if her speech had anything to do with that disease?*

Q3: *What are the cardinal speech signs of myasthenia gravis?*

Testing her speech musculature fails to disclose any evidence of lip, tongue, mandibular, laryngeal, or respiratory weakness. The all-important stress test of counting fails to produce deterioration of her speech. Her cough is normally sharp. You can find no signs of motor-speech disorder. She can lower her pitch level on demand, but she does not maintain it during conversation speech.

Q4:   What would be the next step in your investigation?

The psychosocial history discloses that between the ages of 10 and 17 the patient and both of her parents were alcoholic. She gives a history of physical abuse and psychotherapy on and off since age 13. She says she is just beginning to get hold of her problems with the help of a school counselor. Asked if she would like to have help with her speech, she replies that, for the time being, she would prefer not to because "My voice is me. I don't have a problem; my problem is that other people have a problem with my voice."

Q5:   What do you think is the diagnosis of this person's speech disorder?
Q6:   How would you proceed in handling this case?

DISCUSSION

This is an instance of the relatively rare psychogenic disorder known as childlike speech in adults. Technically, it is not solely a voice disorder, as articulation is integral to the total syndrome. It bears many of the features of a conversion reaction in that the patient's abnormal use of the speech musculature is unconsciously determined, that the childlike speech "selected" serves to communicate something very important about the self, and that the disorder probably affords the patient primary or secondary gain in her daily life. The prior diagnosis of an abnormally small larynx was presumptive; the speech examination proved she was capable of producing a lower pitch appropriate to her age and sex. Nothing in her speech remotely resembled the flaccid dysarthria of myasthenia gravis with its breathy, weak voice, hypernasality, and consonant imprecision that worsen during effortful speaking. Her myasthenia gravis, limited to her ptosis, was completely independent of her speech disorder.

This patient was adamant in her rejection of our offer of speech therapy; in fact, her insight was so poor that she did not even think her speech was abnormal; recall her conclusion was that the problem was other peoples', not hers. Her denial that her speech was abnormal, also common in conversion reaction, and her rejection of help for the "symptom" require respect, for this patient is telling us that she is not ready to relinquish the protection afforded by her childlike speech. Her frankness in disclosing seriously damaging childhood experiences and her acknowledgment that she needs, and is getting, counseling probably indicate that she may one day be well enough to be able to give up her inappropriate speech and return to a normal speech pattern that she once had. We wished her well and sent her on her way.

SUMMARY

1. In actual clinical practice, differential diagnosis of a voice disorder begins with categorizing the abnormal voice and then working backward to its etiology by means of logical correlation with laryngologic, psychologic, and neurologic evidence.

2. Abnormal voices tend to cluster into perceptual groups.

3. Although the voices within these "clusters" may sound similar, they can arise from mass lesions, neurologic diseases, or psychologic disorders which can only be determined by further clinical studies.

4. Interaction between organic and psychogenic factors must be borne in mind in the assessment of all voice disorders.

Chapter Thirteen

DEFINITION AND OBJECTIVES

GENERAL PRINCIPLES

SPECIFIC PRINCIPLES

GENERAL VOICE THERAPY APPROACHES

Auditory Training
Respiratory Control
Relaxation
Optimum Pitch
Trial and Error
Voice Rest
Reactive Anxiety

MANAGEMENT OF SPECIFIC VOICE DISORDERS

Musculoskeletal Tension (Vocal Hyperfunction)
Vocal Abuse
Conversion Voice Disorders
Mutational Falsetto (Puberphonia)
Adductor Spastic Dysphonia
Abductor Spastic Dysphonia
Unilateral and Bilateral Vocal Fold Paralysis

THERAPY FOR PROBLEM VOICE DISORDERS

Neurologic Voice Disorders
Voice Disorders Due to Mass Vocal Fold Lesions

BIOFEEDBACK DEVICES IN VOICE THERAPY

THERAPY FOR VOICE DISORDERS

DEFINITION AND OBJECTIVES

Voice therapy may be defined as an effort to return the voice to a level of adequacy that can be realistically achieved and that will satisfy the patient's occupational, emotional, and social needs. Not everyone, especially not those who have irreversible neurologic or vocal fold lesions, can achieve a normal voice. In such cases, the objective is the best possible voice within the patient's anatomic and physiologic capabilities. It is to the credit of most patients that they understand and accept their voice limitations.

Some voice disorders are so mild that one has difficulty deciding if an abnormal voice actually exists. The patient may be unaware of or unconcerned about the voice. A voice disorder may exist clinically but not therapeutically. Who, finally, is to decide if voice therapy is necessary? If a reasonable effort has been made to increase awareness of the voice, but therapy is declined, such is the patient's right. Where children are concerned, the clinician will usually try more aggressively to obtain the child's cooperation, with the consent of the parents. With experience, clinicians learn that not everyone needs to be helped, can be helped, or wishes to be helped.

GENERAL PRINCIPLES

Principles and methods of voice therapy are continuously evolving. The literature advocates different techniques for the same disorder, and useful therapies have yet to be developed for many disorders. Capable clinicians sometimes are at a loss to say exactly what they do to bring about voice improvement. Reading the literature on voice therapy produces uncertainty as to who is right and which alternatives work. Underneath all of this apparent confusion, however, lie some common principles.

1. Progression from abnormal to normal voice takes place as a product of the patient's conscious, volitional response to the clinician's instruction and encouragement. Yet, at the same time the larynx has a natural propensity toward normal function in nonorganic disorders. There is a sense one has about therapy for nonorganic voice disorders that, rather than the need to teach the patient how to use voice again, the clinician's task is to *remove obstacles* and, by so doing, allow the natural inclination for normal voice to break through. Humans do not have to be taught how to phonate in the first place. There is no reason to believe that our capacity for normal voice does not exist throughout life.

2. Auditory discrimination and feedback occupy a pivotal position in voice therapy, cutting across all voice disorder boundaries, because tactile and proprioceptive feedback is diminished in phonation and cannot be relied upon.

3. Voice disorders resulting from emotional stress ought not be treated as only mechanical problems. Consideration of the patient's self-concept, daily life problems, and dysphoric affect must be incorporated into the therapy. On the other hand, although treating the cause of a voice disorder may be as important as voice production training, the cause may either never be found or may be unalterable.

4. Voice therapy has to be tailored to the individual. Although the fundamental principle of therapy for a given disorder does not vary, differences in age, sex, intelligence, education, culture, occupation, and general health require that techniques be modified to suit these variables.

SPECIFIC PRINCIPLES

For many years, the notion has been fostered that voice disorders follow the same laws of learning as do, for example, articulatory or language disorders, and, as such, are treated in the same way by applying those laws to the larynx and voice. Whereas traditional learning does have application in voice therapy, e.g., practice, targeting, trial-and-error, and the like, special facts about the larynx and voice that do not apply to articulation and language need to be recognized.

1. Phonation is built into the organism as an innate neurophysiologic function. It is not "learned" in the same sense as is articulation or language.

2. In organic disorders caused by airflow disturbances resulting from vocal fold mass lesions or neurologic disorders of paralysis or movement, the main principle of therapy is either muscle strengthening or adaptation to the mechanical problems by means of compensatory phonatory and respiratory maneuvers.

3. Nonorganic voice disorders exist for one or more of the following reasons and often exist in combination.
   a. The vocal folds are adducted with excessive force because of general laryngeal muscle tension, as a reaction to the stress of life, e.g., acute or chronic anxiety. These are called *hyperfunctional or musculoskeletal tension voice disorders*. They are treated primarily according to the principle that when the muscular tension is reduced, the larynx's capacity for normal phonation will fully and normally, return. Voice therapy, then, aims at releasing the inherently normal voice suppressed by excess muscular tension, an objective that can be accomplished in two complementary ways:
      (1) By mechanically relaxing the musculature
      (2) By psychologically releasing the anxiety causing the tension
   b. The vocal folds may fail to adduct (hypoadduct) because they are muscularly flaccid or flabby due to nonuse or incomplete use. These are called *hypofunctional voice disorders* and are usually secondary to prolonged voice rest. These disorders are treated primarily according to the principle of increasing the tonicity of the vocal folds by means of their full employment during phonation.
   c. The vocal folds fail to adduct because, unconsciously, the patient has a need to be partially or completely without voice. These are the *conversion voice disorders*. The original loss or diminution of the voice produces three secondary effects:
      (1) Soon after the aphonia or dysphonia sets in the patient loses the feel for how to produce normal voice, a dissociative type reaction that persists even after the interpersonal or situational conflict causing the voice disorder has resolved.
      (2) Conversion voice disorders are not as passive as their whispering and breathiness suggest, but are actually produced with elevated musculoskeletal tension. In other words, they contain within them a hyperfunctional component involving the extrinsic muscles of the larynx.
      The conversion voice disorders are primarily treated with a combination of therapies directed at exposing and, if possible, resolving the interpersonal or situational conflicts causing them, educating and physically guiding the patient into increasing degrees of phonation, and reducing musculoskeletal tension.
   d. Cultural, personality, and emotional factors can lead to phonation with excessively sharp glottal attack, which traumatizes the vocal fold mucosa, producing general inflammation or discrete lesions. These are the *vocal abuse disorders*. Excess musculoskeletal tension is often a component. They are treated according to the principle of *reducing habits of hard glottal attack, environmental stress, and personality problems.*

GENERAL VOICE THERAPY APPROACHES

Voice therapy is carried out on two planes: (1) A specific one in which techniques are tailored to the requirements of a specific voice disorder type, and (2) a general one, composed of universally applicable methods. Both planes are interwoven in voice therapy, their proportions determined by the patient's requirements.

Auditory Training

Voice lacks finite acoustic boundaries. A mildly defective voice can become incorporated into the self without much notice, especially in children, whose concerns over its acceptability are minimal. Even in severe voice disorders, the person may be upset over the voice but has long forgotten the sound of the normal voice and, therefore, any notion of how it ought to sound again.

For these reasons, auditory training, defined as teaching the identification of and discrimination among different voices, is the staple technique of all voice therapy. Before a better voice can be achieved, the person has to know how his or her voice sounds. Patients of all ages need to hear the differences between normal and defective voices. After comparing them with their own, they should discuss those differences with the clinician.

Of major importance is instantaneous auditory feedback. What is singular about voice therapy is that in the early, critical stages, improved voice will break through suddenly and momentarily, milliseconds in duration; although the clinician may hear and identify these gains, the patient usually does not. Consequently, the clinician needs to listen carefully and, when the voice changes for the better or worse, communicate that information instantaneously to the patient.

Respiratory Control

If expiratory air volume is patently insufficient because of neurologic weakness or incoordination, vocal loudness and steadiness will suffer. In such cases, increasing lung volumes and control of smoother exhalation are desirable ends. However, for the majority of voice patients, respiration is anatomically and physiologically normal. *Any abnormal breathing patterns are probably due to anxiety and tension, which can cause shallow upper chest or clavicular breathing, failing to provide sufficient breath support for optimum voice.* Abdominal or diaphragmatic breathing affords the greatest lung volumes. To encourage maximum air movement, Cooper and Cooper (1977) give the following advice. Lying supine, the patient is asked to:

1. Place one hand on the chest and the other on the abdomen.
2. Inhale easily through the nose and exhale through the mouth, concentrating on inflating and deflating the abdomen but not the chest.
3. Inhale quickly through the mouth only and exhale gradually, using the same abdominal breathing method just described.
4. Repeat these in sitting and standing positions, incorporating the above into phonation at proper pitch and loudness levels.

For development of diaphragmatic-intercostal breathing coordinated with phonation, Greene (1972) advocates the following method.

1. Hand on waist, breathe in slowly and then out, counting in a quiet voice up to four and then gradually increasing the count at a rate of one per second. No breath should escape between each count.
2. Inhale deeply, and, keeping the ribs elevated, count to 15, gradually letting the ribs descend between 15 and 20.
3. Inhale and, on exhalation, sustain /s/ or /f/ steadily, trying not to let it fluctuate or fade toward the end. Feel the gradual contraction of the abdominal wall as breath is exhaled.
4. Repeat this, except with a crescendo and diminuendo or in different rhythmic patterns.

For reinforcing the proper respiratory rhythm for speech, she instructs the patient to:

1. Breathe in and out slowly several times and then imitate the clinician's rapid intake and slow exhalation. The abdomen should jump forward on inhalation and subside gradually on exhalation.
2. Inhale quickly and exhale slowly, counting to six. Gradually increase the count on exhalation to 20.

After many years of experience administering voice therapy and attempting to deal with problems of respiration that often accompany voice disorders, Boone (1988), although he continues to believe in the importance of modifying respiration in voice disorders, has taken a more conservative stand on its relative importance in voice therapy. For the patient who demonstrates faulty respiratory patterns, he believes that some modification of respiration for speech is important, using instrumental feedback and patient education about optimum respiratory actions. However, over the years, he has observed that many patients develop overconcern about how they are breathing, and their attention to the breathing process has actually interfered with a smooth and easy respiratory style, often increasing their laryngeal tension.

> Our thesis might well be that the best respiration training for the patient with a voice disorder is the least amount of training. It would appear that we best alter respiratory patterns by working to extend expiratory control, matching target models, and learning how effortlessly to renew breath.

Relaxation

Relaxation as an adjunct to voice therapy is commonly advocated to combat excessive musculoskeletal tension. It is exemplified by the progressive relaxation techniques of Jacobson (1938, 1964, 1976) and McClosky (1977). These techniques try to teach recognition of the difference between feelings associated with muscular tension and those associated with relaxation by having the patient alternately contract and relax head, neck, thoracic, and abdominal muscles. Biofeedback methods have also achieved relaxation, with the patient auditorily and visually monitoring the degree of muscle tension of the face and neck.

The chewing method of speech muscle relaxation (Froeschels, 1952) is based on the theory that chewing, being a primitive, reflex-like, semi-automatic function, relaxes the lingual, mandibular, hyoid, and laryngeal musculature. The method advocates phonation while performing chewing or munching movements. Its value may be limited in patients who are embarrassed by the unusual nature of this therapy.

Optimum Pitch

Deeply ingrained in the history of therapy for voice disorders is the concept of optimum pitch, i.e., that there is a pitch level best suited to the supraglottic resonators that produces the most resonant voice with the least physical effort, located approximately one-fourth of the total pitch range from the bottom (Fairbanks, 1960). While there is little doubt that pitch level and range are disturbed in virtually all voice disorders, it is not necessary to make a point of finding a correct pitch level and purposefully teaching it to the individual. Each person who has a nonorganic voice disorder has the inherent capacity to phonate at the proper pitch, but the muscular tensions underlying the disorder have pulled the larynx out of optimum position. When the musculature has returned to its normal state, the correct pitch usually follows. When the voice disorder is one of incorrect pitch per se, the clinician can roughly demonstrate both how far off the patient is and the extra effort required to produce voice, by helping the patient find the best pitch level that is physically easiest to produce. The "um-hum" method proposed by Cooper (1973) is ideal for this purpose.

> The patient is asked to say "UM-HUM" using rising inflection with the lips closed, as though he were spontaneously and sincerely agreeing with what was just said. It is vital to underscore the fact that this "UM-HUM" be spontaneous and sincere . . . A natural "UM-HUM," which is easy and gentle, will be felt around the sides and lower portion of the nose and around the lips.
> The optimal pitch will assist the patient in achieving a proper tone focus, which is a balance of oronasopharyngeal resonance in combination with laryngeal resonance.
> To help identify the placement of tone focus (and the optimal pitch), the fingers of one hand should be placed lightly on the bridge and sides of the nose while the other hand is placed lightly on the throat. As one says the "UM-HUM," there should be a slight vibration or tingle in the mask area.

Trial and Error

It may seem paradoxical, but despite established principles and techniques of voice therapy, trial-and-error is an essential methodology. Far from being a science, voice therapy is pragmatic and demands that the clinician take advantage of accidental, unplanned voice improvements during therapy. Boone (1977) states this principle clearly when he says that the clinician must continually "search for the patient's best and most appropriate voice production. This searching is necessary because so much of our vocal behaviors is highly automatic . . . The patient cannot volitionally break vocalization down into various components and then hope to combine them into some ideal phonation. Our therapy techniques are primarily vehicles of facilitation; that is, we try a particular therapy approach and see if it facilitates the production of a better voice. If it does, then we utilize it as therapy practice material. If it does not, we quickly abandon it. As part of every clinical session, we must probe and search for the patient's best voice . . . We use it as the . . . target model in therapy."

Voice Rest

The most common, yet imprudent, advice given to patients with voice disorders is the recommendation of voice rest—to refrain from using the voice, either by not talking at all, whispering, or using breathy quality. The duration of voice rest recommended to patients can range from several days to several weeks. *We are firmly against complete voice rest.* Patients recovering from direct surgery to the vocal folds may be candidates, but even then, not more than a few days of *modified* voice use is advisable.

1. *There are no data that silence has therapeutic value,* and the advice is commonly ignored because of its impracticality. Based on a study of 127 patients who had surgery for vocal nodules, polypoid degeneration, granuloma, cysts, polyps, leukoplakia, and carcinoma, Koufman and Blalock (1989) concluded that voice rest provided no greater protection against postoperative dysphonia than did an alternate program of voice conservation, that is, soft glottal attack, loudness monitoring, and avoidance of abusive vocal patterns.

2. *There is ample evidence that absolute voice rest can do harm.* It implants the idea in the patient's psyche, especially in those who have psychogenic voice disorders, that the larynx and voice are foci of weakness, and that normally energetic voice use is damaging. This idea usually persists beyond the duration of the prescribed voice rest and, unless reversed, can lead to anxiety and to a secondary voice disorder owing to loss of laryngeal muscle tonus. To say it another way, when the recommendation of voice rest creates, perpetuates, or exacerbates a voice disorder, as it often does, voice rest can be considered an *iatrogenic** cause of a voice disorder. *Overcautious voice use is often elected by patients even when not advised to rest their voices. In actuality, the opposite kind of voice use is desired in most patients with voice disorders, that is, rather than voice rest, they need to adopt firm, normally loud voices produced with equally firm exhalatory force.*

Reactive Anxiety

We have, then, the potential for a serious dilemma in the diagnosis and treatment of voice disorders that can get in the way of our helping patients and their helping themselves—the strong tendency for patients to become anxious and overprotective of their larynges as a reaction to the diagnosis of organic or psychogenic voice disorder. The larynx is particularly vulnerable to emotional disequilibrium, mild or severe, transient or chronic. One reason for the oversensitivity of the larynx is its vital importance in everyday life for intellectual and emotional expression. We cannot appreciate the importance of a normal voice until the larynx undergoes structural or physiologic changes producing dysphonia or aphonia. The most stalwart person sooner or later will become frustrated, embarrassed, and hypersensitive to the obstacle that abnormal voice presents.

A second reason for the patient's vulnerability to overconcern and emotional reactivity to dysphonia is that the larynx is a well-known site of malignancy, and the most common concern that patients express when they develop abnormal voice is whether or not they have cancer of the larynx.

So, our problem, diagnostically and therapeutically, is that, despite our best efforts to prevent it, patients will generate overconcern about their larynges and voices. Any advice given to them about

---

*Iatrogenesis is defined as illness induced by unavoidable or improper diagnosis or therapy

the need to avoid certain kinds of abusive vocal activities, or even simply the administration of voice therapy, reinforces the patient's belief that the larynx has to be protected at all costs. This attitude easily translates into anxiety and its associated muscle tensions. The patient elects to phonate with less than normal expiratory effort, breathing shallowly and phonating weakly. That is why the laryngologist and the speech pathologist, who on the one hand need to give advice and therapy for voice improvement, on the other must neutralize the tendency toward the patient's overconcern by not advising it too strenuously and by reassuring the patient that *full voice use* is desirable as soon as possible. Particularly, we need to emphasize that the patient need not protect the larynx by using reduced loudness and respiratory volumes. In many cases the clinician does more for the patient by giving simple advice on proper voice instead of a long series of voice therapy sessions, which risk reinforcement of the patient's apprehensions.

MANAGEMENT OF SPECIFIC VOICE DISORDERS

The remainder of this chapter is devoted to therapy that has evolved for specific voice disorders based on the special requirements of each disorder.

Musculoskeletal Tension (Vocal Hyperfunction)

The majority of cases we shall find suffering from some excess of muscular function (hyperfunction) in various degrees. However, this refers not to the vocal chords themselves but rather to the whole tensor mechanism of the vocal organ which comprises all the muscles surrounding the cartilages of the larynx. We have generally not found it necessary—and often not possible—to decide which specific muscle or muscles were at fault. (Weiss, p. 12).

Life stress elevates general muscle tension, including that of the laryngeal muscles, and can produce an array of voice defects: aphonia, breathiness, hoarseness, or excessively high pitch. No single voice type is associated with musculoskeletal tension. Vocal hyperfunction is the most important concept in the etiology and treatment of nonorganic, and many organic, voice disorders. Intrinsic and extrinsic laryngeal muscle tension expresses anxiety, depression, or anger. In organic voice disorders it may occur as a result of efforts to compensate for the organic deficit. *All patients with voice disorders, regardless of etiology, should be tested for excess musculoskeletal tension, either as a primary or as a secondary cause of dysphonia.* The degree of voice improvement following therapy for musculoskeletal tension is proportional to the reduction of musculoskeletal tension.

Following are the principles basic to therapy for musculoskeletal tension associated with vocal hyperfunction.

1. Extrinsic and intrinsic laryngeal muscle cramping is responsible for the abnormal voice. Reducing musculoskeletal tension releases the inherent capability of the larynx to produce normal voice.
2. When gently rubbed or kneaded, muscles relax and become less painful.
3. Lowering laryngeal position in the neck permits more normal phonation.

The first procedure for implementation of these principles is to assay signs of musculoskeletal tension. Its presence is suspected when patients complain of spontaneous pain in the region of the larynx shooting up to the ears and down to the chest and a feeling of a lump, a ball, or tension in the larynx or pharynx. Testing for muscle tension is subdivided into determining three things: (1) extent of laryngeal elevation, (2) pain in response to pressure in the region of the larynx, and (3) extent of voice improvement following tension reduction.

Referring to Figure 13-1*a* and *b* one should:

1. Encircle the hyoid bone with the thumb and middle finger, working them posteriorly until the tips of the major horns are felt.
2. Exert light pressure with the fingers in a circular motion over the tips of the hyoid bone and ask if the patient feels pain, not just pressure. It is important to watch facial expression for signs of discomfort or pain.

3. Repeat this procedure with the fingers in the thyrohyoid space, beginning from the thyroid notch and working posteriorly.

4. Find the posterior borders of the thyroid cartilage just medial to the sternocleidomastoid muscles and repeat the procedure.

5. With the fingers over the superior borders of the thyroid cartilage, begin to work the larynx gently downward, also moving it laterally at times. One should check for a lower laryngeal position by estimating the increased size of the thyrohyoid space.

6. Ask the patient to prolong vowels during these procedures, noting changes in quality or pitch. Clearer voice quality and lower pitch indicate relief of tension. Because these procedures are fatiguing, rest periods should be provided.

7. Once a voice change has taken place, the patient should be allowed to experiment with the voice, repeating vowels, words, and sentences.

Rate of improvement varies. If the dysphonia has been due to musculoskeletal tension alone and has been present only a short time, the voice may become normal within minutes. Those who have been dysphonic longer may require several hours of therapy administered in separate sessions. *The voice rarely changes from aphonia or dysphonia to normal without first passing through several dysphonic stages.* The clinician should not hesitate to attempt normal voice within one session, for the majority of patients can be helped considerably, if not completely, within that time. Patients whose voices fail to improve despite the above ministrations may not be ready to relinquish the abnormal voice because of musculoskeletal tension secondary to conversion reaction. One should watch for the first signs of improvement. Recovery takes on its own momentum. A switch then, should be made from repetitions of speech sounds to spontaneous speech beginning with more automatic responses such as the patient's name, address, and occupation.

Once the normal voice has returned, most patients ask why it did and why they were not able to accomplish this themselves. The clinician explains the effects of muscle tension on voice in terms the patient can understand. Often, after voice improvement the patient recalls unpleasant life situations giving rise to the voice disorder. A frank and open discussion of such situations and the extent of their seriousness is necessary in order to determine whether more intensive psychologic investigation and therapy are necessary. Commonly, musculoskeletal tension is not due to a specific problem but is the patient's lifelong way of reacting to stress. Such patients overdrive themselves, and changing daily habits may serve to preclude future abnormal voice episodes. Realistically, the normal voice may be short-lived, and the dysphonia may return when the tension returns. Not much is known about the long-term fate of such therapy or ways to prevent further occurrences.

The literature on voice therapy is replete with advocacy of chewing therapy, progressive relaxation, and biofeedback for vocal hyperfunction. These therapies have the same objective as the method just described. However, musculoskeletal tension is a powerfully resistive force, and less aggressive methods often fail. Here, as elsewhere, the best approach is trial and error.

Maneuvering the patient's laryngeal and hyoid anatomy as just described is safe as long as it is performed with good judgment. This technique is not offered as an alternate therapy but as a primary one. It is hard work for both clinician and patient and would not be advocated were it not useful in achieving its aims. Patients will complain of soreness in the region of the larynx following such therapy, but they can be assured that it will disappear within a day or two.

Finally, in addition to elevation of the larynx and hyoid bone, the tongue may be elevated, integral with the total pattern of extrinsic laryngeal muscle contraction. The tongue is carried high in the mouth, and the submental musculature is tense and painful. The tongue should be pressed down along with the hyoid bone and larynx, either with the finger or with a tongue depressor, while simultaneously listening for voice improvement.

Vocal Abuse

VOCAL NODULE IN CHILDREN

In children and adults, vocal abuse produces general inflammation or focal lesions that result in breathiness, huskiness, or hoarseness. Musculoskeletal tension is often the physiologic basis of the abuse, and emotional factors are its driving force. Vocal abuse in children takes the forms of loud

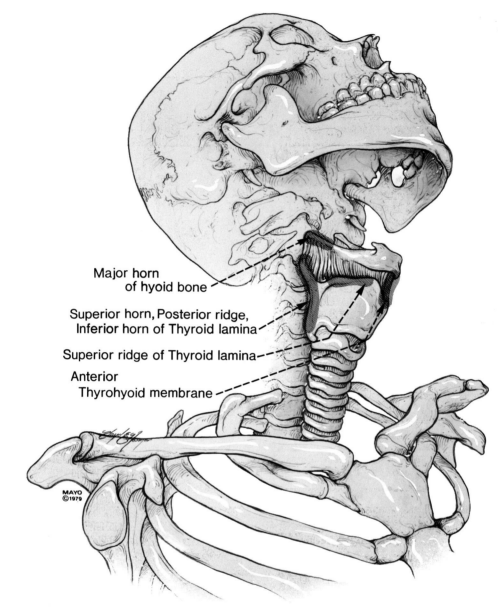

Major horn
   of hyoid bone

Superior horn, Posterior ridge,
   Inferior horn of Thyroid lamina

Superior ridge of Thyroid lamina

Anterior
   Thyrohyoid membrane

MAYO
©1979

Figure 13–1a   Loci of laryngeal and hyoid bone pain from digital pressure (shaded areas).

talking, shouting, screaming, coughing, or throat clearing. The purposes of therapy are to reduce vocal fold trauma through re-education and to reduce or eliminate emotional and environmental stress.

The therapy of choice in children and adults who have vocal nodules is vocal re-education rather than surgical removal of the nodules, which will only return if vocal abuse is not reduced. Surgery without treating vocal abuse is now recognized as ineffective, or worse, in the treatment of vocal nodules except in cases of chronic, advanced, mature, fibrous nodules. Patients who have not had speech therapy show a higher recurrence rate (Barnes, 1981).

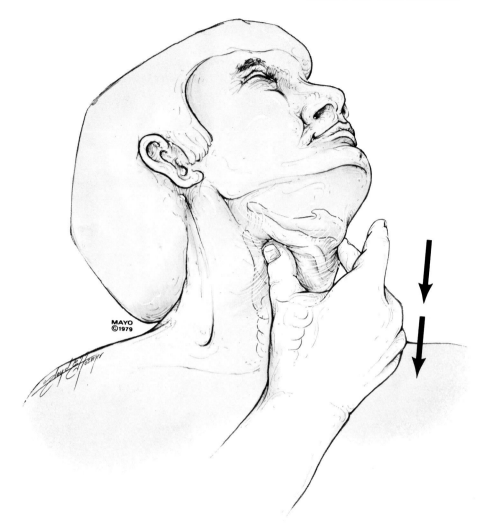

Figure 13–1b   Maneuvering the larynx to a lower position in the neck.

Von Leden (1988) has written that:

the presence of vocal nodules is not an automatic indication for surgery, particularly in patients who use their voices professionally, and if nodules do not respond to conservative treatment and if surgery is necessary, all efforts must be made to preserve healthy mucous membrane covering the vocal folds. "Stripping" has no place in the removal of vocal nodules because this procedure includes removal of healthy mucous membrane, denuding the vocal folds likely causing scarring, fibrosis, restricted vibratory excursions and permanent dysphonia. The vocal folds may *appear* normal on laryngoscopic examination even with magnification; however, stroboscopic examination has shown limitations in the vibratory motions of the vocal folds that are typical in patients who have fibrotic changes. This same precaution to preserve the mucous covering of the vocal folds applies to other benign lesions.

In a survey of 535 otolaryngologists, Moran and Pentz (1987) found that 59 percent of otolaryngologists expressed preference for voice therapy as the *sole* mode of treatment for vocal nodules in children; less than 1 percent preferred surgery as the sole treatment; 9.4 percent recommended surgery to be followed by voice therapy; 50 percent of otolaryngologists indicated that voice therapy is frequently or always effective in the treatment of vocal nodules in children.

Voice therapy for children who have vocal nodules can be conducted either individually or in small groups. Group therapy has the advantage of heightening competitiveness and, consequently, motivation.

Informational Phase.   The child should be given simplified information on the structure and function of the larynx. Drawings, color photographs, slides, models, and motion pictures of the larynx can be used for this purpose. One should explain why the voice is defective by comparing photographs or drawings of the normal vocal folds with those of vocal nodules or general inflammation.

Auditory Discrimination Phase.   Using audiotape recordings, one can compare children's normal voices with those who have dysphonia as a result of vocal abuse and can discuss in detail how the voices differ. In group therapy, the children can evaluate each others' voices as compared with the normal. Children can use severity rating scales or other means of documenting their reactions.

Voice Production Phase.   By now, the child should know the reason for the voice disorder and its characteristics. Two considerations in the voice production phase are: (1) Situations in which vocal abuse is most likely to occur. The child needs to be made aware of situations in which vocal abuse is likely to occur, for example, yelling during sports activities and other forms of play, airing of conflicts among friends and family, and uncontrolled coughing and throat clearing. (2) Training the child to reduce vocal loudness and glottal attacks is central to direct voice therapy.

a. Reduce vocal loudness. The child's loudness discrimination abilities can be increased by recording voice at various loudness levels. One should identify a comfortable loudness level and get the child to agree not to exceed this level in outside situations. The child should be told to use alternate signaling devices instead of yelling.

b. Reduce sharpness of glottal attack. The child should be taught to produce words beginning with vowels by using a gentle vocal attack. The difference between the sharp or abrupt coup de glotte and the easy onset of voicing should be demonstrated. This technique can be illustrated by asking for phonation during sighing, leading into vowels produced with a breathy attack, i.e., beginning with the /h/ phoneme. The child should be made kinesthetically aware of relaxed, easy exhalation along the entire respiratory-laryngeal tract. One should teach the child to be aware of muscle sensation as well as the sound of the voice while developing new habits of phonation.

c. Discuss personal and family problems. As in all voice disorders, one should try to eliminate underlying causes or aggravating factors. Clinical research has shown that children abuse their voices in the process of acting out their aggressions, thereby discharging emotional tensions. Although many children are insufficiently aware of the emotional aspects of their lives, others have considerable insight and can talk about unpleasant situations, feelings, and attitudes toward friends and family. Time should be given for discussion of anxiety, frustration, anger, and unpleasant experiences. Group therapy is an excellent vehicle for generating discussion among children about their feelings and attitudes. Such discussions can be conducted maturely and without guilt about disclosing personal and family problems. To do so is valuable for the clinician in order to judge the extent to which the vocal abuse is a component of a larger emotional problem. Discussion with parents, school psychologists, and other professionals in a position to help may be necessary.

Parent Counseling Phase.   Parents are an important part of the therapy for vocal abuse. They should be informed as to why voice therapy is being given their child. They should know the rationale and the methods being used and, especially, what is expected from the child in the way of self-control. Parental interviews are superior to communicating by letter or telephone. Parents differ in their attitudes toward voice therapy for their children. Many are not aware of the voice disorder—to them the child always sounded that way; that's just his voice. Others may not be convinced of the need for a change, and resent that their child has been singled out for voice therapy. It is useful, therefore, to clarify objectives and to allow parents to express their attitudes.

Notwithstanding the time-honored concept of vocal nodule as a simple vocal abuse disorder, research studies have now established unequivocally that children who develop vocal nodules have aggressive personality traits and are often in conflict with family members and peers at school. The speech pathologist must weigh the factor of vocal acting out because of personality problems as a cause of the vocal abuse, investigate psychosocial forces at home and at school, and consider appropriate psychologic referral if indicated. One should discuss with parents, as with the child, sources of personal or family conflict that might be producing emotional distress leading to vocal abuse.

Parents want to know whether or not they should remind the child at home about not abusing the voice. There is no firm rule except that the child is responsible for the voice, and the burden of that responsibility needs to be placed primarily on the child. If reminders are necessary, they should be infrequent and should never take the form of nagging. As reminder devices, the child can be given a calendar or other charting device on which to record gradations of voice use and abuse during each day. The child rates the voice according to how much and how loudly it was used. While such devices are useful as reminders, they should be kept simple. Rewards for progress should be given.

VOCAL NODULE IN ADULTS

Vocal nodules in adults produce dysphonia similar to that found in children. It is husky, breathy, hoarse, and of lower than average pitch. Because the cause of vocal nodules in adults is basically the same as in children, so are the principles of therapy. Adults need to be informed of the reasons for the nodules. Graphic illustrations and technical explanations should be tailored to the patient's background. Advice to reduce abuse of the voice during speaking and singing is usually accepted and implemented by most adults. When singing is suspected as a major or contributory cause, the patient should be taken off all singing activities until the nodule has disappeared. Then a reassessment needs to be made as to how the voice ought to be used during singing, e.g., loudness, background accompaniment (which may be excessive), and appropriate pitch range. After disappearance of the nodule, singing on a modified scale can be resumed. Whether or not the patient will remain free of nodules cannot be determined beforehand; this must be assessed on a trial-and-error basis.

Emotional problems paralleling the development of the nodules should be investigated. Many patients develop nodules even though they have not changed their singing or speaking habits. What often emerges during a thorough voice evaluation is that they have experienced an emotional upset in their lives that increased their musculoskeletal tension to the point of adding enough frictional trauma to the vocal folds to produce nodules. These problems may be minor—transient emotional stresses from situational problems at work or at home—or more severe chronic stresses which seriously interfere with the person's sense of well being. The speech pathologist needs to determine how serious these background factors are, and if the patient cannot manage them, he might need to be referred for psychologic or psychiatric consultation.

Adult females with vocal nodules are characteristically active, talkative people. They openly, smilingly, and with a tincture of pride admit they have always liked to talk. They do readily accept advice to limit the amount of their speaking, however. As in children, adults should be taught to produce voice with less forceful stress or emphasis patterns and with easy onset of phonation rather than with a hard glottal attack. Some speech clinicians advocate reducing the pitch level of the voice to an "optimum pitch"; however, the location of optimum pitch is impossible to find in someone who has a lesion of the vocal folds causing the latter to vibrate abnormally. The necessity for finding an optimum pitch for reduction of nodules is controversial. The clinician should help the patient find a *comfortable* pitch level. The "um-hum" method described previously can be used for this purpose.

If vocal abuse has been the true cause of the nodules, as it is in most cases, the voice modifications already mentioned should reduce the size of the nodule and even eliminate it within several weeks, depending upon its size. Except for encapsulated nodules, which many laryngologists believe should be removed surgically, voice re-education is the therapy of choice and should be attempted first. Patients should be seen periodically on return visits for both laryngoscopic and speech pathology re-evaluations to determine the effects of therapy.

One should not hesitate to involve family members in discussions with the patient about habits of voice use and implementation of therapy. Parents, spouses, siblings, and even children can provide objectivity for the adult and can help effect the clinician's recommendations by understanding the objectives of such therapy and feeling like a part of the therapy process.

An electronic device for monitoring vocal loudness has been used successfully in the treatment of vocal abuse disorders and is described later in this chapter.

CONTACT ULCER

Vocal abuse can produce a contact ulcer, resulting in hoarseness and excessively low pitch. Therapy aims at reducing vocal fold trauma through vocal re-education and eliminating emotional and environmental stress. Prognosis is excellent if the patient is able to produce voice consistently in the manner prescribed. Surgical removal of a contact ulcer is contraindicated; clinical evidence shows that healing is best achieved with vocal re-education. Voice therapy begins with an informational phase, during which the patient is given an understanding of the mechanics by which the ulcer has formed, using graphic illustrations. During the auditory discrimination phase, comparisons between the abnormally low-pitched, hoarse dysphonia and the normal voice are made via audiotape recordings. The vocal production phase concerns modification of voice use in daily life. After a thorough analysis of daily voice use and abuse, the patient needs to be informed that until the ulcer heals, the quantity and intensity of voice use has to be reduced approximately 50 percent for one month, eliminating all but necessary speaking. *Silence or whispering is definitely contraindicated.* Patients can return to normal voice use afterward provided that they follow the additional instructions detailed next. Careful analysis of abnormal vocal use often reveals shouting under tension or anger and attempts to communicate over long distances.

The physiology of vocal abuse in patients who develop contact ulcer is abnormal and needs to be treated in the following ways.

1. Because words beginning with vowels may be produced with an explosive glottal attack, which augments the force of vocal fold adduction and the frictional trauma to the vocal folds, the patient must be trained to produce words beginning with vowels by means of an *easy or aspirate vocal attack.* The patient should be taught to recognize and to feel the difference between hard and soft glottal attacks. Explosive speech ordinarily used for emphasis needs to be modulated.

2. Because trauma may result from excessively low pitch, employed because the patient believes it is more authoritative or impressive in the classroom, courtroom, or salesroom, a more appropriate pitch level will need to be taught. The "um-hum" method is advocated for obtaining the most comfortable pitch.

3. Because frequent coughing or throat clearing not only is damaging to vocal folds but also retards healing of the contact ulcer, the patient needs to reduce these activities. Patients can be taught to swallow when they feel the need to bring up material, or to clear the throat or cough with an easier, more aspirate approach rather than with an explosive glottal attack, i.e., the "silent cough."

4. Because trauma is aggravated by alcohol consumption and smoking, the patient needs to be informed that both substances irritate the vocal folds. For the initial period of one month, both drinking and smoking need to be eliminated completely.

5. Because patients with vocal abuse disorders have increased musculoskeletal tension, the speech pathologist needs to work on reduction of those tensions. (See section on voice therapy for musculoskeletal tension.)

6. Interpersonal problems and environmental stress are commonly associated with the development of contact ulcers. The evidence is clear that these patients are hard driving, competitive, angry, and aggressive, traits which may be modifiable if the patient is concerned enough about their effects on the voice. If such tendencies are mild, they can be dealt with by the speech pathologist, but in more severe cases, referral for professional psychotherapy needs to be considered. Vocal abuse often occurs in fundamentally well-balanced people who have allowed themselves to be subjected to tremendous environmental stresses, such as an intensive schedule of speaking under adverse conditions at work, and burdening extracurricular activities. There needs to be discussion with the patient about refusing to participate in such a vocally demanding schedule. Heavy work schedules that place the patient under extreme pressures resulting in irritability and leading to anger are precursors of the vocal abuse that leads to contact ulcer. The modification of the psychologic environment of the contact ulcer patient is as important as direct voice therapy, and, in fact, one without the other may prove ineffectual.

Conversion Voice Disorders

Conversion reactions produce diverse voice signs: muteness, aphonia, intermittent aphonia, breathiness, hoarseness, excessively high pitch, and falsetto. The abnormal voice, a sign of emotional or interpersonal conflict, has served or continues to serve the purpose of enabling the patient to avoid confrontation with an unpleasant life situation. The voice may be serving the purpose of primary or secondary gain. Conversion aphonia or dysphonia may continue even after conflict resolution.

The voice disorder exists on an unconscious level; the patient is not willfully or volitionally producing the abnormal voice, and he consciously believes that the disorder is organic, not psychogenic. Even though the neuromuscular system is intact, the patient is unable to phonate voluntarily and is convinced of this inability. The interpersonal problems causing the voice disorder remain unexpressed to the parties concerned, including the clinician from whom the patient has sought help. The likelihood of complete return of the voice via symptomatic voice therapy is excellent if the patient is ready to relinquish the voice sign and to bring the problem causing it into the open. The prognosis is also excellent if the original problem has disappeared, leaving the residual voice sign. The prognosis is poor for patients who are unwilling to face and deal with the underlying problem causing the voice disorder, in which case either it will be impossible to improve the voice by means of any therapy or, if improvement does take place, it will be incomplete or short-lived.

Symptomatic voice therapy is subdivided into the following phases: patient education; symptom removal by means of direct voice therapy; catharsis; and psychotherapy when indicated. The efficacy of symptomatic voice therapy is predicated on the following principles:

1. Reduction of laryngeal musculoskeletal tension.
2. Evoking voice by any one of a variety of means to convince the patient of phonatory capability.

THERAPY RATIONALE

Successful therapy for conversion voice disorders begins with the speech pathologist taking primary responsibility for patient management. The history of speech pathology's attitudes toward the treatment of patients with conversion voice disorders has been one of avoidance of this responsibility. It is often reasoned, erroneously, that because the disorder is primarily psychogenic, its treatment should be left in the hands of the psychiatrist or clinical psychologist. Another time-honored belief held by clinicians of all specialties is that symptom removal in a conversion reaction is dangerous if its underlying cause is not treated and that the conversion sign will crop up someplace else. This idea dies hard despite the fact that psychiatrists no longer subscribe to it. Hundreds of cases of symptom removal in many different body parts without adverse effects or subsequent conversions have been documented. The worse result will be failure to relieve the voice sign because of patient unreadiness, undoubtedly a defense mechanism. Psychiatrists now believe that reported adverse reactions to attempted symptom removal were caused, not by the removal of the conversion itself, but by the precipitous and traumatic manner by which it was removed.

Experience with conversion voice disorders shows that premature referral of the patient to the psychiatrist or psychologist is almost a guarantee of failure to improve the voice. The validity of this statement is based upon the following reasons:

1. The voice disorder, a somatic sign, is, in the patient's mind, dissociated from conscious awareness of any emotional problem. This is the reason why most patients whose voices have been treated through traditional "interview" psychotherapy alone have not improved.

2. Symptom removal in conversion voice disorders requires laryngeal muscular alterations simultaneous with auditory feedback, i.e., treatment directed at the larynx itself.

3. Despite what might be excellent training in psychodiagnostics and psychotherapy, most psychologists and psychiatrists are not trained to deal with voice disorders.

4. The unavailability of psychiatric and psychologic personnel and their lack of interest in voice disorders because of the relative mildness of the psychologic problems that underlie most of them make conversion patients less acceptable to such specialists. The psychiatrist and psychologist become important only after the voice disorder has been eliminated or improved. Then, if the emotional factors are sufficiently severe, referral is warranted.

5. The patient with a conversion voice disorder who is convinced that the disorder is organic more often than not refuses referral to a psychologist or psychiatrist, in the beginning. Only after the voice has returned do such patients become aware of psychologic causes; they are then more receptive to referral.

There is, then, a proper sequence of clinical events that needs to take place in the treatment of conversion voice disorders: laryngologic clearance of organic laryngeal disease and systemic illness; symptomatic voice therapy coupled with ventilation and elaboration of emotional problems, if the patient is capable of doing so; and referral to the psychologist or psychiatrist in order to achieve a more enduring stabilization of the patient's life adjustment. A mature, cautious, and well-trained speech pathologist will not harm the patient. On the contrary, the opportunity given the patient to discuss emotional problems simultaneously while undergoing the more mechanical aspects of voice therapy can only serve to provide that patient with new hope for a better voice. It is for patients such as these that we advocate so strongly the interdisciplinary practice of speech pathology in settings that bring psychologist, psychiatrist, laryngologist, and speech pathologist together, for such relationships provide a feeling of greater confidence on the part of all clinicians treating such patients.

PATIENT EDUCATION

As in other voice disorders, the first phase of therapy for conversion voice disorders is patient education. After obtaining a complete history and after deciding that a conversion voice disorder exists, if the voice has not improved spontaneously during the history—as it sometimes does as the patient reveals underlying emotional stresses for the first time—the first necessity in therapy is to educate the patient about the cause of the aphonia or dysphonia. Almost universally characteristic is their initial insistence that the disorder is organic. This denial will delay, in many cases, and prevent, in others, successful voice therapy. Time needs to be taken to discuss the beliefs of both laryngologist and speech pathologist that the voice disorder is not due to infection, tumor, or other organic cause and that it is due to emotional stress. How the speech pathologist handles this informational phase can determine the difference between continuation on to success and early failure. *The difference lies in the manner by which this information is communicated.* Many patients previously seen by other clinicians have been told pointblank that they needed to see a psychiatrist. Such precipitous revelation of what may be essentially true is almost always indigestible by the patient. On the other hand, a gradual, sympathetic unfolding of this fact through discussion can make the difference between acceptance and rejection of the idea.

The first step is to divest the patient of the notion that the voice disorder is organic by reviewing the laryngologist's findings with the patient. Firmly and authoritatively, the clinician should tell, or preferably read aloud, the laryngologist's report—that the larynx was normal on laryngoscopic examination, that no lesions or paralyses were noted, and that the patient has the capability to produce normal voice. This information not only serves to start the patient thinking about emotional factors but also relieves anxiety about threatening laryngeal disease, namely, cancer. Patients show visible signs of relief upon hearing this report. Their anxieties about laryngeal disease are real, and with the restatement about the normal laryngologic examination, the patient's mind is cleared of fears of serious illness. The germ of the idea that perhaps the voice is due to emotional causes after all is thus planted. The next step is to present the concept, in language appropriate to the patient's educational background, that the larynx is a common site for the expression of emotional problems. Most people are already aware of this fact on the basis of lifelong experience. It can be pointed out to them how, in everyday life, we express our emotions—anger, fear, grief—through the larynx, and how it sometimes undergoes violent, uncontrollable muscular reactions that can be felt as well as heard during transient emotional states. The rate of informational exchange, the pacing, and the clinician's finesse develop with practice. It is wise to stop at various points along the way to sample the patient's reactions to this new knowledge. It is always interesting to see how different patients with conversion voice disorders react to the idea of psychogenicity. Some are so threatened and incensed by the idea that they refuse to continue the interview, grabbing for their coats and purses in preparation for terminating the session. Fortunately, although most patients react at first with skepticism, they are willing to listen. Some amiably agree. They "knew it all the time" but needed someone else to confront them with the facts. Once the patient is willing to consider the possibility that the voice disorder is related to emotional conflict or stress, the stage is set for the next phase.

The clinician proceeds to inform the patient that there has been a loss of contact between the desire to produce voice and the voluntary muscular ability to do so. After working with several patients who have conversion voice disorders, the clinician will eventually become convinced that they are genuinely under the impression that they are unable to phonate more than they do at the time of examination, even though they have been making audible sounds via throat clearing and coughing, thus failing to appreciate the relationship between those signals and the potential for normal voice.

DIRECT VOICE THERAPY

All attention is now paid to the larynx and voice, and psychologic considerations are set aside. One should test first for the presence and extent of musculoskeletal tension, which almost invariably accompanies conversion voice disorders. The identical procedures for the relief of isolated musculoskeletal tension are employed at this time. Incorporated into the manual relief of such tension are the clinician's instructions to the patient to produce various laryngeal noises—coughing followed by an extension of coughing into continuous voicing, throat clearing, and humming. The purpose of this activity should not be lost on either clinician or patient: *It is to convince the patient that there is more voice capability than the patient realized.* When increased laryngeal sound occurs, it should be pointed out instantaneously.

Patients vary in their rate of voice improvement and in the acoustic characteristics that accompany such improvement. Those who have had aphonia or dysphonia for long periods of time will go through several stages of dysphonia, which may require as much as an hour of therapy before normal voice is approached. These dysphonic transitional stages can take the form of raucous hoarseness or harshness. They must be recognized as transitional stages and must be worked through to normal voice. Patients react early to voice improvements with much surprise, proving their obliviousness to their actual voice capabilities. Their voice improvements should be met with the clinician's approval and pleasure. Patients who have had conversion voice disorders for shorter periods will often shift from severe dysphonia or aphonia to normal voice within minutes. Others who are not ready for symptom removal either will fail to respond with any voice improvement or will produce varying degrees of voice improvement short of normal and then plateau despite continued efforts at therapy. Such patients are not candidates for further therapy at that point and ought to be asked to return for a second or third try. Some will fail to keep future appointments, for obvious reasons.

CATHARSIS AND COUNSELING

The next phase of therapy is catharsis and discussion of emotional causes. Upon experiencing a return of their voices, most patients will express emotional relief, usually a mixture of smiling and weeping, which they attribute to their happiness for having been relieved of the burden of the abnormal voice. Such emotional reaction is healthy and is to be encouraged, despite the patient's protestations of embarrassment. One should discuss with them their feelings about the return of the voice while at the same time encouraging them to use the voice to its fullest. This is a good time to get the patient to talk about the frustration, embarrassment, and other effects of the voice disorder. Most will describe considerable inconvenience that they and their families have suffered as a consequence of the disorder. The patient's change of facial expression and general attitude should be noted. The face is less tense, less frowning; there are fewer signs of distress around the mouth and eyes and a general impression of happiness. The patient's attitude will change to one of increased openness, a willingness to talk more freely, and, most important, an apparent improvement in insight and memory for the events, feelings, and attitudes that gave rise to the voice disorder in the first place.

For patients who are receptive to discussion of psychogenic causes, despite earlier denial of them, this is an excellent time to reopen the subject. It is a never-ending source of wonder how often patients become aware of emotional conflicts only *after* the voice has returned, and how they go on to describe acute or chronic stresses and conflicts in their lives, usually of an interpersonal nature and having to do with a breakdown in communication with persons close to them and in whom they have much ego investment. The speech pathologist will discover that quite ordinary irritations are, to many patients with psychogenic voice disorders, monumental. One quickly learns that each person responds to life's problems with different degrees of emotional reactivity. Here are some examples: loss of voice following an argument with a relative or friend; loss of voice because of feelings that one's position of authority has been usurped in an office setting; a feeling of having been wronged in the settlement of a family estate; inability to tolerate personal habits in one's spouse and to confront that person with one's feelings; deep frustration, disappointment, or job dislike that one is unable to change for fear of repercussions from employers or family; an engagement or marital relationship that has gone sour in which the patient is unable to express the wish that the relationship be discontinued. *A common denominator runs through these themes despite the differences in their specifics: The need to express anger, dissatisfaction, or grief, but an inability to do so.* Lifelong, these individuals have never been able to express their feelings openly and directly. Often, the speech pathologist is the first person to whom they have had an opportunity to reveal these unspoken and sometimes unspeakable ideas.

REFERRAL

Finally, the speech pathologist and patient need to talk about the future. They need to decide whether the original emotional problem is still operative or whether it has been resolved or is resolving. With clinical experience, a certain practical sense develops in judging whether or not the patient can benefit from further professional psychotherapy. The decision for referral to a psychologist or a psychiatrist should be bilateral. The patient, however, must make the final decision. Does he or she feel happy or satisfied with life? Is this someone who has long felt the need for professional help but has been too shy, indecisive, or confused as to how to obtain it? Realistically, not all patients with conversion voice disorders are candidates for psychotherapy. Many are superficial and denying; they either reject such therapy on the grounds of not needing it or, once begun, discontinue. Sometimes all one can do is carry the person over the crisis by being a listener and a friend. Although speech clinicians do not practice psychotherapy, they have a responsibility for being the "advanced party," for breaking new ground, and for helping the patient to discover, perhaps for the first time, that further help is needed. An impressive number of patients, upon learning that their abnormal voice was a primitive substitute for a more mature solution, will then attack their problems directly. Often, patients will obtain enough insight from voice therapy and discussion alone to make effective changes in their lives, usually those who have sufficient ego reserve and aggressiveness. The passive and dependent types, overwhelmed by life's punishments, cannot seem to get out from under, and for them psychiatric consultation and therapy are indicated and should be advocated as strongly as possible.

The evolution of therapy for conversion voice disorders has arrived at the point where it is now known that mechanical, symptomatic voice therapy must be cradled in kindness, psychotherapeutic counseling, and respect for the unusual nature of conversion itself. The history of treatment of this disorder has been brutal and ineffectual because of the failure to respect and recognize the patient's potential for insight and growth.

The following case studies show the interaction between patient and speech pathologist during interviewing and voice therapy for conversion voice disorders.

*   *   *

A 26-year-old police officer, on the force for three years, had never been happy in his work. He had never told anyone about his feelings for fear of disappointing his parents, who were very much in favor of this vocation. He had always been a quiet, unaggressive person who found it difficult to lose his temper, but when he did, he shook and became livid with rage. He found it difficult to reprimand motorists or pedestrians because of a strong need to be liked by everyone. The patient had had several previous episodes of aphonia and dysphonia which, heretofore, had cleared up spontaneously. At the time of interview, he was aphonic. Laryngologic examination was normal.

C: What brings you to this clinic?

P: (Patient's voice is a complete whisper.) My voice. I haven't been able to talk. It started April 9th; it came back for a few days and then it was gone again. But it was all high-pitched. And then, finally, that went away again. And it has been like this for the last three or four weeks now. I had a bad cold. It started with laryngitis. And my voice started to come back again. Then, all of a sudden it was gone, just like it is now—completely. Altogether it was about four or five weeks that I lost it.

C: How did it come back?

P: I coughed and I had a voice back. The next time, it was in either September or October of last year, I had a slight cold—no sore throat or anything—but the next day my voice was gone again. And that lasted only for about nine days.

C: How did it come back?

P: I can't remember exactly how that one did come back.

C: Are you able to make any sound at all?

P: Once in a while a sound will come out.

C: Before we go any further, I wonder if you would read this aloud for me. (Just before beginning, the patient coughs audibly, but reads the passage in a completely whispered voice.) Now would you cough for me? (Patient coughs repeatedly, each time with an excellent glottal attack and brief audible voicing.)

C: What kind of work do you do?

P: Police officer.

C: How long have you been doing that?

P: Since January of last year.

C: Have you been happy in your work?

P: I wonder . . . if I actually do like the work that I am doing, or if I am just saying I do because I don't want to tell everybody that I would like to quit and that I don't want the Police Department.

C: Disregarding what other people think, how do you actually feel about the job?

P: Well . . . I have trouble giving somebody a ticket. I have trouble talking to a person.

C: What is there about talking to people that is so difficult?

P: I get nervous. I am always afraid that I am going to say something or do something wrong . . . that's going to get either me or somebody else in trouble. Because if you do one thing wrong in the Police Department, you might as well forget your job.

C: In other words, when you are talking to a motorist who may have violated a law, you feel under pressure to be correct.

P: I can tell them what they have done wrong, and if they don't start arguing I am all right . . . But once they start arguing, then, well, if I get mad I start to shake when I get nervous like that. Then my words start to get mixed up. I know I shouldn't get nervous. That is our job, and people expect it. It's just something that happens to me. The worst time I got angry, I actually saw red. I got mad once, really mad, while I was in a fight, and a guy bit me; and then I really got mad. I didn't think it was possible to see red, but I saw red.

C: That must have been very frightening.

P: I shook for about an hour and a half after it.

C: Does being a policeman make you uncomfortable because you are in the position of being a disciplinarian?

P: I never thought of that. I don't like people to dislike me. .

C: Well, let's say that you have to apprehend a motorist for speeding or some other violation. What are your feelings? What goes through your mind?

P: If we see someone we think is speeding, we get in behind him and clock him with our speedometer . . . If he is speeding, we'll stop the clock which locks the speedometer so that we know what speed he is still going at, and stop the car and go over and tell him, you know, that he has been speeding. Once in a while, you will get a guy who will argue, but usually they will go along with you. Once in a while, you find a guy who is never wrong. His car can't go that fast. And then, we start to argue and then I . . . I don't know, I get flustered. . .

C: You have the evidence there. . .

P: I have the evidence, but yet, I . . . I know I am right and that's what I don't get. I know I am right and yet I am the one that gets nervous. When actually he should be the one. He is getting the ticket . . . I know I am sensitive to other people's feelings about me . . . how people think of me . . . what they think of me. (At this point, discussion was discontinued and voice therapy begun.)

C: I would like to explain something to you. You haven't really lost your voice. You have temporarily lost the knowledge of how to make it function again. But the voice is there, and through certain activities there is a good likelihood that we can get it back. First of all, hum for me. (Clinician demonstrates. Patient does not seem to know how to go about producing a humming noise.) Make a coughing noise. (Patient coughs audibly.) Now do it again, except prolong it this time. (Patient prolongs the cough into a predominantly breathy dysphonia.) Now, did you hear that voicing? That's the voice. And I would like you to keep it going. Try it again. (Patient repeats the cough with the breathy prolongation.) Now, try it without the cough. Hum. (Patient begins to produce an intermittent, weak humming noise.) Yes, I hear it now. Again. (Patient repeats. After approximately 15 seconds of humming at the weak, high pitches, the pitch drops with a marked tremor, at the same time becoming increasingly louder. Suddenly, the patient speaks in a normal voice.)

P: It's back!

C: Well! . . . Very good.

P: Huh! . . . It's back. (Voice quality and loudness are normal.)

C: How does it feel?

P: It feels all right (tentatively). It's not normal. It's higher. A little more gravelly.

C: This is fairly common, and it will come down to where it should be in a reasonably short time.

P: Because, this happened to me before. It was real high, and then it went away again. But it's not as high as it was then.

C: Would you read this out loud for me, to strengthen it a little bit? (Patient reads the passage.)

P: Wonderful! . . . A little funny . . . that it was that easy to get back . . . Would it have come back like this if I had just walked in here, without talking to you fellows? Or is it because I've talked to you and the other doctor?

C: What do you think?

P: I think so . . . I mean I think that I might not have gotten it back.

C: Why do you think that talking to us has played a part in your getting your voice back?

P: Because I know when I was talking to the other doctor (the psychiatrist), there is something that I brought up, that I started feeling funny.

C: What was that?

P: It was about the Police Department. He asked me about . . . that "you don't really like your job and you are afraid to tell your family this." And I agreed with him, but I felt real funny.

C: Was it true?

P: Yes . . . I have never told anyone.

C: Having talked about it with somebody, how does it make things different?

P: I shouldn't be afraid to tell my family. It's my life. I should enjoy what I am doing. I shouldn't be working for something because they all think I should be working there. I should be doing something that I want to do. And not what they want me to do. That's what I feel, anyway.

C: You feel, then, that having said this *to someone else* has changed your attitude.

P: Right. Because I had thought of it before, but I had never mentioned it to anybody. You two fellows are the first people I ever told it to.

C: Was it hard for you to think about? To admit it to yourself?

P: Uh huh. I didn't want to admit to myself, you know, that I didn't like the job. Like, me, I am a constant daydreamer, and I dream about it.

C: What would you like to be doing?

P: My old job.

C: Which was. . .

P: Textile chemist.

C: Tell me about that.

P: I'd mix the chemicals, bleach the cloth, dry the cloth . . . I don't know, I just enjoyed working. It was long hours. The pay wasn't that great. But I enjoyed working there.

C: What did you enjoy the most about it?

P: I don't know if it was because I worked alone. I'd maybe say ten words a day. I didn't mind it. I sing a lot. I'd sing all the time. And I enjoyed it. Or if I wanted to daydream, I could daydream.

C: What do you daydream about?

P: You name it (laughs). Mostly about, oh I don't know, money, being strong, you know, crazy things.

C: How could your loss of voice be related to . . . all this?

P: Well, I don't know . . . Subconsciously, it was the only way I knew of getting away from there . . . maybe rebelling.

C: What do you think would be the solution to the problem of the voice loss?

P: I think it's the job that's causing it. Maybe I'm wrong. Maybe I'd get another job, and it would go away again. I don't think so.

C: Do you really think that you will be able to put into action what you would really like to do?

P: Well, I think that now that I have talked to you fellows, and I know that it's because I don't want to tell my parents, maybe now I can tell my parents. Because I was always shutting it out before. I never wanted to think about it. Maybe it wouldn't bother them half as much as I think it would.

* * *

A 46-year-old cosmetologist had been under chronic stress resulting from several sources: her concern about her son, a rebellious, belligerent young man of 25; her unspoken rage at her husband, who had never supported the family completely and usually didn't work at all; and her chronic irritation with her cosmetology-salon employees. She insisted on perfection from them, yet was never able to voice her irritations when they fell short. Instead, her voice faltered into an intermittent hoarseness and whisper, and she was overwhelmed with fatigue and usually forced to go home and take to her bed. Her marginal insight into all this was evidenced by her statement that "I am afraid my employees think that I am angry with them when I lose my voice and can't talk." The patient had had many previous brief episodes of dysphonia and aphonia which had cleared up spontaneously. The most recent one brought her to this clinic because of its unusually long duration (nine weeks). At the time of interview, her voice was an intermittent dysphonia-aphonia. Results of laryngologic examination were negative.

C: Is this your first loss of voice?

P: No, I've had it many times, but I've never had it for more than 14 days.

C: But this last time it's been longer.

P: Started my ninth week yesterday. I know one thing, it seems that I always lose my voice in October. One of my problems is that I have trouble hiring efficient help.

C: Have you felt at all depressed or unhappy whenever you have lost your voice in the past?

P: I've tried to analyze that myself, and I don't come up with the answer. A couple of my better employees say that they think that this directly follows mental strain—if I become upset over something—but I haven't been able to look back and prove to myself that that's true.

C: Does it create any problems, your not being able to use your voice normally?

P: Yes, it makes it so that I'm not really able to cope with my business activities. You can't answer a telephone, people just hang up on you . . . I can't conduct extracurricular activities.

C: What else?

P: (With great emphasis) *I can't express myself at all.* There is no intonation in your voice at all. You sound like you are angry all the time.

C: Well . . . we would like to help you get your voice back, but we would also like to learn more about you. Would you have any objections to staying on for a few days and being interviewed by some of our psychiatrists?

P: Not at all (surprised). You're not a psychiatrist?

C: No. I am a speech pathologist.

P: You're certainly putting a lot into it, psychology-wise (embarrassed laughter).

C: It's all interrelated, isn't it? Before we arrange these interviews, we would like to help you get your voice back, and I think we can start right away. Would you open your mouth, now, wide as you can? Now say /a:/. (Patient produces a weak, high-pitched, scratchy voice.) Make it louder. Now stick your tongue out. Again, now, /a:/. (Patient produces a harsh voice a shade louder which has a rapid tremor.) Kind of a tremorous voice, isn't it, but it's there. Try it again. Let's do something else now. Tilt your head back, now open your mouth as wide as you can and stick your tongue way out. Now say /a:/ and keep that up. I want you to listen for that sound and try to keep it going. Try it again, real sharp now. (Patient produces slightly louder tone, momentarily, and is encouraged to listen for it and repeat it.) It sounds worse than it is, doesn't it?

P: It doesn't hurt . . . at all.

C: Can you hum for me? (Patient produces a very clear high-pitched tone on humming.) Oh, very good. Take a deep breath and do that again. Can you do that a little louder? (Tone clearer this time.) Now try /m:a:/. (Patient produces a high-pitched, breathy voice which is an improvement over previous productions. She is asked to repeat this several times.) Let's try /m:a:/ again. (Patient produces this equally well.) It's still too high, isn't it? That's not your normal voice.

P: No. But I've never been able to sing for years. (Patient continues to produce a variety of vowels with gradual reduction of breathiness. However, there is a great deal of quavering or tremor to the voice on vowel prolongation.)

C: Let's go down one tone, now. (Patient complies, and the vowel /a:/ is produced at progressively lower pitches. Vocal loudness is also increasing. There is a strained, harsh quality, nevertheless.) Very good. Continue. Not let's make it real smooth . . . Let's try it again. Do you hear the way your voice catches now and then? Do you feel a tightening whenever that happens?

P: I'll . . . take . . . better notice.

C: Now I want you to say this: M-o-n-d-a-y. (Clinician produces it in a monopitch. Patient repeats, "Monday," in a monopitch with fairly good clarity, although with some harshness and voice tremor. She is asked to produce this word at successively lower pitch levels. As she repeats this word, and as the voice quality and loudness improve, she becomes increasingly tearful, and the voice begins to crack.) This improvement in the voice seems to have affected you. True?

P: Yes . . . It relieves me.

C: You notice how your voice has dropped down to a lower pitch? I think that's where it wants to settle. Let's see if it gravitates down in that direction. Try it again. (Patient repeats sentence.) Yes, there it goes down to the lower pitch. That's fine. Continue. (She is then given a passage to read aloud. She does so in a nearly normal voice. As she is reading, the clinician intersperses requests that she speak louder at various points in her reading. With that last reading of the passage, it is apparent to both clinician and patient that the voice is normal or near normal.) How do you feel now?

P: Tired . . . sore . . . but good!

C: Go on.

P: How do I feel? . . . I feel . . . uh . . . sort of exuberant, I am sure . . . it's . . . been a long . . . long time. I feel good. Now my voice sounds more normal. I feel nice. I feel good. (Gives a great sigh.) Now what happens? . . . Is this going to happen every once in a while? When I started talking again, I always just started talking. I never had to struggle like this. I would all of a sudden realize I was talking. I would be whispering and all of a sudden I would be talking. That feels better. It sounds better, too, doesn't it?

C: Is it completely back to normal? Or does it have a way to go yet?

P: Well, I am afraid I have a way to go. My normal voice doesn't take any effort.

C: Does it still take some effort now?

P: Yes, it still takes effort. (Patient resumes practice. Pitch of voice is gradually decreasing, loudness is increasing, and quality is clearing. After this, she is asked to employ spontaneous speech in an effort to enable her to use her voice in more automatic speech situations. She describes the furnishing of her business establishment.)

C: Let's talk about these voice losses. Do you have any warning that you are going to lose it?

P: I do seem to have a warning when I am going to lose my voice . . . I have this tight feeling in my chest. However, I have never associated it with any happening in my life. These are such common, everyday things that it might just take an accumulation to make a person, all of a sudden, fight back some way or another, you see?

C: By "fight back," what do you mean?

P: Well, my husband says, and I think he has got it pretty straight, maybe, that I get so sick and tired of talking to women day in and day out . . . I like my work, but he says I get so sick of women talking and yakking and the daily noise around me, that finally I make up my mind I'm just not going to talk. Well, he might have something there. I don't know. Maybe things pile up on me or something, 'til I'll just fight back by not talking. I'll show them. I don't know. Day in and day out, we have to talk to people and be nice to them, which, of course, we want to be, and, uh, if someone comes in and throws themselves into your chair, starts to be a little bit obnoxious, she's had an argument with her husband, or she didn't like the news on the radio, or one of her children acted up before he got on the school bus . . . You know there is something in the back of her mind, so the first thing you do is try to kind of butter her up a little bit. Now, it's a very very trivial thing, but uh . . . when you've done this about ten times in one day you get sort of sick of it after a while . . . and there is one thing that I cannot do when I don't have a voice, I can't do that!

C: Do you think that your voice loss comes about after a series of stressful events?

P: I have asked myself this same question many times before. As I have said, one of my valuable employees has told me that she has noticed over the years that every time I have a real nervous spell . . . not every time . . . when I have a real nervous time, perhaps not just one day of it, that I oftentimes get laryngitis. So, since she told me that, and I had never heard her voice this until this last siege of laryngitis, I have been trying to think that through and see if she is right. If this is true, I still don't know how to keep from having it happen again. (Patient sent for psychiatric consultation at this point. Resumes next day.)

C: Tell me, what did you do after your appointments yesterday?

P: (Patient's voice virtually normal. She is in good spirits—almost childlike attitude; many pitch and inflectional changes; generally a great deal of melody to the voice.) Well (laughs), we went down to one of the restaurants, had a bit piece of cake, and celebrated, and we made up our minds to hunt for one of my husband's friends living near here. I was tempted to go back to my room and go to bed, but I didn't think that would be smart. I felt that I should keep talking, and driving in my husband's truck I would have to talk loud and keep talking, and so, I just talked over the noise of the motor, and I think my husband helped me along. He asked me everything twice (laughs), on purpose, I think.

C: Is he pleased with your voice?

P: Yes! I should say so.

C: So, you feel that your voice is normal now?

P: Uh huh.

C: You feel well?

P: Uh huh.

C: Is there anything that you would like to ask about?

P: No . . . uh . . . I would like to know about . . . about my psychoanalyst (sic) yesterday . . . I find that very interesting. I'd just like to know a little bit more about myself.

C: I talked with him (psychiatrist), and he confirmed what we had discussed yesterday, that your voice loss is related to your way of reacting to the stresses around you. He thought that you have the habit of bottling up your emotions, instead of allowing yourself to express how you feel, like blowing off steam.

P: That I know about myself.

C: Do you have any idea why you can't?

P: I have always wondered about myself in this respect. I never can express love or emotions of that sort, either, without forcing myself. That's probably why I don't blow up, too . . . Now, I am sure that I feel just as deeply as anyone, but I just don't talk about it.

C: Do you know why this is true?

P: No, unless it's my upbringing. My parents were very close to each other, and they never argued. I never heard them argue in my whole life. I see this as something unusual. However, neither did I ever see my father kiss my mother more than maybe a couple of times in my life. I mean, there was no outward expression of love. I think maybe I was sort of ashamed to express myself. I wasn't brought up to wear my emotions on my sleeve.

C: How do you feel toward people who do express themselves in these ways?

P: Oh! I think it's wonderful! I really do. That is the only way to live.

C: Do you wish, perhaps, that you could live that way?

P: Yes, I think maybe that those around me would like me better.

C: Which of your parents do you think kept their feelings to themselves more?

P: Mother did. Very much.

C: Were you close to your mother?

P: (Emphatically) Yes! My father was 20 years older than my mother. He just worshipped me; I know that. But I was still closer to my mother.

C: Do you feel that you're like your mother?

P: Yes. Uh huh. Everyone does. I mean, in appearance, and they say the older I get the more I look like her and the more I act like her. I always felt that I couldn't be any better than that.

C: Do you think that you are like her also in the respect that you don't show your feelings externally?

P: I suppose you are right! You know, I never thought of that? I never thought of being emotionally like my mother. I presume that I have often expressed the desire to be. Because she was a person who was always so well liked and never seemed to resent anyone. I never heard her say anything unkind about anyone in my whole life. Women would come to our house and gossip, sometimes, and mother would clam right up and not say a word. For a woman not to ever gossip is almost unheard of.

C: Do you think she allowed herself to be taken advantage of?

P: Yes, I think she did.

C: Do you think you are like that?

P: Not as much as she was. I let people run over me at times. That's probably half my trouble in my business. I will let someone keep getting away with something until it builds up too much, I suppose. I should not have let them get away with it to start with. But rather than putting my foot down and saying, "Now look, we don't do things that way," that this is it, I would let them get off easy.

C: Well, why don't you?

P: (Laughs.) I am going to try, I'll tell you.

*   *   *

Mutational Falsetto (Puberphonia)

Despite anatomically and physiologically normal respiratory and phonatory structures, mutational falsetto is produced with the larynx positioned excessively high in the neck and vocal folds lax and stretched thin anteroposteriorly. Phonation is produced with abnormally reduced infraglottal air pressure caused by shallow respiration. The voice is high or intermediate in pitch, weak and thin, breathy, hoarse and gives the impression of immaturity, passiveness, and effeminacy.

Voice therapy begins with asking the patient to *breathe in deeply* and to produce a vowel or cough with a *sharp glottal attack,* as demonstrated by the clinician. The pitch will break abruptly to a lower level. If the sharp glottal attack is unsuccessful, one should manually pull the larynx downward as the vowel is being produced. If these measures fail, while holding the larynx down, one should depress the tongue with a tongue depressor as the patient produces the sharp glottal attack.

The low-pitched voice should be identified immediately for the patient. If the disorder is actually mutational falsetto, it is important to explain early in therapy that the low-pitched voice is the normal one and that the patient must learn to think of it as the target voice in therapy. This information must be conveyed persuasively, because the patient will not be completely convinced until after habituation of the low-pitched voice.

As soon as the low-pitched voice is produced, it should be maintained through repeated vowel production using a sharp glottal attack. *The therapy is not a gradual stepwise progression from the high to the low pitch. The break must be sudden and complete. Phonation must be forceful and vigorous.* The voice will want to shift up to the falsetto, in which case the patient will need to be reminded to breathe in deeply and then phonate sharply. Increased depth of breathing is fundamental to success in therapy, and the patient needs practice in phonating after deep inhalation. The clinician judges on a moment-to-moment basis how long to remain on vowels before attempting words, sentences, and conversational speech.

In a study of the pitch and quality characteristics of 10 adolescent males aged 13 to 18 years and two adult males, 26 and 29 years old, who had mutational falsetto, Hammarberg (1987) found that the mean change in fundamental frequency in 10 of the subjects between 13 and 18 years of age before and after therapy was 221 Hz (range, 168 to 288 Hz) and 119 Hz (range, 105 to 135), respectively. In the two males 26 to 29 years of age, the mean fundamental frequency prior to therapy was 198 Hz and after, 100 Hz.

A reasonably stabilized voice should be achievable within an hour. Three to five additional therapy sessions are usually necessary to effect habituation. The most difficult phase of the therapy for mutational falsetto is getting the patient accustomed to the low-pitched voice. Gradual guidance into outside activities is necessary. Embarrassment upon returning to school is common among adolescents with mutational falsetto, and for that reason, therapy during vacation is desirable.

Patients who have mutational falsetto, for reasons of immaturity, lack insight into the reason for their voice disorders and make poor candidates for counseling and psychotherapy. Fortunately, in most cases the psychologic cause is no longer operative by the time the patient comes for voice therapy. A complete and permanent low pitch can be attained without delving into the psychologic reasons for the failure of voice change. Occasionally, despite their ability to produce the low-pitched voice, certain patients will refuse to proceed with the therapy because they are threatened by the prospect of a masculine voice. Discussion with the patient and parents may result in a referral for psychologic or psychiatric therapy. Such patients, however, often return for therapy later after having become accustomed to the idea of the lower pitch.

The typical sequence of events in therapy for mutational falsetto is given in the following study of a 21-year-old male college student.

* * *

P: I guess it was in the ninth grade when my voice first started changing. Seems like it started growing in spurts. The first time I was really aware of it was in stressful situations. We had an English class where you did a lot of book reports, and I'd try to get up and give a report and it would be long periods where it wouldn't break and I couldn't get anything out. I just kept getting worse and worse. At first, it would crack a lot. And a lot of people would say it was so shrill. It would sound just like a girl's, that high. Then through high school, in the tenth grade, it was still the same way, but in the twelfth it got to where it wasn't as shrill and it didn't break quite as much. Like, when a substitute would come and call the roll, and I'd yell "here," it wouldn't even come out; I'd have to try it twice. One guy where I work said, "Whenever you get excited you sound just like a girl." When I was relaxed, it would be hoarse. After swimming, if I was cold, tired, or really nervous, it would get much worse. When I got to college I could try to make it where it wouldn't crack, but it still sounded hoarse.

C: Do you have some confusion in your mind as to which is the right voice?

P: Yea. But the cracking didn't bother me a great deal. We'd moved about six or seven times, and in the seventh grade it was really traumatic. I was extremely shy. I was so shy it was really incredible. I don't think I ever went anywhere in the seventh grade except to school and then straight home. In the eighth grade, I had a pretty low self-image. But I think I've grown out of it a lot. I had a low self-image in the seventh and eighth grades and I was shy, and then it began cracking in the ninth grade and that about shot me down. There wasn't a lot of schoolground taunting, but, like, if you'd answer the telephone, you'd know what people were really thinking.

I put up with it through the whole ninth grade, and then we ended up going to about three or four throat specialists, and they said the voice would change. The last doctor I saw was a year and a half ago; he said it would change, too. Physically I was in real good shape, and I had a real good home life; it was my only refuge. I always wanted to be like my father. Do you think it was a fear of the cracking that made me stay at the high pitch? I think it is possible.

(Therapy)

C: Have you ever noticed that when you shout, your voice will drop to a lower pitch?

P: Yes, sir, when I shout I've noticed it. I have trouble shouting, though.

C: The first thing I think you ought to know is that the low-pitched voice is the normal voice. For some reason you haven't been using enough muscular effort in exhaling for voice, and if you have a weak flow of air when you speak, it has a tendency to produce this high pitch. But when you get good pressure under it, the voice will go down. There is a second factor—how forcefully you are bringing the vocal folds together. And I'll show you how we can accomplish that. I want you to sit up straight and do this for me. (Clinician demonstrates a sharp glottal attack. Patient repeats, and the voice drops to a low, masculine pitch.) See what I mean? Do it again. Now I want you to hold it out as long as you can. Now produce the old voice. (Patient does at the high pitch level.) Hear the difference? Do you notice how much less effort you have to exert in order to make the high-pitched voice? Try the low one again, sustaining the vowel. There is an interesting little quiver or warble to the voice which may be a sign that you haven't been using the vocal folds and they are a little bit flabby. Now say "Monday." (Patient says the word, the first syllable at the low pitch, the second at the high. With slightly more effort on the second trial, the entire word is produced at the low pitch.) Say "one Monday," sharply. Now, "one Monday morning"; take a deep breath first. Now we'll do some exercises. (Examiner demonstrates five vowel sounds in short succession, each produced with a sharp glottal attack. Patient repeats all at a low pitch level. This exercise is repeated for several minutes. Following that, the patient is asked to count to ten sharply.) Sound all right? It didn't crack, did it? Now say the days of the week the same way. Notice that when you slack off on the effort, the pitch goes up? Get into the habit of breathing deeply and putting forth effort when you talk. Now, pick up that card and start reading with that voice. (Patient does so with very few falsetto pitch breaks.) Not bad. All right, now let me hear you start counting and see how far you can go. Now I'm going to ask you some questions, and I want you to answer in a low-pitched voice. Remember, sharp and loud. How old are you? (Patient answers 21 in a falsetto voice.) Let's go back to the vowels. Produce them sharply. Now, how old are you? (Patient responds in the low-pitched voice.) Are you getting the feel of it? Now tell me about school, where you go, what subjects you're taking, and so on. (Patient begins to describe his college experience somewhat hesitantly, but in the low-pitched masculine voice.)

C: Well, what do you think of your voice now?

P: Strange. I just can't believe that was it.

C: It sounds completely normal to me, but I know it sounds peculiar to you. It's not cracking, is it? Do you like the new voice?

P: Yeah (somewhat tentatively and quizzically).

C: Well, just keep talking and get some experience with it.

P: I love to play handball. I'm starting to get halfway decent in gymnastics. At first, I was going to be a business major, but it wasn't for me. So I decided on physical therapy. I think I'll be real good at that.

C: A while back you said your mother was an unusual person. Could you tell me more about that?

P: I guess I consider her pretty unusual. I've had a pretty warped view of people in general, twisted, well, not really warped; I saw a lot of cruel things. My mother is real sensitive. She teaches children with learning disabilities. And I think she is probably one of the best in the state. People can be callous and they can be cruel, at school, mostly toward me, but to other people who were shy too. She has a great deal of empathy. She's kind of headstrong though. My father, he didn't have a lot of time, say, when we were growing up. You know, the old deal about making money. And about two years ago, he changed more than any person I'd ever seen. He was pretty dogmatic and rigid, and he became more understanding and more open, just less structured, kind of seemed more human. He'd played on a basketball scholarship and I really wanted to be like him, quite a bit. With my sister, we fought a lot. She is real pretty. The guy she married, we just don't make connections. I'm not kidding, he's really a strange character. (All the above is produced in the low-pitched masculine voice, with few pitch breaks. His rate of speech progressively increases as he becomes more comfortable with the new voice.) We got real close since she has been married. We really have fun with her now. Except, I think she could have reached a higher potential if she had married someone else. She could really write. In English classes, her name would come up a year later when I would take those classes, and her teachers would say, "She could really write. I hope you're as good as she is."

C: You sound as if you are a sensitive person and that you have high standards.

P: I'd like to believe that.

C: Do you think that you're oversensitive?

P: Definitely. As a matter of fact, about three months ago, I finally told mother—like that one doctor, he's crazy, thinking that my voice was still going to change, and it got to where I was becoming callous. I'd put up with the voice for seven years, and I didn't have too much patience with people. It might be that I didn't try to understand them because I was too wrapped up in my own problem. Like the first two doctors, I thought they had to be right, and then the best one in the state said that at 19 I just needed more time! I was pretty well disgusted. Mother asked me once if I ever forgot about my voice, and I said, "No way." (At this point the session was terminated, and the patient was asked to return the following day.)

C: What were your parents' reactions to your voice?

P: Well, I called my mother on the phone and I didn't tell her who I was at first, and when she realized who I was (laughs), she broke down and started crying quite a bit and said that she didn't think she would even recognize me until I told her. I almost didn't sleep last night, and when I woke up this morning I had to concentrate quite a bit to get the voice started. My dad said it was deeper than it was yesterday, and we were outside shopping and it was cold and I said a few words and they came out the old way, but I caught it right away. That was the only time it ever slipped.

C: Does it sound more normal to you now?

P: Yeah. I went over to start talking to Daddy and I almost got lightheaded; I wasn't used to breathing that deeply. I used it in restaurants and shopping. It was fun.

C: Do you have any other impressions of the voice?

P: Not really. I told Daddy the whole story. I just told him I couldn't believe it, and I don't guess he could either. Even he said he couldn't hope for that much. Because they had both been preparing me for partial improvement, maybe having to go home and work at it, and it would take maybe a few months. I thought to myself that I don't know if I'm going to be able to go back and talk to my friends and relatives. I guess it was concern about the hassle of drawing attention to it. Then, I thought that after talking to Mother and Dad, that that's the farthest thing I should be worrying about. In fact, all my aunts and uncles and cousins are coming over Friday, and I can hardly wait. But I had thought about it, that it would be some hassle.

C: Do you feel satisfied?

P: Totally. It's more than you could really hope for in your wildest dreams. When I was in high school, people would treat me like I was a poor little kid. You know, I can't go back to it, but I really could have been a fantastic basketball player. I could have been on a scholarship now, but you know, I just kind of copped out. You know, my mother told me once that she thought I'd gotten used to the voice, and I just couldn't believe it. And I said, "Mother, you've never been to a place where you have to give a speech or talk to a stranger." For a while it dictated my whole life, what I'd do and what I'd try.

The patient's father wrote two months later:

Prior to the change in Mike's voice, I felt that he was a shy, sensitive person with a very poor self-image. During Mike's early years, I believe he was what I would call "painfully shy." Mike was not a confiding person, and it was difficult to get him to engage in an open-ended discussion, what I would call a "bull session."

The change in Mike's voice has brought about a profound change in his view of himself and his relationship to other people. Since things are now so much more positive, Mike opens up much more easily and is quite willing to discuss anything and everything.

Prior to Mike's session with you, I was very concerned about his future. I now feel that his confidence and self-image have improved so sharply that he will reach his potential as a person and will have a rewarding life.

Mike now participates in class discussions. He had told us that during four years of high school and three years of college, he had never before done so.

* * *

The patient wrote the following letter three months after acquiring his masculine voice.

Most things don't measure up to their expectations. My new voice was one that did. I was in a state of bliss when I returned to _____. When I got home my mother and sister were the first people I talked to. I described every detail and emotion of my trip to the Clinic.

When I first came in contact with people outside my family, it was an almost laughable situation. I'd say something and their faces would register shock, but they'd never comment about my changed voice. I assume that in the past, by my action and behavior, it was well understood that my voice embarrassed me and not to mention it. But it was so unusual to me that not a *single* person outside of my family has ever mentioned or commented on my new voice. And for once in my life I was more than willing to discuss it. As a matter of fact, I wanted to talk about it. I have finally come out and said a few things to my friends, who would immediately be full of questions. We ended up having very enlightening conversations.

The peer pressure was incredible. I've never even so much as flinched before it. Nothing could force me back to the misery that was before my trip. But I can see how powerful role expectations are and to have such a major change in not only voice but identity. Because, too often after hearing my voice people tacked on behavior traits to me as well. They expected me to act gimpy, since I talked gimpy. I don't know if anyone else can understand how all-encompassing my voice was to me. My father asked me when I had returned if I thought my change of voice would have a very major effect on my life. I could have cried. It was not part of my life, it *was* my life. Every action I made, every decision, opinion, all of my behavior was what it was because of my voice.

It takes a long time to get everything straightened out. To this day if a phone rings and I'm by myself I'll find myself trying to warm up my vocal cords by talking to myself. The behavior patterns don't fall by the wayside as rapidly or as painlessly as did my voice. There's a whole way of life involved in coping with my voice since it bothered me so much. And it takes effort and desire to overcome that way and replace it with another. In a class once a fellow student made a comment that no one knew what Hell was like. I smiled to myself, because in all honesty and sincerity I felt I was living a Hell and nothing could be worse.

I'll be going to a new school this semester. My whole life is one uphill swing since the Clinic. Everything keeps getting better. After visiting four specialists who did nothing, I had a very low opinion of doctors. You raised that opinion, and I thank you for your competence. After saying that it was a living Hell I must also say that my voice gave me a unique perspective on life. I'm glad that I am what I am. I'm thankful that I can relate to unfortunate people—to someone with a handicap. That I'm not someone who has only tunnel vision because they can't see outside of their own experiences.

Adductor Spastic Dysphonia

Any consideration of therapy for adductor spastic dysphonia must account for the following realities: (1) Not one, but several, different types of the disorder exist. Therefore, no single therapy can be recommended for all types. (2) Adductor spastic dysphonia is notorious for its fluctuations in severity in response to mood and environment. Therefore, valid, reliable assessment of the effectiveness of therapy cannot be made on the basis of office sampling alone, but needs to be based on a cross-section of communicative experiences. (3) Clinicians differ among themselves in their criteria for improvement, because the results of therapy are more often partial than complete. (4) Clinicians differ from patients in their criteria for improvement owing not only to differences in their expectations, but also because improvement in the amount of physical effort required to phonate can only be evaluated by the patient and cannot be judged by an observer. (5) Studies of the effectiveness of therapy are difficult to compare owing to different methodologies, e.g., decision as to what constitutes adductor spastic dysphonia, failure to consider etiology with respect to homogeneity or heterogeneity of the patient population, method of measurement of the effects of therapy, and type and duration of follow-up.

DIFFERENTIAL DIAGNOSIS

Establishment of the different etiologic types of adductor spastic dysphonia has been based on after-the-fact research findings. However, in actual clinical practice, although etiology can be apparent in the evaluation, a differential diagnosis among psychogenic, neurologic, or idiopathic types may be difficult and not apparent until the patient is well into therapy. For example, dysphonias that disappear for extended periods of time in response to symptomatic voice therapy or psychotherapy are not likely to be neurologic etiology. For this reason, in the interest of conservative patient care, it is wiser to begin with a trial of symptomatic voice therapy and to reserve more risky types of therapy for intractable patients.

What seems to be emerging as experience with voice disorders accumulates, but in particular with adductor spastic dysphonia, is that therapy is more often successful when it is based upon a solid foundation of diagnostic examinations. The information obtained is obviously of primarily differential diagnostic value, but not entirely. If the clinician assumes that all patients who have adductor laryngospasms are alike, the probability is high that the wrong therapy will be selected, and, because patient education is indispensable, the clinician will not be in a very comfortable position to convey sufficient or correct information. The prematurely informed, and therefore, the often misinformed patient is unusually common in cases of adductor spastic dysphonia. If at all possible the following examinations should be collaborative.

Laryngologic Examination. At the earliest opportunity the patient should be scheduled for a thorough laryngologic examination. Although the signs of adductor spastic dysphonia are easily identifiable through listening, the ear, nose, and throat examination is important for several reasons: (1) The patient expects, and needs to be reassured by, a physical inspection of the interior of his or her larynx. (2) The clinician cannot confidently divest patients of their commonly held beliefs that tumors or other structural lesions are causing their dysphonias unless the clinician is convinced on the basis of firsthand information that such lesions are absent. (3) A minority of adductor spastic dysphonic patients have vocal nodules, polyps, or contact ulcers traumatically induced by their adductor laryngospasms, which contribute to the severity of their dysphonias. (4) Rhythmic adduction of the vocal folds producing voice tremor and rhythmic hyperadduction producing voice arrest can be viewed on laryngoscopic examination and is important diagnostically.

Speech Examination. A thorough speech examination is a necessity and should include a motor speech test for dysarthria. The reason for this prescription will be apparent if it will be recalled that spastic dysphonia may be of the neurologic type, and signs, often quite subtle, of tremor or movement disorder of the oral musculature may reveal information that can be of use to the neurologist.

Of all the speech tests that are usually administered during such an examination, none is more critical than vowel prolongation. The reason is that irregular laryngospasms during contextual speech may become regular or rhythmic during vowel prolongation, revealing that the patient's spastic dysphonia is of the essential (organic) tremor type. Also of particular importance is to obtain baseline audiotape and, if possible, videotape recordings for a more detailed study of the patient and for comparison with subsequent recordings, especially during and after therapy.

Musculoskeletal tension testing and brief efforts to reduce such tension through laryngeal manipulation, as described elsewhere in this book, is another indispensable portion of the examination. Patients who have such tension associated with psychogenic forms of the disorder will often respond with enough voice improvement for a sufficient length of time during the examination to convince the clinician, and the patient, of a nonorganic form of the disorder, thereby approximating the diagnosis and indicating the direction that therapy should most likely take.

Psychosocial Examination. No patient with the voice signs of adductor spastic dysphonia should be denied the benefit of an exploration of possible psychologic causes, precipitants, or effects of the voice disorder. As noted elsewhere in this book, a preliminary psychosocial history surrounding the onset and development of the dysphonia deserves careful investigation, preferably by the examining speech pathologist or by a psychiatrist, psychologist, or psychiatric social worker of known qualifications. This examiner should collaborate with the laryngologist and speech pathologist. Here, again, the patient will often reveal the etiologic diagnosis by providing psychodynamic information to help explain the voice disorder and, during the course of such revelations, demonstrate diminution or disappearance of the spastic dysphonia.

Neurologic Examination. Referral of the patient for a neurologic examination is not routinely warranted, but if there is any doubt about the patient's neurologic status, such referral can be highly clarifying, for example, when tremor or movement disorders are suspected of being related to the spastic dysphonia.

Armed with data from these different disciplines, the speech clinician, alone if necessary, or, better, in collaboration with the other specialists, particularly the laryngologist, can chart a plan of action to help the patient with this most incapacitating of all voice disorders. A review of the findings with the patient is always a wise decision. Information itself is therapeutic beyond question even when nothing can be done for the voice for the time being. Based on all of these data, the speech clinician must decide whether symptomatic voice therapy alone, psychotherapy alone administered by a qualified therapist, or both in parallel are warranted, with the idea held in reserve that should these fail, more drastic measures may have to be considered.

Symptomatic voice therapy as the first stage in attempts to alleviate the disorder should be started with all patients except those in whom a neurologic type has been definitely established. The voices of patients who have the tremor and dystonic types do not respond well to attempts to alter their control over their spasms. Although there is no harm in trying such therapy with patients whose dysphonia is neurologically related, especially if the clinician is not sure about the etiology, expectations of improvement should be guarded. These patients often give the impression of being able to alter their voices during therapy, but their ability to sustain less spastic voice in their daily lives usually breaks down.

Musculoskeletal Tension Reduction.   In patients who have nonorganic forms of adductor spastic dysphonia, muscle tension reduction, as described elsewhere in this book, will often yield normal or nearly normal voice within a brief period of time. If the muscle tension is associated with an active conversion reaction, such physical manipulation will be only partially successful or totally unsuccessful, pending resolution of the underlying emotional conflict. However, even in cases in which conflict is active, considerable voice improvement can be expected. However, such patients will also require psychologic counseling.

Voice Quality and Pitch Modification.   Paradoxically, normal or nearly normal voice under certain conditions of phonation becomes apparent to most clinicians as they investigate patients who have adductor spastic dysphonia, except the essential tremor type. A patient may have a severely strained voice during contextual speech most of the day, but, it may be normal on arising, when shouting, laughing, crying, or singing. It may also be free of spasm during vowel prolongation even though not during conversation. It may be nearly normal at higher pitch levels or when phonating with a breathy voice quality.

These conditions of improved voice often give promise of relief, suggesting to the clinician that if the patient can phonate more easily at a higher pitch or using a breathy voice during vowel prolongation, or during reading of practice material in the clinic, the patient consciously ought to be able to sustain spasm-free voice during daily conversational speech. And, in many patients, such improvement has been effected. Cooper's (1980) therapy program for adductor spastic dysphonia is an example of the school of thought that believes voluntary alteration of phonation, and respiration, can benefit these patients. He advocates as individual and group therapy (1) re-establishment of natural or optimum pitch and "tone focus in the mask area" using the spontaneous "um-hum" method, (2) correct breath support using gentle, abdominal breathing, (3) "peripatetic" voice therapy during which the clinician works with the patient at the actual site and under actual speaking conditions.

As a means of alleviating adductor spastic dysphonia, historically psychotherapy has been highly suspect. This attitude may have developed due to a failure to separate the neurologic from the psychogenic types. Adductor spastic dysphonia due to conversion reaction or to depression or anxiety often yields to the emotional catharsis and discussion and resolution of emotional conflict. Often, the spastic dysphonia, whatever the cause, produces such withdrawal and depression that psychologic help is warranted on that basis alone.

The first person to perform surgery to alleviate sphincter laryngospasm responsible for spastic like disturbances of voice was Réthi (1952), who blamed the disorder on the stylopharyngeus muscle and divided it in one such patient. Twenty years later Hannebert (1972) advocated injecting either the posterior wall of the pharynx or the stylopharyngeus muscle to anesthetize these sphincters, describing the effect of the injection as highly favorable, the voice recovering in quality and volume and even persisting after the novocaine had worn off. Neither surgery to the stylopharyngeus muscle nor injection of the pharynx ever became popular as a therapy for adductor spastic dysphonia. What did was a surgical approach in which one of the recurrent laryngeal nerves in the neck is severed, paralyzing one vocal fold and thereby reducing the degree of adductor force, allowing a freer flow of air through the glottis during phonation. Called the *recurrent laryngeal nerve section,* the procedure was first introduced in 1976 by Dedo. After first temporarily paralyzing one vocal fold by injecting one recurrent laryngeal nerve with lidocaine and listening for improvement in the voice,

> Under general anesthesia a collar incision is made one finger-breadth below the cricoid cartilage. Dissection is carried down to the anterior surface of the trachea and around its right side to the tracheoesophageal groove. The recurrent nerve is identified ordinarily at the level of the inferior pole of the right thyroid gland 1 cm lateral to the trachea . . . Direct laryngoscopy is then performed so that the right vocal cord can be observed while an assistant crushes the presumed recurrent nerve with a hemostat. If the vocal cord contracts abruptly at the instant of crushing, the structure is presumed to be the whole recurrent nerve and is ligated . . . A 1 cm segment is then removed adjacent to the inferior pole of the thyroid gland about 3–4 cm below the cricoid (Dedo, 1976, pp. 454–455).

The history of the results of this surgery and estimates of its value reported by different investigators requires careful reading and thought because of differences in philosophies and methods of postsurgical follow-up. All the references on the surgery cited at the end of this chapter under Suggestions for Additional Reading ought to be carefully scrutinized. When the findings from all of these studies are weighed, they demonstrate:

1. The immediate postsurgical effects on the voice are overwhelmingly favorable, and for the following reasons. The voice is freed of the strained, hoarse quality and the often fatiguing physical effort to produce it. Facial grimacing and other body movements associated with the spasms diminish or disappear. Patients experience a reversal of their depression and withdrawal.

2. The voice quality during the early postsurgical period tends to be breathy, weak, and hoarse. With time, the voice becomes clearer and louder. However, only a minority of patients can be said to achieve a completely normal voice. Some degree of breathiness or hoarseness remains in patients regarded as successful.

3. With the passage of time, many patients experience partial or complete return of their adductor spastic dysphonia to presurgical levels of severity or worse. The percentage of patients who fail depends upon which studies are consulted. They range from 15 to 64 percent failure after three years postsurgery.

4. Return of the spastic dysphonia is usually not due to reactivation of the paralyzed vocal fold but to compensatory hyperadduction of the opposite vocal fold, ventricular folds, or supraglottic pharyngeal constrictors.

5. Females experience a higher failure rate than males for unknown reasons.

6. There is no way of predicting who will succeed in the longer term and who will fail.

7. Patients have a greater tendency than clinicians to rate the postsurgical voices as better (Sapir et al, 1986).

8. To the patient, the reduction of effort and fatigue of phonation is as important as improvement in the sound of the voice.

9. Many patients who have failed within three years of the surgery say they were grateful for whatever relief they had from the spastic dysphonia.

10. Postsurgical voice therapy may help patients destined to remain improved to maintain a smoother, clearer voice but will probably not prevent recurrence of the spastic dysphonia in patients whose voices are destined to deteriorate.

11. Side effects of the surgery are minimal. Some patients experience a temporary need to swallow fluids carefully to avoid minor dysphagia, but this is not a serious or long-term complaint.

12. Patients who have experienced a return of the spastic dysphonia are sometimes helped by further surgery, consisting of vocal fold thinning with carbon dioxide laser.

13. Patients whose voices have remained excessively breathy for a long period after surgery owing to an excessively wide glottis may benefit from injection of Teflon into the paralyzed vocal fold.

14. An alternate surgical procedure in which the laryngeal nerve is crushed instead of severed is not recommended owing to the unusually high failure rate, greater than 85 percent, within 10 months, and is probably due to reinnervation of the nerve.

What can clinicians conclude about the wisdom and advisability of performing recurrent laryngeal nerve section on adductor spastic dysphonia patients? How should they counsel their patients when the subject of surgery is raised? A conservative answer is to advise them of the results of studies that show a degree of risk of return of the voice, but that there should be no fear that they would be worse off from the surgery than if they had not elected it. The positive aspects of the surgery need to be presented as well; that successful patients can experience excellent voice and are grateful for the benefits of the surgery. The lidocaine block as a preliminary procedure to allow the patient, family, and clinician to evaluate the simulated effects of surgery is a highly useful way of eliminating patients who are poorly motivated or who have excessively high expectations from the surgery. Allowing prospective patients to evaluate the audiotape and videotape recordings of patients who have had the surgery is another useful way of educating the patient as to the effects of surgery. The most balanced view of the surgery would be that, while it is not the solution for all patients, it can afford value for others. It should be carefully offered as a temporary benefit for highly motivated patients who have severe adductor spastic dysphonia and who have seriously suffered psychologically and vocationally from their disorder.

BOTULINUM TOXIN INJECTION

A treatment for adductor spastic dysphonia that has shown considerable promise is the injection of botulinum toxin (Botox) directly into the thyroarytenoid muscles, which produces partial paralysis, preventing spastic hyperadduction of the vocal folds.

Botulinum toxin is a potent neurotoxin produced by the bacteria *Clostridium botulinum* found in one form of food poisoning. Of eight known strains, the type A botulinum toxin is the most potent and the only one capable of being crystalized in stable form. When injected in low doses, it binds firmly to muscle and is rapidly fixed at the terminal nerve fibers with little remaining toxin allowed to pass into the general circulation, accounting for its relative safety (Cohen and Thompson, 1987).

Physiologically, botulinum toxin blocks the release of acetylcholine from the nerve ending, interfering with calcium metabolism and, in effect, denervating muscle fibers for months; because the motor end plate does not release acetylcholine, the muscle fibers cannot contract. When denervated, the muscle atrophies but then develops new nerve sprouts, reinervating the muscle, reversing the weakness over a period of approximately three months.

The toxin is injected percutaneously through the cricothyroid membrane into the thyroarytenoid muscle by means of a syringe with a monopolar Teflon-coated hollow electromyographic recording needle. The hypodermic needle functions as an electromyographic electrode in order to locate the thyroarytenoid muscle before the toxin is injected into it.

The toxin has been injected in patients' vocal folds unilaterally and bilaterally. Experience has shown that bilateral vocal fold injection is preferable to unilateral for the reasons that bilateral injections require considerably less toxin, and there is evidence to suggest that a better voice can be achieved (Blitzer et al., 1988). Patients who have had a return of their spastic dysphonia after recurrent laryngeal nerve resection have also benefited from the procedure.

The toxin takes effect within 24 to 72 hours, during which the voice becomes breathy. However, patients' voices respond differently because of differences in the severity of their spastic dysphonia and because the amount of toxin needed depends on the individual patient. Laryngoscopic examination after the induced weakness of the vocal folds discloses that they are not completely paralyzed but appose each other with less than full closure, revealing a slight glottal opening during phonation. The initial breathiness disappears within days and a smoother, nearly normal voice, can last from three to six months, toward the end of which the strained voice gradually returns to its preinjection status signaling the need for reinjection.

Injections are performed on an outpatient basis with a minimum of discomfort. The degree of weakness can be controlled by the administration of low doses of the toxin in the beginning and by adjusting the dose until the proper amount for producing optimum voice is found.

The voice quality achieved from the botulinum toxin injection has been found to be at least as good as, and in some cases better than, the voice quality obtained from recurrent laryngeal nerve resection (Miller et al., 1987). In addition to the improved voice, as in recurrent laryngeal resection, patients also report reduced physical effort to phonate, corroborated quantitatively by a considerable reduction in pre- and postinjection intrathoracic pressures. For example, in a study reported by Miller et al. (1987), in one patient the preinjection intrathoracic pressure was 22 to 23 cm H_2O and 5 cm H_2O after injection, and in a second patient, it was 75 cm H_2O preinjection and 3.5 cm H_2O postinjection.

In summary, the botulinum toxin injection for adductor spastic dysphonia promises to be the therapy of choice for intractable adductor spastic dysphonia that is refractory to other therapies. The voice quality obtained is as good or better than the recurrent laryngeal nerve resection, the injection can be given as an outpatient procedure rather than under general anesthesia, and the toxin does not produce a permanent paralysis of a vocal fold. The latter advantage is especially attractive to patients and practitioners alike who are reluctant to paralyze a vocal fold permanently if it can be avoided. Repeated injections produce similar or identical results. The main disadvantage to the procedure is that the patient needs to be reinjected within three to six months. However, highly motivated patients have reported that this is a minor inconvenience considering the relief from the laryngospasms and improvement in voice and ease of phonation. Because the long-term effects of repeated injections have not yet been determined, it is not known for how many months or years patients will continue to derive benefit from repeated injections or whether the immune system will eventually negate the effects of the toxin over time (Brin et al., 1987; Blitzer et al., 1988).

Abductor Spastic Dysphonia

Resistance to therapy is as true for abductor spastic dysphonia as it is for the adductor type. The approach to therapy should take a form similar to that for adductor spastic dysphonia.

1. First, it is necessary to determine if the disorder is primarily psychogenic by means of a thorough psychosocial history. As in other psychogenic voice disorders, disclosure of personal problems may be accompanied by improvement or disappearance of the dysphonia.
2. Symptomatic voice therapy should always be tried. For abductor spastic dysphonia specifically, the abductor laryngospasms and breathy air release will diminish or disappear if the clinician teaches the patient to *voice all unvoiced consonants*. For example, saying the phrase "*c*offee *c*ream" will produce severe breathy air releases in most abductor spastic dysphonic patients. If the clinician then tells the patient to substitute the /g/ for the /k/ phoneme as in "*g*offee *g*ream," the breathy air releases will be diminished. In the same way, if the patient is taught to voice all of the remaining voiceless consonants, it is possible that the abductor spastic dysphonia will either diminish considerably or disappear completely. Telling the patient to keep the vocal cords vibrating through all of connected speech will accomplish the same objective.

Unilateral and Bilateral Vocal Fold Paralysis

Incomplete glottic closure during phonation because of unilateral or bilateral adductor vocal fold paralysis produces variously, aphonia, breathiness, hoarseness, excessively low volume, diplophonia, and high-pitched falsetto. Therapy is based on the principle of compensatory glottic closure by capitalizing on the primitive effort closure capabilities of the larynx. In unilateral paralysis, the normal vocal fold is encouraged to cross the midline and contact the paralyzed fold. In bilateral, both folds are forced toward the midline. Voice recovery depends upon the etiology of the paralysis and the position of the paralyzed vocal fold(s). Patients who have degenerative peripheral nervous system diseases are poorer risks than those with static lesions. Those who have unilateral vocal fold paralyses are better therapy risks than those who have bilateral paralysis. The closer the paralyzed vocal fold is to the midline, the better the prognosis. Patients who have idiopathic vocal fold paralysis may experience spontaneous return of voice.

Voice Therapy

Voice therapy for vocal fold paralysis is based primarily on the patient's potential to compensate by means of adduction of the intact vocal fold. The following methods have found widespread support among clinicians.

1. Effort closure techniques. In the chapter on normal laryngeal physiology, effort closure was described as a primitive reflex mechanism. Stronger glottic closure is facilitated by capitalizing on the effort closure reflex by means of grunting, controlled coughing, laughing, pushing, and lifting. Linking the fingers and pulling in opposite directions while phonating the vowel /i/ and pushing against a table or pulling up on a chair synchronously with phonation are activities that were originally advocated by Froeschels et al. (1955). Vowels are introduced with the vowel /u/ having particular value in producing better voice. Progression from vowels to syllables, words, and sentences follows. Singing and humming are additionally helpful. Not all patients who have vocal fold paralysis require strenuous pushing, for many clinicians report that initiating vowels with an abrupt, sharp, or hard glottal attack is often sufficient.

2. Excessive musculoskeletal tension which may have developed as a secondary reaction should be eliminated. (See section on therapy for musculoskeletal tension voice disorders.)

3. A trial-and-error search should be conducted for a pitch and loudness level that will yield the best voice quality with the least physical effort. Pinching the wings of the thyroid cartilage together gently during phonation will bring the vocal folds into closer proximity, producing improved voice, which may then be repeated without the therapist's help. Turning the head to the right or left may also improve the voice by increasing the tension on the paralyzed vocal fold.

4. Sensitizing the patient to improvements in voice during trial-and-error procedures should be emphasized. Moment-to-moment voice changes during therapy need to be pointed out to the patient instantly; otherwise, they will escape notice.

5. Attention should be paid to secondary personal and emotional problems arising from the voice disorder. One should provide time during each therapy session for discussion of the patient's voice experiences in everyday life, encouraging ventilation of frustrating experiences. It is important to be attentive to more severe emotional reactions, particularly depression, and be ready to consult with appropriate mental health personnel.

Teflon Injection

An alternative for patients with unilateral vocal fold paralysis who do not respond to voice therapy is injection of the paralyzed vocal fold with a Teflon-glycerine suspension, which increases the bulk of the fold and narrows the glottis. With the patient under either local or general anesthesia, the paste is injected into the middle third of the fold just above the vocal process of the arytenoid cartilage. Some patients respond with virtually normal voice. In others, the voice is minimally adequate, and in still others it can be worse if the injection has been done improperly. Overinjecting, injecting too close to the vocal margin, or injecting too deeply are errors that can produce worse voice. According to Rubin (1975), the high-risk patient is one whose voice prior to injection is only mildly to moderately breathy, with good quality.

> Virtually every study that has ever been done on the efficacy of Teflon injection to improve voice in unilateral vocal fold paralysis has proved the virtue of this procedure. Lewy (1976) reported a 96 percent success rate in a survey of studies that represented 1,139 injection procedures. Hammarberg et al. (1984) judged voice improvement in 75 percent (12 of 16 patients) based on perceptually and acoustically documented evidence. Their report stated that injection was most successful in patients who had very breathy voices with diplophonia, whereas in patients with only slight degrees of breathiness Teflon injection often led to an "overtight," vocal fry voice quality, the result of overinjection.

Following are typical experiences with patients who have had vocal fold paralyses.

* * *

A 45-year-old widowed mother of three children, a clerk in a department store, had no previous history of voice disorders, when she awoke one morning with marked hoarseness.

After two weeks she consulted a laryngologist, who found a right unilateral vocal fold paralysis. She had no history of upper respiratory infections or trauma. Neck palpation and chest radiographs failed to reveal any masses. Remaining cranial nerves were normal. The laryngologic diagnosis was idiopathic unilateral vocal fold paralysis.

Her voice was hoarse and diplophonic. Glottal attacks on vowels and coughing were weak. Peripheral speech musculature examination failed to disclose any other abnormalities; neither did the motor speech evaluation. Her voice had not improved during the two weeks since onset, and she had taken leave from her job because of difficulty in communicating with customers, especially in noisy settings. She became easily fatigued, both because of the increased vocal effort and because of the need to breathe more frequently owing to air wastage during phonation. She was having trouble talking to her three active children.

A series of voice therapy sessions was begun, stressing sharp glottal attack activities. She began to show reduced hoarseness and diplophonia while phonating at slightly higher pitch levels. However, when she increased her loudness level beyond a certain point at those pitch levels, diplophonia reappeared, so that therapy necessitated that she learn to modulate the loudness of her voice. A home therapy program was outlined, and the patient was seen biweekly. During the first month of therapy, her voice underwent stepwise improvements, the first observable change being a disappearance of diplophonia. She returned to work at that point, enduring without undo concern the well-meaning remarks of fellow employees and customers concerning her voice. She managed to communicate with others by standing closer to them while speaking.

Her voice continued to improve during the next three months, and four months following the beginning of therapy, she was dismissed with mild residual breathiness. Loudness and pitch range had become acceptable, if not normal. The final laryngoscopic examination showed normal bilateral vocal fold movements.

* * *

Spontaneous return of voice is common in patients with idiopathic unilateral vocal fold paralysis, although voice therapy may facilitate such recovery. The decision to begin therapy in this case was a precautionary measure predicated on the assumption that the patient might not have had spontaneous improvement.

An experience totally different from the above study is the following.

* * *

A 53-year-old housewife and cashier at a coffee shop emerged from anesthesia for thyroidectomy with a severely breathy-hoarse voice that did not improve during the two-month postoperative period. She returned for laryngologic examination and was found to have a fixed left vocal fold. She returned to work a month following surgery but met with considerable difficulties in her job, being unable to make herself heard in the noisy restaurant and becoming increasingly self-conscious about the steady stream of comments from customers regarding the sound of her voice. She and her husband made no attempt to conceal their hostility and were determined to get help for the voice.

The laryngologist, after explaining to the patient the unavoidability of the paralysis, and after demonstrating much concern over her welfare, referred the patient for voice therapy. On evaluation, she was breathy, bordering on aphonia. She broke down several times during discussion of the effects of her voice on her job and home life, stressing the embarrassment it caused her and how it made her feel self-conscious and "peculiar."

During four months of voice therapy, her voice failed to improve. Finally, one day the patient's husband called, saying that his wife had gone on an extended leave of absence from her job and was showing signs of increasing depression and withdrawal.

The patient was referred to a psychiatrist, who believed that the depression was a reaction to her illness, surgery, and voice disorder and placed her on antidepressant medication, agreeing to see her periodically for support. Voice therapy was continued simultaneously, and although she appeared less depressed, her dysphonia failed to improve.

Review of her case with the laryngologist led to the decision to do a Teflon injection of the paralyzed vocal fold. She underwent general anesthesia, during which the left vocal fold was injected. Upon recovery and re-examination 24 hours after surgery, her voice was virtually normal in quality, loudness, and pitch. Her response was ecstatic, her depression had lifted almost instantaneously, and comparison of pre- and postsurgical videotape recordings showed an indescribable difference in facial expression.

The patient returned to work immediately, and her husband reported that her mood had changed back to normal. Six-month and one-year follow-up examinations showed continuation of normal voice and personal adjustment.

* * *

In contrast to the first patient, whose personality strengths and somewhat better voice enabled her to tolerate her dysphonia, the second patient fared less well. In addition to her increasing depression over her voice loss, necessitating psychiatric treatment, her normal vocal fold gave little indication that it intended to compensate. The effects of the Teflon injection, affording a new voice and its concomitant emotional benefits, illustrate the virtue of this procedure.

On the pitfalls of injecting Teflon into *mobile* vocal folds such as for the correction of atrophy and bowing of the folds, Kaufman (1988) wrote:

> Teflon in the mobile vocal cord diffuses and produces a stony-hard cord. The resultant voice may be temporarily improved, but with the passage of time, the voice becomes very poor, indeed worse than prior to injection. Over the past 5 years I have attempted to surgically remove Teflon in six such cases, using the CO_2 laser. The diffusion of the Teflon makes this impossible, and the vocal improvement following removal is modest at best . . . no matter how appealing it may seem to use that technique to correct such cordal defects, no available data supports that practice. Furthermore, irreversibility once Teflon is introduced makes such injections ill advised . . . at present there is no surefire method to correct bowing of the vocal cords, least of all Teflon injection.

THERAPY FOR PROBLEM VOICE DISORDERS

The therapy principles and methods already described are for those voice disorders about which there is a moderate amount of knowledge and certainty. In this section are discussed voice disorders about which less or little is known.

Neurologic Voice Disorders

Aside from therapy for unilateral and bilateral vocal fold paralysis resulting from lesions of the Xth nerve, which are amenable to surgical and behavioral therapy, most voice disorders due to central nervous system diseases are resistant to modification. In the majority, the dysphonia does not exist alone but is a component of a dysarthria involving resonation and articulation as well. Respiratory weakness and incoordination are inseparable from these defects of phonation and contribute heavily to the voice disorder.

MYASTHENIA GRAVIS

Improvement of the breathiness, hoarseness, and insufficient loudness associated with this disease is directly dependent upon alteration of the neurochemistry at the myoneural junction. Patients who respond successfully to the administration of anticholinesterase drugs or to thymectomy will correspondingly experience an improvement in their voices. The velopharyngeal insufficiency of myasthenia gravis can be considerably improved and even eliminated with the use of a palatal-lift prosthesis. Symptomatic voice therapy for patients on maintenance doses of anticholinesterase drugs has not been advocated because of questionable effectiveness; however, more knowledge is needed in this area, and the effects of voice therapy need to be clinically investigated.

PSEUDOBULBAR PALSY

The strained-strangled hoarseness and excessively low pitch of spastic (pseudobulbar) dysphonia, a component of spastic dysarthria, can be a serious obstacle to speech intelligibility. The dysphonia is especially severe when accompanied by a flaccid component in amyotrophic lateral sclerosis. The accumulation of saliva in the pyriform sinuses of the larynx in ALS worsens the dysphonia.

PARKINSONISM

The breathiness, monopitch, and especially the inadequate voice volume can severely compromise speech intelligibility in this disease. The value of voice therapy is limited; it is more effective for the mildly impaired. Many patients undergoing drug therapy with L-dopa experience an improvement in their voices along with other signs of parkinsonism. A portable, body-worn sound amplifier has been used, as has a vocal intensity controller, with variable success. Some patients can become aphonic. Here, as in other very severe communicative disorders, consideration of a communication aid should be given.

ESSENTIAL (VOICE) TREMOR

Although they suffer social embarrassment, patients who had mild to moderate essential (voice) tremor do not usually have an intelligibility problem. Voice therapy is ineffective in reducing the tremor, which is unfortunate, because the tremor is socially restricting for many patients.

MOVEMENT DISORDERS

The waxing and waning laryngeal spasms and uncontrollable pitch changes, which are slower in the dystonias and faster in chorea, have not been treated successfully with symptomatic voice therapy.

GILLES DE LA TOURETTE'S SYNDROME

The laryngeal components of this syndrome have been reduced and even eliminated with the administration of the drug haloperidol. The value of voice therapy has not been assessed.

APRAXIA OF PHONATION

Muteness or aphonia as a component of apraxia of speech can be successfully treated by working from primitive, reflexive coughing and throat clearing into humming, vowel production, and, ultimately, word formation, the latter being dependent upon the severity of the apraxic articulatory component.

Voice Disorders Due to Mass Vocal Fold Lesions

HYPOTHYROIDISM

The hoarse, low-pitched voice of hypothyroidism improves with the administration of thyroid replacement drugs administered for treatment of the total illness. The pitch of the voice increases and the severity of hoarseness decreases as the patient's thyroxin level approaches normal.

NEOPLASMS

No rational disorder-specific therapy exists for benign lesions, and therapy depends upon individual circumstances. With this group of patients more than any other, trial-and-error therapy is the order of the day. Different pitch and loudness levels, head positions, and varieties of glottal attack all need to be tried to determine which modes of phonation yield the most audible and aesthetically acceptable voice. Clinician and patient need to be realistic about accepting less-than-desired results.

In patients who possess only one vocal fold because of removal of the other for carcinoma, and in others with severe atrophy, scarring, or other lesions of the vocal folds, ventricular phonation may yield a better voice than voice production with the true vocal fold.

A serious problem is the child who is unable to phonate because of chronic laryngeal obstruction due to congenital or acquired laryngeal stenosis, papilloma, trauma, or subglottal stenosis. A substitute form of communication is mandatory. Children who have had glottic stenoses for long periods, preventing conventional phonation, often spontaneously acquire pharyngeal and buccal speech, gestures, and abnormal breathing patterns. Kaslon et al. (1978) advocate alternative approaches to communication, such as sign language, an artificial larynx, communication boards, and esophageal speech. The need for some form of substitute laryngeal sound is especially critical in the very young who are undergoing normal language development, for failure to provide substitute voice will almost assuredly result in delayed speech and language.

BIOFEEDBACK DEVICES IN VOICE THERAPY

It cannot be overstressed how important feedback from the voice is, because there is minimal tactile and proprioceptive sensation arising from the larynx during phonation. Audition is the primary channel through which voice is monitored, as proven by the congenitally deaf who are known for their severely aberrant voices, which are typically monopitched, poorly modulated in loudness, and abnormal in nasal resonance. When voice becomes defective, intensification of its parameters during therapy is needed. The tape recorder is the most common feedback device used by the clinician to enable the patient to examine voice after it has been produced. Instantaneous feedback is also necessary. Amplification of the voice, fed back through earphones, is one means. Even simpler is cupping the hand around the ear or phonating while facing the corner of a room, where the voice rebounds off the walls. Biofeedback devices should be considered as adjuncts to therapy, but should not be substituted for the interpersonal and environmental techniques integral with the mechanical aspects of therapy.

One specially devised instrument for vocal abuse disorders is the Voice Intensity Controller (VIC), which instantly warns the speaker when vocal intensity becomes excessive. Worn like a hearing aid, with the microphone attached to the base of the neck anteriorly and an earphone in the ear, the device can be set so that when the speaker's voice exceeds a certain intensity, a warning tone is triggered. Holbrook et al. (1974) reported on the complete resolution of vocal nodules, polyps, and contact ulcers in 32 patients who used this device, the mean treatment time being 5.3 weeks. The sound spectrograph or sonograph is a visual feedback device that displays voice spectra, intensity, and duration. We have already been introduced to this device as a clinical evaluation and research instrument, but it also has therapeutic applications, especially those models that provide an instantaneous visual display on a video screen. Because the sonograph is most sensitive to noise in the voice spectrum, this device is especially useful for the treatment of voice quality disorders.

The ability to monitor voice pitch is visually afforded by fundamental frequency indicators. A typical one is a microphone attached to the neck adjacent to the thyroid cartilage; fundamental frequency is read on an attached meter.

SUMMARY

1. The objective of voice therapy is to return the voice to a level of social and occupational adequacy within the patient's anatomic, physiologic, and psychologic capabilities.

2. Voice therapy revolves around the general principles of instantaneous auditory feedback, is tailored to the voice and personality of the patient, and pays attention to emotional as well as the mechanical and acoustic aspects of abnormal voice.

3. General principles of voice therapy are blended in with the principles and techniques devised for specific voice disorders.

4. Voice therapy for excess laryngeal musculoskeletal tension is based on the principle of muscle tension reduction and is accomplished by kneading the laryngeal musculature, reducing the elevated position of the larynx, encouraging general relaxation, and alleviating environmental stress.

5. Voice therapy for vocal abuse is based on the principle of patient re-education to use the voice more judiciously in everyday life and to reduce those stress factors that drive the patient into patterns of vocal misuse. These principles are implemented by increasing patient awareness of abnormal modes of phonation, teaching modified voice use, and discussing sources of emotional tension.

6. Conversion aphonia and dysphonia are treated according to the principle of re-establishment of the patient's conscious awareness of greater phonatory capability and discussing the emotional conflicts that have generated the voice disorder, continuously monitoring the possibility of referral for deeper psychotherapy. These principles are implemented by musculoskeletal tension reduction, evocation of increased glottal activity, and encouragement of patient awareness and disclosure of interpersonal conflicts and life stress.

7. Therapy for mutational falsetto is based on learning to inhale with increased air volume, and to exhale with increased force simultaneous with a sharp glottal attack.

8. Voice therapy for adductor spastic dysphonia has limited value. Phonation with a breathy vocal attack and at elevated pitch can yield reduced laryngospasm under less socially pressured speaking conditions. The recurrent laryngeal nerve resection procedure is the most promising approach to alleviation of this disorder, but its long-term value is unpredictable.

9. Therapy for unilateral vocal fold paralysis is based on compensatory glottic closure by the intact vocal fold. Therapy for bilateral paralysis is based on residual adductor vocal fold ability. Both are implemented by effort closure exercises through phonation with a sharp glottal attack during lifting, pushing, and grunting activities.

10. Several voice disorders resulting from central nervous system disease and vocal fold mass lesions are minimally responsive to voice therapy; further research is necessary.

SUGGESTIONS FOR ADDITIONAL READING

Blitzer, A., Brin, M.F., Fahn, S., and Lovelace, R.E.: Localized injections of botulinum toxin for the treatment of focal laryngeal dystonia (spastic dysphonia). Laryngoscope, 98:193–197, 1988. The technique of botulinum toxin injection for adductor spastic dysphonia in five cases is reported and voice effects described.

Boone, D.R.: The Voice and Voice Therapy, Englewood Cliffs, N.J., Prentice-Hall, 1977. Contains excellent advice on general and specific therapies for virtually all voice disorders.

Brin, M.F., Fahn, S., Moskowitz, C., Friedman, A., Shale, H., Greene, P.E., Blitzer, A., List, T., Lange, D., Lovelace, R.E., and McMahon, D.: Localized injections of botulinum toxin for the treatment of focal dystonia and hemifacial spasm. Mov. Disord., 2:237–254, 1987. An excellent review of the use of botulinum toxin for the treatment of a variety of dystonic movement disorders in addition to adductor spastic dysphonia, namely, torticollis, blepharospasm, oromandibular dystonia, limb dystonia, and lingual dystonia.

Greene, M.C.L.: The Voice and Its Disorders. Philadelphia, J.B. Lippincott Co., 1972. Voice therapy from the viewpoint of a British speech pathologist. Organized and authoritative.

Hammarberg, B., Fritzell, B. and Schiratzki, H.: Teflon injection in 16 patients with paralytic dysphonia: Perceptual and acoustic evaluations. J. Speech Hear. Disord., 49:72–82, 1984. Probably the most comprehensive and objective analysis available on the effects of Teflon injection on voice in patients with unilateral vocal fold paralysis.

Lancer, J.M., Syder, D., Jones, A.S., and Le Boutillier, A.: Vocal cord nodules: A review. Clin. Otolaryngol. 13:43–51, 1988. This article on vocal nodules is an excellent review of its histology, symptoms, incidence, age and sex distribution, hypothesized causes, occupational background, psychologic factors, and treatment.

Special Readings on Recurrent Laryngeal Nerve Resection

The following articles should be read to grasp the similarities and dissimilarities in methodology used to study the effects of surgery for adductor spastic dysphonia and the interpretation of results.

Aronson, A.E.: Neurologic and Psychiatric Aspects of Adductor Spastic Dysphonia and the Effects of Recurrent Laryngeal Nerve Resection. Transcripts of the Twelfth Symposium Cure of the Professional Voice. New York, The Voice Foundation, 1983, pp. 184–191.

Aronson, A.E., and DeSanto, L.W.: Adductor spastic dysphonia: 1½ years after recurrent laryngeal nerve resection. Ann. Otol. Rhinol. Laryngol., 90:1–6, 1981.

Aronson, A.E., and DeSanto, L.W.: Adductor spastic dysphonia: Three years after recurrent laryngeal nerve resection. Laryngoscope, 93:1–8, 1983.

Barton, R.J.: Treatment of spastic dysphonia by recurrent laryngeal nerve section. Laryngoscope, 89:244–249, 1979.

Biller, H.F., Som, M.L., and Lawson, W.: Laryngeal nerve crush for spastic dysphonia. Ann. Otol. Rhinol. Laryngol., 92:469, 1983.

Dedo, H.H., and Izdebski, K.: Intermediate results of 306 recurrent laryngeal nerve sections for spastic dysphonia. Laryngoscope, 93:9–15, 1983.

Dedo, H.H., and Izdebski, K.: Problems with surgical (RLN section) treatment of spastic dysphonia. Laryngoscope, 93:268–271, 1983.

Fritzell, B., Feuer, E., Haglund, S., Knutson, E., and Scheratzki, H.: Experiences with recurrent laryngeal nerve section for spastic dysphonia. Folia Phoniatr. 34:160–167, 1982.

Izdebski, K., Dedo, H.H., Shepp, T., and Flower, R.M.: Postoperative and follow-up studies of spastic dysphonia patients treated by recurrent laryngeal nerve section. Otolaryngol. Head Neck Surg., 89:96–101, 1981.

Levine, H.L., Wood, B.G., Batza, E., Rusnov, M., and Tucker, H.M.: Recurrent laryngeal nerve section for spasmodic dysphonia. Ann. Otol. Rhinol. Laryngol., 88:527–530, 1979.

Salassa, J.R., DeSanto, L.W., and Aronson, A.E.: Respiratory distress after recurrent laryngeal nerve sectioning for adductor spastic dysphonia. Laryngoscope, 92:240–245, 1982.

Stoicheff, M.L.: The present status of adductor spastic dysphonia. J. Otolaryngol., 12:311–314, 1983.

Wilson, F.B., Oldring, D.J., and Mueller, K.: Recurrent laryngeal nerve dissection: A case report involving return of spastic dysphonia after initial surgery. J. Speech Hear. Disord., 45:112–118, 1980.

REFERENCES

Barnes, J.E.: Voice therapy for vocal nodules and vocal polyps. Rev. Laryngol. Otol. Rhinol., 102:99–103, 1981.

Blitzer, A., Brin, M.F., Fahn, S., and Lovelace, R.E.: Localized injections of botulinum toxin for the treatment of focal laryngeal dystonia (spastic dysphonia). Laryngoscope, 98:193–197, 1988.

Boone, D.R.: The Voice and Voice Therapy. Englewood Cliffs, N.J., Prentice-Hall, 1977.

Boone, D.R.: Respiratory training in voice therapy. J. Voice, 2:20–25, 1988.

Brin, M.F., Fahn, S., Moskowitz, C., Friedman, A., Shale, H., Greene, P.E., Blitzer, A., List, T., Lange, D., Lovelace, R.E., and McMahon, D.: Localized injections of botulinum toxin for the treatment of focal dystonia and hemifacial spasm. Mov. Disord., 2:237–254, 1987.

Cohen, S.R., and Thompson, J.W.: Use of botulinum toxin to lateralize true vocal cords: A biochemical method to relieve bilateral abductor vocal cord paralysis. Laryngoscope, 96:534–541, 1987.

Cooper, M.: Modern Techniques of Vocal Rehabilitation. Springfield, Ill., Charles C Thomas, 1973.

Cooper, M., and Cooper, M.H. (Eds.): Direct vocal rehabilitation. In Approaches to Vocal Rehabilitation. Springfield, Ill., Charles C Thomas, 1977.

Cooper, M.: Recovery from spastic dysphonia by direct voice rehabilitation. Proceedings of the 18th Congress of the International Association of Logopedics and Phoniatrics, Washington, D.C., 1980, pp. 579–584.

Dedo, H.H.: Recurrent laryngeal nerve section for spastic dysphonia. Ann. Otol. Rhinol. Laryngol., 85:451–459, 1976.

Fairbanks, G.: Voice and Articulation Drillbook. New York, Harper & Row, 1960.

Froeschels, E.: Chewing method as therapy. Arch. Otolaryngol., 56:427–434, 1952.

Froeschels, E., Kastein, S., and Weiss, D.A.: A method of therapy for paralytic conditions of the mechanisms of phonation, respiration, and glutination, J. Speech Hear. Disord., 20:365–370, 1955.

Greene, M.C.L.: The Voice and Its Disorders. Philadelphia, J.B. Lippincott Co., 1972, pp. 169–170.

Hammarberg, B.: Pitch and quality characteristics of mutational voice disorders before and after therapy. Folia Phoniatr., 39:204–216, 1984.

Hammarberg, B., Fritzell, B. and Schiratzki, H.: Teflon injection in 16 patients with paralytic dysphonia: Perceptual and acoustic evaluations. J. Speech Hear. Disord., 49:72–82, 1984.

Hannebert, P.E.: L'Injection de Réthi dans certaines dysphonies par spasme des bandes ventriculares. Acta Otorhinolaryngol. Belg., 26:801–805, 1972.

Holbrook, A., Rolnick, M., and Bailey, C.: Treatment of vocal abuse disorders using a vocal intensity controller. J. Speech Hear. Disord., 39:298–303, 1974.

Jacobson, E.: Progressive Relaxation, 2nd ed. Chicago, University of Chicago Press, 1938.

Jacobson, E.: Anxiety and Tension Control, A Physiologic Approach. Philadelphia, J.B. Lippincott Co., 1964.

Jacobson, E.: You Must Relax, 5th ed. New York, McGraw Hill Book Co., 1976.

Kaslon, K.W., Grabo, D.E. and Ruben, K.J.: Voice speech and language habilitation in young children without laryngeal function. Arch. Otolaryngol., 104:737–739, 1978.

Koufman, J.A.: Avoidance and treatment of complications of Teflon injection of the vocal cord. J. Voice, 2:269, 1988.

Koufman, J.A., and Blalock, P.D.: Is voice rest never indicated? J. Voice, 3:87–91, 1989.

Lewy, R.B.: Experience with vocal cord injection. Ann. Otolaryngol., 85:440–450, 1976.

McCloskey, D.G.: General Techniques and Specific Procedures for Certain Voice Problems. In Cooper, M. and Cooper M.H. (Eds.): Approaches to Vocal Rehabilitation. Springfield, Ill., Charles C Thomas, 1977.

Miller, R.H., Woodson, G.E., and Jankovic, J.: Botulinum toxin injection of the vocal fold for spasmodic dysphonia. Arch. Otolaryngol. Head Neck Surg., 113:603–605, 1987.

Moran, M.J., and Pentz, A.L.: Otolaryngologists' opinions of voice therapy for vocal nodules in children. Lang. Speech, Hear. Serv. Sch., 18:172–178, 1987.

Réthi, A.: Role des stylopharyngealen muskelsystems in krankheitsbild der taschenbandstimme und der dysphonia spastica. Folia Phoniatr., 4:201–216, 1952.

Rubin, H.J.: Misadventures with injectable polytef (Teflon). Arch. Otolaryngol., 101:114–116, 1975.

Sapir, S., Aronson, A.E., and Thomas, J.E.: Judgment of voice improvement after recurrent laryngeal nerve section for spastic dysphonia: Clinicians versus patients. Ann. Otol. Rhinol. Laryngol., 95:137–141, 1986.

von Leden, H.: Legal pitfalls in laryngology. J. Voice, 2:330–333, 1988.

Weiss, D.A.: Introduction to Functional Voice Therapy. Basel, S. Karger, 1971.

Chapter Fourteen

INTRODUCTION

ANATOMY OF EXTERNAL RESPIRATION

Trachea
Lungs
Thoracic Cage
Muscles of Respiration

PHYSIOLOGY OF EXTERNAL RESPIRATION

The Larynx in Respiration
The Respiratory Cycle
Pressure, Volume, and Flow Changes During the
    Respiratory Cycle
Flow-Volume Curve
Recoil Tendency of the Lungs
Compliance
Pulmonary Volumes
Practical Significance of Pulmonary Volumes

NEUROPHYSIOLOGIC AND CHEMICAL CONTROL
OVER RESPIRATION

The Respiratory Center
Chemical Control Over Respiration
Pulmonary Stretch Receptors

ANATOMY AND PHYSIOLOGY OF RESPIRATION

The lighted candle respires and we call it flame
The body respires and we call it life
Neither flame nor life is substance, but process
The flame is as different from the wick and wax
As life from the body, as gravitation from the falling apple,
Or love from a hormone

—Severinghaus

INTRODUCTION

Without respiration, life would be snuffed out like a flame without oxygen. There could be no exchange between oxygen and carbon dioxide in the lungs and, therefore, no metabolism to sustain life. However, respiration for life has to be changed for speech: (1) The larynx changes from a valve for protection of the lungs to a mechanism for sound production; (2) respiratory rhythm is changed to rapid inhalation of a large quantity of air and prolonged exhalation for sustained speaking; (3) during expiration, the inspiratory intercostal and abdominal muscles are balanced to control transglottic pressure in order to maintain steadiness of voice during constantly changing subglottic and supraglottic air pressure; and (4) automatic, reflex chemical control over respiration for life is temporarily overridden by cortical control.

Respiratory insufficiencies are directly responsible for phonatory disorders causing disturbances in voice quality, loudness, pitch, and emphasis patterns. Neurologic diseases, for example, interfere with the ability to inhale sufficient quantities of air, shortening duration and reducing force of exhalation. Respiratory deviations are almost always present in psychogenic voice disorders; the same muscle tensions that cause hyperadduction of the vocal folds spread to the thoracic and abdominal musculature producing shallow breathing.

Respiratory disorders not only cause voice disorders; they are caused by voice disorders due to overconstriction and underconstriction of the glottic and supraglottic musculature. Vocal fold overconstriction leads to excess, compensatory forcing of exhaled air through the glottis. Underconstriction allows excessive airflow through the glottis, prematurely depleting air from the lungs.

In hospitals and medical clinics we are confronted daily by patients who have respiratory disorders from neurologic and obstructive lung diseases. When mild, they barely interfere with speech. When extreme, as in patients who are still in intensive care, tracheostomized, and on respirators, they are balancing on the threshold between life and death where the distinction between respiration for speech and respiration for life no longer exists.

The intent of this chapter is to establish the beginnings of a foundation for the understanding of normal respiratory anatomy and physiology and to show how respiration for speech is compromised in certain illnesses. It will explain how and why dysphonia results from respiratory disorders.

The subject of respiration is immensely complex. To understand it even at an elementary level requires some preparation in physics, biochemistry, and physiology. Entire textbooks have been written on the subject, and a select few are listed in the Suggestions for Additional Reading section at the end of this chapter.

ANATOMY OF EXTERNAL RESPIRATION

Respiration is subclassified into external and internal respiration. *External respiration* is the exchange of air between the lungs and the outside atmosphere produced by expansion and contraction of the thoracic cage. *Internal respiration* is the exchange of oxygen and carbon dioxide between the blood and the alveolar air sacs of the lungs and between the blood and the cells of the body. This chapter will dwell almost entirely on external respiration.

The anatomic structures of external respiration are subdivided into: (1) the airway, consisting of the larynx, trachea, and lungs; (2) the thoracic cage; and (3) the muscles responsible for expanding and contracting the thoracic cage.

Trachea

The uppermost part of the airway is formed by the larynx and trachea. The airway is designed for gas exchange only and will not tolerate the intrusion of liquids or solids. The trachea is a tube about 10 cm long. It is composed, on the average, of 20 horseshoe-shaped *cartilaginous rings* held together posteriorly and superiorly by *fibroelastic tissue* (Fig. 14–1). The first tracheal ring lies immediately beneath the cricoid cartilage of the larynx. Each tracheal ring is about 2.5 cm in diameter, is not quite cylindrical, and is flattened posteriorly. The trachea extends inferiorly to the level of the fifth thoracic vertebra. There it divides into two bronchi, one for each lung.

Lungs

The two lungs are cone-shaped, spongy, light, and elastic (Fig. 14–1). The *left lung* is divided into *two lobes* and the *right* into *three*. Within each lung the two *bronchi* subdivide into smaller *primary*, *secondary*, and *tertiary* bronchi (Fig. 14–2). These further divide into progressively smaller

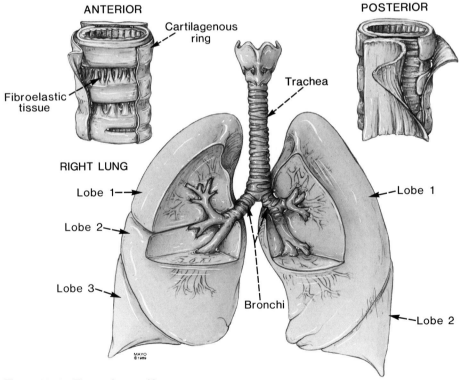

Figure 14–1 The trachea and lungs.

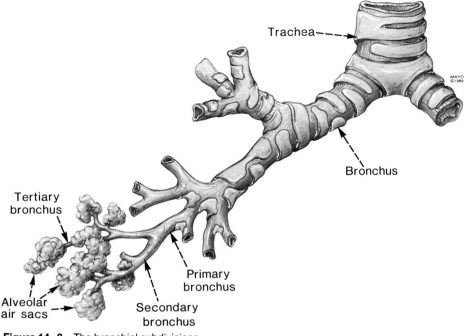

Figure 14–2   The bronchial subdivisions.

primary lobules, respiratory bronchioles, alveolar ducts, atria, and *alveolar air sacs*. The alveolar air sacs are the ultimate divisions of the lungs. Their walls interface with blood capillaries through which oxygen and carbon dioxide are exchanged by a process known as *diffusion*.

Thoracic Cage

The lungs are enclosed by the thoracic or rib cage (Fig. 14–3). The rib cage consists of 12 ribs bilaterally. They are attached to the *sternum* anteriorly and to the *vertebrae* posteriorly. The *first rib* is different from the others because it is rigidly attached to the sternum. On inhalation, it moves as a single unit, its anterior part raised and carried forward. Its movement *increases the anteroposterior and transverse diameters of the upper region of the chest*.

The *second rib* is attached anteriorly to the sternum and, therefore, is prevented from moving forward. Its sternocostal articulation, however, allows the middle of the body of the rib to be drawn up. Its purpose is to *increase the transverse thoracic diameter*.

Elevation of the *third, fourth, fifth, and sixth ribs* raises and thrusts their anterior portions forward. This thrust causes the body of the sternum to move forward and upward. The movement of these ribs *increases the anteroposterior thoracic diameter*.

The costal cartilages of ribs *7, 8, 9, and 10* articulate with one another in such a way that when they are raised each pushes the one above it upward. In this way, the lower end of the sternum is pushed upward and forward. Movement of these ribs *enlarges the thorax in the region of the upper abdominal space*. In addition to their shafts being elevated, the ribs move upward and backward. This movement *increases the lateral and anteroposterior diameters of the thorax*.

Ribs *11 and 12* are free at their anterior ends and capable of minor movements in all directions. Figs. 14–4a and 14–4b illustrate the effects of rib cage elevation on the anteroposterior and transverse diameter of the thoracic cage.

In summary, each rib has its own range and variety of movements, which combine with the others to act as a unit for the purpose of enlarging the thoracic diameters during inhalation. Because the anterior ends of the ribs lie in a lower plane than the posterior ends, when the body of the rib is

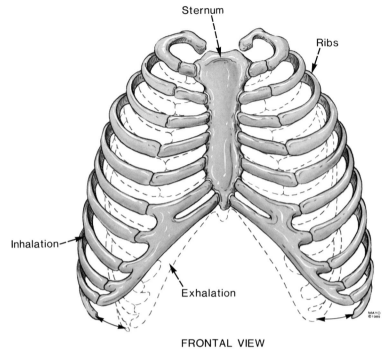

FRONTAL VIEW

Figure 14–3   The rib cage during inhalation and exhalation (frontal view).

elevated its anterior end is thrust forward. Simultaneously, the rib is carried outward from the median plane of the thorax. Each rib forms the segment of a curve greater than that of the rib immediately above it. Therefore, elevation of a rib increases the transverse diameter of the thorax in the plane to which it is raised. The upper ribs increase the anteroposterior dimension of the thorax by elevating the sternum. The lower ribs increase the transverse or lateral diameters primarily by

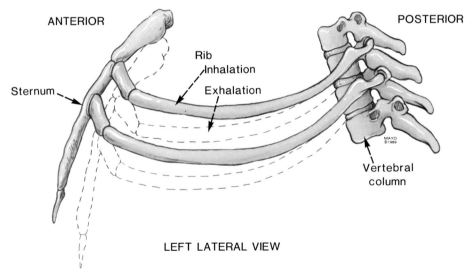

LEFT LATERAL VIEW

Figure 14–4a   The rib cage during inhalation and exhalation (lateral view).

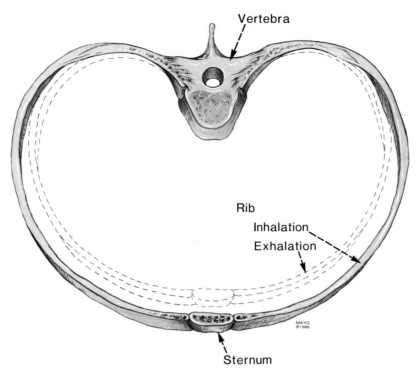

Vertebra

Rib

Inhalation

Exhalation

Sternum

SUPERIOR VIEW

Figure 14–4b   The rib cage during inhalation and exhalation (superior view).

outward rotation. The lower ribs expand the thorax more than the upper ribs so that the lower regions of the lungs are ventilated more than the upper regions.

Muscles of Respiration

Two modes of external respiration are recognized, quiet and forced. *Quiet respiration* is defined as inhalation and exhalation while the organism is silent and in repose, when the metabolic requirements for oxygen-carbon dioxide exchange are minimal. *Forced respiration* is defined as the conscious effort to inhale and exhale a greater volume of air than required during quiet respiration. This mode of breathing is used during increased metabolic demands for oxygen-carbon dioxide exchange, as in heavy work and during speech.

MUSCLES OF QUIET RESPIRATION

Quiet Inhalation.

   1. The *diaphragm* is the most important muscle of inhalation, is *exclusively a muscle of inhalation,* and has no active function during exhalation. It moves a greater volume of air into and out of the lungs than any other single muscle or group of muscles. It is responsible for most of the increase and decrease in the vertical dimension of the thorax. During quiet breathing, the level of the diaphragm descends about 1 cm, but during forced inhalation and exhalation, its descent may increase up to 10 cm., as shown in Fig. 14–5.

   The diaphragm is a thin sheet of muscle that, when at rest, is dome-shaped. It is attached to the lower part of the *sternum,* to the cartilaginous and bony portions of *ribs 7 to 12,* and to the lumbar vertebrae. These portions of the diaphragm converge and insert into the *central tendon.*

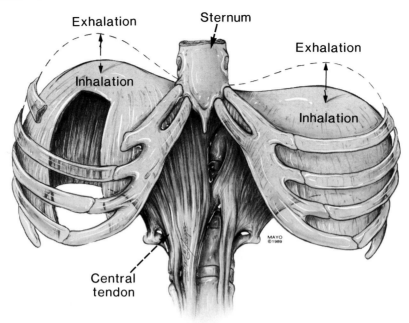

Figure 14–5   The diaphragm.

When the diaphragm contracts, its central tendon is drawn down, increasing the volume of the thoracic cavity. As it contracts and flattens, it presses downward against and displaces the abdominal viscera, distending the abdomen. In addition, the rib margins move upward and outward. This action of the ribs may appear contradictory when one considers that it happens when the diaphragm is depressed. However, the ribs expand because of the leverage brought about by the force of the diaphragm against the abdominal contents.

Each half of the diaphragm is innervated by one *phrenic nerve*, which contains fibers of cervical nerves 3, 4, and 5. Should one half of the diaphragm become paralyzed due to unilateral phrenic nerve damage, it will move up instead of down on inhalation when there is a drop in intrathoracic pressure.

2. The *scalenus anterior* is attached to the 3d, 4th, 5th, and 6th cervical vertebrae and to the inner border of the *first rib*. It fixes and raises the first rib, slightly bending and rotating its neck. This muscle is innervated by branches of the *lower cervical nerves*.

3. The *scalenus medius* is attached to the lower cervical vertebrae and to the upper surface of the first rib. It fixes and raises the first rib and bends and slightly rotates its neck. It is innervated by the *lower branches of the cervical nerves*.

4. The *scalenus posterior* is attached to the lower two or three cervical vertebrae and to the outer surface of the second rib. It fixes and raises the second rib and bends and rotates its neck. It is innervated by the *phrenic nerve* and fibers from the *3rd, 4th, and 5th cervical nerves*.

5. The *intercostales externi* are attached to the borders of the ribs and separate them. They maintain a constant distance between the ribs in order to prevent bulging or retraction during changes in intrathoracic pressure. They also regulate the distance between the ribs during postural changes. They are innervated by the *intercostal nerves*.

6. The *intercostales interni* are attached to the inner surfaces of the ribs at their upper and lower borders in the direction opposite to the internal intercostals. They maintain a constant distance between the ribs in order to prevent bulging or retraction during changes in intrathoracic pressure. They regulate the distance between the ribs during postural changes. They are innervated by the *intercostal nerves*. Table 14–1 summarizes the muscles of quiet inhalation, their attachments, actions, and innervation.

Table 14-1   Muscles of Quiet Inhalation

NAME	ATTACHMENTS	INNERVATION	ACTION
1. Diaphragm	1. Sternal: dorsal surface of lower part of sternum 2. Costal: cartilaginous and bony portions of ribs 7–12 3. Lumbar: Lumbar vertebrae. All converge and insert into central tendon	Phrenic nerve from cervical plexus; contain fibers from 3rd, 4th, and 5th cervical nerves	Draws central tendon down; increases volume, decreases pressure in thoracic cavity; presses against abdominal viscera protruding anterior abdominal region
2. Scalenus anterior	From anterior tubercles of transverse processes of 3rd, 4th, 5th, 6th cervical vertebrae to scalene tubercle on inner border of first rib	Branches of lower cervical nerves	Fixes and raises first rib; bends and slightly rotates the neck
3. Scalenus medius	From posterior tubercles of transverse processes of lower six cervical vertebrae to upper surface of first rib	Branches of lower cervical nerves	Fixes and raises first rib; bends and slightly rotates the neck
4. Scalenus posterior	From posterior tubercles of transverse processes of lower 2 or 3 cervical vertebrae to outer surface of 2nd rib behind attachment of serratus anterior	Phrenic nerve from cervical plexus; contain fibers from 3rd, 4th, and 5th cervical nerves	Fixes and raises second rib; bends and slightly rotates neck
5. Intercostales Externi	From lower borders of first 11 ribs to upper borders of last 11 ribs	Intercostal nerves	Maintains constant distance between ribs in order to prevent bulging or retraction during changes of intrathoracic pressures. Alter distances between ribs during postural changes
6. Intercostales interni	From ridge on inner surface of a rib or the corresponding costal cartilage to upper border of rib below	Intercostal nerves	Maintains constant distance between ribs in order to prevent bulging or retraction during changes of intrathoracic pressure. Alter distances between ribs during postural changes

Quiet Exhalation.   Quiet exhalation is brought about mainly by *passive forces* that cause the rib cage and muscles of inhalation to return to their resting positions, thereby decreasing the thoracic dimensions. The passive forces behind quiet exhalation are:

1. *Gravity.* When the muscles of inhalation relax, the elevated rib cage falls of its own weight.

2. *Elastic recoil of ribs.* The ribs and costal cartilages, displaced during inhalation, recoil to their original rest positions.

3. *Untorquing of ribs and costal cartilages.* The ribs and costal cartilages, twisted under rotational stress during inhalation, exert their inherent tendency to return to their original untorqued positions.

4. *Elastic recoil of lungs.* The lungs possess a natural elasticity that contributes to their collapse during deflation as the thoracic cage returns to rest position.

5. *Elastic recoil of viscera.* The abdominal contents, displaced by downward movements of the diaphragm during inhalation, and pressing against the abdominal muscles, are moved back to their original position when forces displacing them cease.

MUSCLES OF FORCED RESPIRATION

Forced Inhalation.   In addition to the muscles of quiet inhalation, the following are added during forced inhalation:

1. The *sternocleidomastoid* is attached to the mastoid process of the skull, the front of the sternum, and the inner surface of the clavicle. It lifts the sternum when both act together while the head is erect. It is innervated by the spinal portion of the *accessory nerve* and branches of the *2nd and 3rd cervical nerves.*

2. The *serratus posterior superior* is attached to the 7th cervical and the upper two or three thoracic vertebrae and to the borders of the 2nd to 5th ribs. They assist in raising the ribs. They are innervated by T1, T2, T3, and T4.

3. The *pectoralis minor* is attached to the scapula and 2nd, 3rd, 4th, and 5th ribs. They raise the ribs and are innervated by C7 and C8.

4. The *pectoralis major* is attached to the humerus, sternum, clavicle, and costal cartilages. They raise the ribs and are innervated by C6, C7, C8, and T1.

5. The *latissimus dorsi* is attached to the humerus, lower six thoracic vertebrae, lumbar, and sacral vertebrae, ilium, and four lowest ribs. They raise the ribs and are innervated by C6, C7, and C8.

The *accessory muscles* of inhalation that fix the shoulder girdle, thereby aiding in forced inhalation, are the *trapezius, rhomboideus major, rhomboideus minor, levator scapulae,* and

Table 14-2   Muscles of Forced Inhalation

NAME	ATTACHMENTS	INNERVATION	ACTION
1. Sternocleido-mastoideus	From mastoid process of skull to front of sternum and inner surface of medial third of clavicle	Spinal portion of accessory nerve and branches from anterior rami of 2nd and 3rd cervical nerves	Lifts sternum when both act together and when head held erect; flexes neck; rotates head to opposite side
2. Serratus posterior superior	From ligament of neck and spinous process of 7th cervical vertebra and 1st three thoracic vertebrae	Branches of anterior rami of upper four thoracic nerves	Exact function not determined; position and attachment would suggest it to be elevator of ribs 2, 3, 4, 5
3. Pectoralis minor	From outer surfaces of 3rd, 4th, and 5th ribs at point lateral to junction of ribs with costal cartilages, to end of coracoid	Medial anterior thoracic nerve originating in brachial plexus. Fibers are from 8th cervical and 1st thoracic nerve	Tends to lift scapula away from ribs, but if scapula is fixed it may lift the middle ribs
4. Pectoralis major	From anterior border of clavicle, sternum, cartilages of 1st six ribs, to ridge of outer border or bicipital groove of humerus	Medial and lateral anterior thoracic nerves from brachial plexus. Fibers from 5th cervical to 1st thoracic nerves	Is believed that if arms are fixed, will raise ribs. Also flexes, adducts, and rotates arm medially; draws arm or shoulder forward, medially, or downward
5. Latissimus dorsi	From spinous process of lower six thoracic, lumbar vertebrae, back of sacrum, crest of ilium, and lower three ribs	Thoracodorsal nerve from brachial plexus; fibers come from 6th, 7th, and 8th cervical nerves	Is believed to elevate lower ribs if arm fixed; also extends, adducts, and rotates arm medially; draws shoulder downward and backward

deltoideus. Table 14–2 summarizes the muscles of forced inhalation, their attachments, actions, and innervation.

Forced Exhalation.   Forced exhalation not only capitalizes on the return of the thoracic cage to its normal resting position due to such passive forces as untorquing of the ribs and the pull of gravity on the chest cage but is augmented and supplemented by active contraction of the following muscles:

1. The *rectus abdominis* attaches to ribs 5 and 7, the xyphoid process of the sternum, and pubis. It compresses the abdominal contents and is innervated by T7, T8, T9, T10, and T11.

2. The *transversus abdominis* is attached to the ilium, lower six costal cartilages, lumbar fascia with fibers of the diaphragm, and pubis. It compresses the abdominal contents and is innervated by T7, T8, T9, T10, T11, T12, and L1.

3. The *obliquus internus abdominis* is attached to the ilium, inguinal ligament, pubis, 7th, 8th, and 9th costal cartilages, and the costal cartilages of the lower three ribs. It depresses the thorax and is innervated by T9, T10, T11, T12, and L1.

4. *Obliquus externus abdominis* is attached to the ilium, pubis, and the lower eight ribs. It compresses the abdominal contents and depresses the thorax. It is innervated by T5, T6, T7, T8, T9, T10, T11, and T12, and by L1.

Forced exhalation is also aided by the *subcostal, quadratus lumborum,* and *intercostales interni muscles.* Table 14–3 summarizes the muscles of forced exhalation.

PHYSIOLOGY OF EXTERNAL RESPIRATION

The Larynx in Respiration

The larynx can be considered as an organ of respiration as well as phonation. The vocal folds abduct during inspiration and partially adduct during expiration. Vocal fold abduction is wider with deeper, more vigorous inspiration. The respiratory positions of the vocal folds are shown in Fig. 14–6. In the figure, A shows inspiration at rest, B shows relatively deep or forced inspiration, and C shows deeply forced inspiration in which the vocal folds are abducted all the way to the lateral walls of the larynx for maximum air intake.

In addition to a widening and narrowing of the glottis during inhalation and exhalation, the entire larynx moves downward on inspiration and upward on expiration. The range of these excursions is proportional to the depth of inspiration. The downward excursion of the larynx can be detected during quiet and forced inhalation by placing the index finger on the thyroid notch during inhalation.

Table 14–3   Muscles of Forced Exhalation

NAME	ATTACHMENTS	INNERVATION	ACTION
1. Rectus abdominis	Ribs 5 and 7, xyphoid process of sternum	T7, T8, T9, T10, T11	Compresses abdominal contents
2. Transversus abdominis	From lower six ribs, lumbar fascia, ilium, and fascia of thigh to fellow of opposite side	Branches from 7th to 12th intercostal, the iliohypogastric, and ilioinguinal nerves	Constricts and compresses abdominal contents
3. Obliquus internus abdominis	Lumbar fascia, ilium, fascia of thigh to cartilages or 8, 9, or 10 ribs	Branches of 8th to 12th intercostal nerves. The iliohypogastric and ilioinguinal nerves	Compresses abdominal contents
4. Obliquus externus abdominis	From ilium, fascia from thigh, and pubis to lower eight ribs in alternation with those of serratus anterior and latissimus	Branches of 8th intercostal nerves. The iliohypogastric and ilioinguinal nerves	Compresses abdominal contents

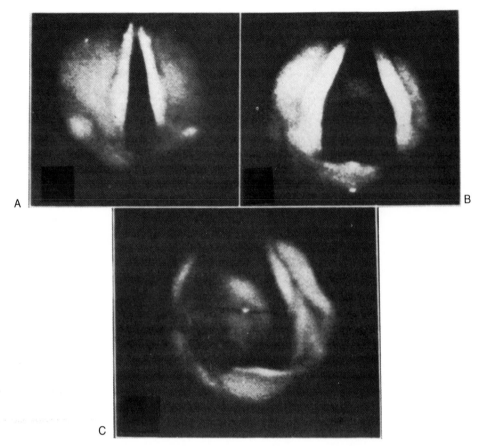

Figure 14-6   The respiratory positions of the vocal folds. A: quiet inspiration; B: deep inspiration; C: extremely forced inspiration. (*From* Pressman, J.J.: Physiology of the Vocal Cords in Phonation and Respiration. Arch. Otolaryngol., 35:355–398. Copyright 1942 by American Medical Association.)

Fig. 14–7 is a lateral roentgenogram of the neck showing the higher position of the hyoid bone and larynx in the neck during quiet inspiration and the descent of these structures to a more caudal position during forced inhalation.

The Respiratory Cycle

The respiratory cycle refers to airflow into and out of the lungs. Air flows in and out of the lungs because of positive and negative air pressures within the lungs produced by changing the thoracic diameters. The sequence of events and air pressure changes during inhalation and exhalation in Figure 14–8 are explained as follows:

1. *The respiratory system at rest* (Fig. 14–8a)
   a. The respiratory muscles are at rest. The recoil of the lung and chest wall are equal and opposite. Because the pleural space is always closed to the outside atmosphere, pleural pressure is slightly negative to atmospheric pressure—approximately -1 mm. Hg. This area of lower pressure with respect to atmospheric is designated in the figure by *minus signs*.
   b. Alveolar pressure within the tracheobronchial tree, continuous with the outside atmosphere, is at atmospheric pressure.

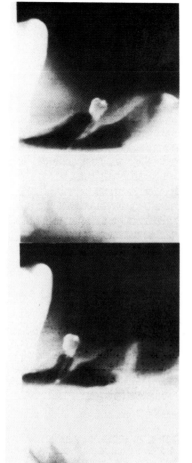

Figure 14–7 Positions of the larynx and hyoid bone during quiet inspiration (A) and forced inspiration (B). (*From* Fink, B.R.: *The Human Larynx.* New York, Raven Press, 1975, p. 62.)

    c. At this point in the respiratory cycle, the respiratory muscles are at rest, and there is no airflow into or out of the lungs.

  2. *The respiratory system during inhalation* (Fig. 14–8b). As the muscles of inhalation contract enlarging the thoracic diameters, the volume of the sealed-off pleural spaces increases.

    a. Pleural pressure becomes increasingly subatmospheric. The lung expands due to the drop in pleural pressure, indicated by the darker minus signs in the figure.

    b. Alveolar pressures become subatmospheric with respect to higher atmospheric airway pressure and, consequently,

    c. Air flows into the lungs.

  3. *The respiratory system during exhalation* (Fig. 14–8c). Relaxation of the muscles of inhalation and the elastic recoil of the lungs allow the thoracic cage to collapse and, along with it, the lungs to their original size.

    a. Alveolar pressure at this point exceeds atmospheric pressure and,

    b. Air is forced out of the lungs.

Pressure, Volume, and Flow Changes During the Respiratory Cycle

A more detailed analysis of the changes in volume, pressure, and flow that occur during the breathing cycle is found in Fig. 14–9. This figure shows the quantitative changes in *air volume,*

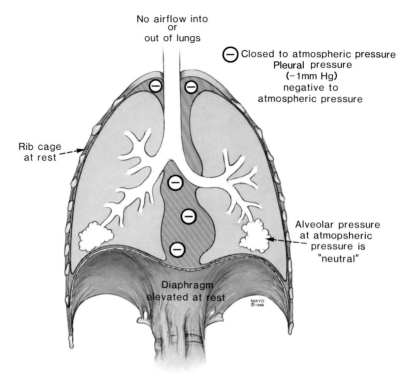

Figure 14–8a The respiratory system at rest.

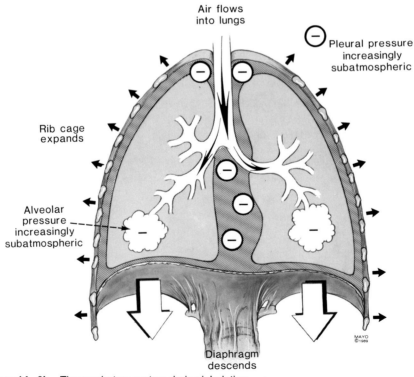

Figure 14–8b The respiratory system during inhalation.

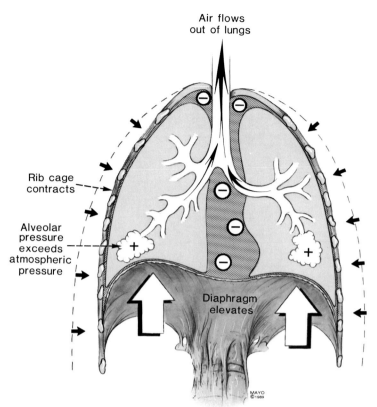

Figure 14–8c   The respiratory system during exhalation.

intrapleural pressure, airflow, and *alveolar pressure* that take place during the inhalatory-exhalatory cycle. Referring to the figure:

1. *Air volume.* As the subject begins to inhale, the curve descends, showing a peak inhalation of 0.4 liters of air.
2. *Intrapleural pressure.* As the lung expands, intrapleural pressure falls from a resting pressures of −5 to −8 cm. H_2O because, as the lung expands, its elastic recoil, or tendency to retain its original shape, increases, causing intrapleural pressure to follow the broken line ABC. However, the pressure drop along the airway is also related to a decrease in intrapleural pressure, shown by the hatched area. Consequently, the actual path of the pressure drop is AB'C.
3. *Air flow.* Expressed in liters per second, airflow increases from 0 to a maximum of 0.5 liters/sec. by the middle of the inhalatory cycle and drops back to 0 by its termination.
4. *Alveolar pressure.* Alveolar pressure begins at 0 and falls to −1 cm. H_2O by the middle of the inhalatory cycle and returns to 0 by its termination, shadowing the airflow curve already noted.

Flow-Volume Curve

A *flow-volume curve* is obtained when a subject inhales maximally and then exhales as forcefully as possible. Fig. 14–10 illustrates flow-volume curves under three different conditions of exhalation in a normal subject. Curve A shows that flow increases rapidly to maximum but then diminishes over most of exhalation. In healthy persons it does not matter whether the person inhales slowly and then accelerates inhalation, as in B, or exhales less vigorously, as in C; the descending portion of the flow-volume curve remains the same.

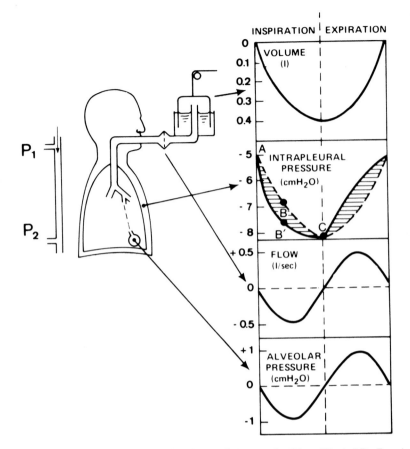

Figure 14–9   Pressure changes during the respiratory cycle. (*From* West, J.B.: Respiratory Physiology. Baltimore, Williams & Wilkins, 1985.)

Recoil Tendency of the Lungs

Elasticity of the lungs is indispensable to the respiratory cycle. The reason for this statement is that the increase and decrease in the thoracic diameters would have little or no effect on the lungs unless they were able to expand and contract along with intrapleural pressure changes. When not inflated, the lungs collapse, pulling away from the chest wall. This characteristic is called the *recoil tendency* of the lungs. This recoil tendency owes its existence to a vast network of *elastic fibers* in the lungs, which are stretched by lung inflation, and to *surface tension* of the fluid lining the alveoli, which has

Figure 14–10   Flow-volume curves. A: maximum inspiration followed by forced expiration; B: expiration initially slow, then forced; C: expiratory effort, submaximal. Note how, in all three, the descending portions of the curve are almost superimposed. (*From:* West, J.B.: Respiratory Physiology. Williams & Wilkins, Baltimore, 1985.)

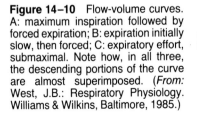

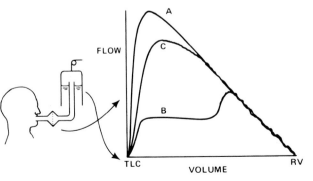

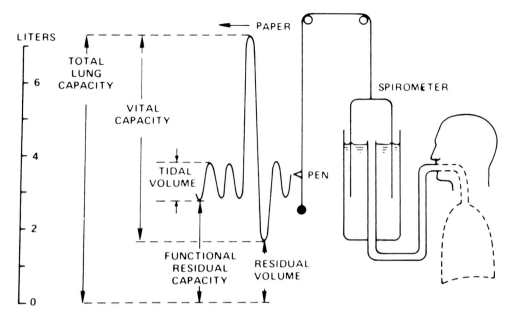

Figure 14–11   Spirometric measures of pulmonary volumes and capacities. (*From* West, J.B.: Respiratory Physiology. Williams & Wilkins, 1984.)

an elastic tendency to contract. It has been estimated that the elastic fibers of the lungs account for approximately one third of the recoil tendency of the lungs and the surface tension for about two thirds.

Compliance

The expansion and contraction of the lungs during inhalation and exhalation, following along with increases and decreases in the thoracic diameters, is called *compliance,* defined as *the volume increase in the lungs for each unit increase in alveolar pressure or for each unit decrease in pleural pressure.* The compliance of the normal lung and thorax combined is 0.13 liters/cm. H_2O, that is, each time alveolar pressure is increased by 1 cm. H_2O the lungs expand 130 ml.

We can see, then, that several kinds of energy in the form of work has to be expended during breathing:

1. *Compliance or elastic work* to overcome the existing forces during lung expansion

2. *Tissue resistance work* needed to overcome the viscosity of the lung and chest wall structures

3. *Airway resistance work* required to overcome resistances to airflow as it is being moved into the lungs

Pulmonary Volumes

The air that passes into and out of the lungs during external respiration can be subdivided into *lung volumes.* Lung volumes are determined by *spirometry.* As shown in Fig. 14–11, a spirometer is a drum inverted over water and counterbalanced by a weight. Air, or an oxygen mixture, is contained within the drum. A tube connects the subject's mouth to the cylinder chamber. When the subject breathes into and out of the tube, the pen rises and falls, respectively. The left side of the spirogram in the figure shows normal tidal breathing; inhalation is up and exhalation is down. This volume is called *tidal volume,* which is about 500 ml. in the young adult male. The subject next inhaled maximally; this volume is known as *total lung capacity,* about 6000 ml. The subject then exhaled maximally; this volume is known as *vital capacity,* about 4500 ml.

We should note that when the subject exhaled maximally, not all of the gas was expired from the lungs. The volume remaining in the lungs is known as the *residual volume,* which averages 1500 ml. The volume of gas in the lung after normal exhalation during tidal breathing is called *functional residual capacity,* which is about 2500 ml. (Neither functional residual capacity nor residual volume can be measured by this type of spirometry.)

The volume of gas that can be exhaled from functional residual capacity down to residual volume is called the *expiratory reserve volume,* which is about 1000 ml. The volume of gas that can be exhaled from the end of normal tidal inspiration to total lung capacity is known as the *inspiratory reserve volume,* which is about 3000 ml.

In *clinical* spirometry, the two most important measures of lung function are *forced vital capacity* (FVC) and *forced expiratory volume* in 1 sec. (FEV_1). FVC is the volume of air exhaled during a forced expiratory maneuver. FEV_1 is the average flow rate during the first second of the FVC maneuver. A reduced FVC indicates a restrictive respiratory disorder. FEV_1 is reduced with airflow limitation or obstruction. All pulmonary volumes and capacities are approximately 20 to 25 percent less in females than in males, and they are higher in larger athletic individuals compared with smaller and more sedentary people. Respiratory volumes and capacities also change, depending on body position. They are decreased when lying down compared with standing up.

Practical Significance of the Pulmonary Volumes

The implications of respiratory volumes for everyday life might be stated in the following way. *Residual volume* is the air that cannot be removed from the lungs even during forced exhalation. Its purpose is to supply the alveoli with reserve air in order to aerate the blood between breaths. Were it not for residual volume, oxygen and carbon dioxide concentrations in the blood would fluctuate excessively with each respiration. Availabilities of residual air between breaths enables us to maintain a constant level of these gases within the blood. *Vital capacity* is affected by the position of the individual during its measurement, respiratory muscle strength, and distensibility of the lungs and thoracic cage.

The average vital capacity in young adult males is approximately 4.6 liters and in females 3.1 liters (4600 cc. and 3100 cc., respectively). Paralysis of the respiratory muscles can profoundly influence vital capacity, reducing it to as low as 500 to 1000 ml. This level is borderline for sustaining life, although it is still adequate for conversational speech. Vital capacity also can be decreased due to reduced pulmonary compliance, as in tuberculosis, asthma, lung cancer, bronchitis, and pulmonary congestion from left heart failure or other diseases that cause pulmonary vascular congestion and edema. Vital capacity is reduced because excess fluid in the lungs decreases lung compliance.

NEUROPHYSIOLOGIC AND CHEMICAL CONTROL OVER RESPIRATION

The central nervous system has the responsibility for matching the rate of alveolar ventilation to the metabolic demands of the body by ensuring that *pulmonary blood oxygen pressure (PO2)* and *pulmonary carbon dioxide pressure (PCO2)* are minimally altered during exercise, speech, and other forms of respiratory demand.

The Respiratory Center

The respiratory center consists of several widely distributed groups of neurons in the *medulla* and *pons* of the brainstem (Fig. 14-12). These bilaterally localized nuclei are subdivided into the following neuronal collections:

1. The *dorsal respiratory group.* Dorsal respiratory neurons extend the entire length of the medulla. Most of them are located within the *nucleus of the tractus solitarius.* However, additional neurons can be found in the adjacent reticular formation of the medulla. This nucleus also serves as

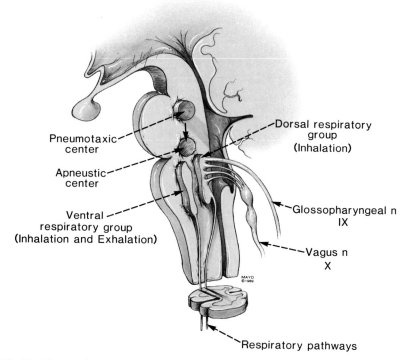

Figure 14–12 The respiratory centers in the pons and medulla.

the termination point of vagal and glossopharyngeal sensorineurons, which transmit signals to the respiratory center from peripheral chemoreceptors, baroreceptors, and several types of receptors within the lung. Stimulation of the dorsal respiratory neurons produces *inhalation only*. The basic rhythm of respiration is controlled by dorsal respiratory neurons.

Nerve impulses transmitted by dorsal respiratory neurons, instead of being bursts of action potentials, begin weakly at first and then steadily increase in a ramplike fashion for approximately 2 sec. Stimulation then abruptly ceases for about the next 3 sec. Stimulation then begins again for still another cycle and continues in the same sequence as before. This pattern of inspiratory neuronal impulses is called a *ramp signal*. Its purpose is to generate a graded increase in volume of the lungs during inspiration rather than sudden inspiratory gasps.

2. The *ventral respiratory group*. This group of neurons is located in the *ventrolateral portion of the medulla*. It is capable of stimulating either *exhalation* or *inhalation,* depending on which neurons of the group are stimulated. It is located approximately 5 mm. anterior and lateral to the dorsal respiratory group and is found along the entire length of the medulla. It is clustered mainly in the *nucleus ambiguus* rostrally and the *nucleus retroambiguus* caudally. The ventral differs from the dorsal respiratory group in the following ways: 1. Ventral respiratory neurons are almost completely inactive during quiet respiration. 2. When respiratory drive exceeds normal for increased ventilation, respiratory signals spread into the ventral neurons, which contribute to the respiratory drive. and 3. Electrical stimulation of some neurons in the ventral group causes inhalation, whereas stimulation of other neurons causes exhalation. In other words, neurons in the ventral group contribute to both phases of the respiratory cycle, but, they are alleged to be primarily responsible for providing powerful expiratory forces during exhalation. The area is believed to function as an overdrive mechanism during requirements for high pulmonary ventilation.

3. The *apneustic center*. This center is located in the lower region of the pons. Its function can be demonstrated only when the vagus nerve to the medulla has been sectioned. When this happens, the apneustic center sends signals to the dorsal respiratory group, which prevents switching off of inspiratory ramp signals. In this way the apneustic center might be considered to provide an extra drive to inspiration.

4. The *pneumotaxic center*. This center is located in the upper pons. Its function is to inhibit inhalation, thereby regulating inspiratory volume.

Chemical Control over Respiration

The ultimate purpose of respiration is to maintain proper oxygen, carbon dioxide, and hydrogen ion concentration in the body fluid. The respiratory centers in the brain, therefore, need to be highly sensitive and responsive to these gases and ionic concentrations. Excess carbon dioxide or hydrogen ions mainly *excite* the respiratory center, producing an increase in the strength of signals to the respiratory muscles. During increased respiratory activity and ventilation, carbon dioxide is eliminated from the blood. Also removed are hydrogen ions, because decreased carbon dioxide also decreases blood carbonic acid (HCO_3). Oxygen, on the other hand, does not directly affect the respiratory center of the brain controlling respiration. Rather, oxygen acts almost entirely on the *peripheral chemoreceptors* located in the *carotid* and *aortic bodies*, which, in turn, transmit appropriate nerve impulses to the respiratory center (Fig. 14–13). The carotid bodies are located at the bifurcation of the common carotid artery and the aortic bodies at the aortic arch. The dorsal,

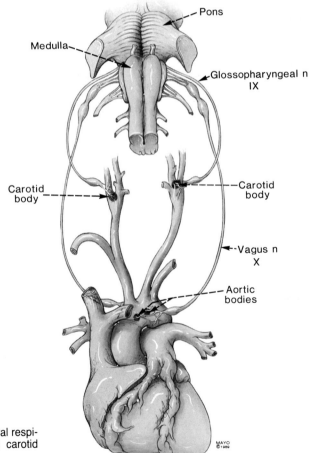

Figure 14–13 The peripheral respiratory chemoreceptors. The carotid and aortic bodies.

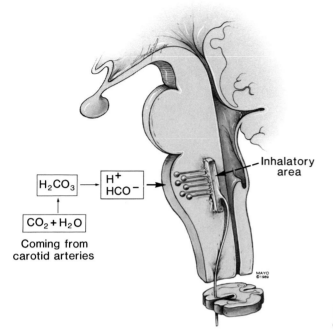

$$H_2CO_3 \rightarrow \begin{array}{c} H^+ \\ HCO^- \end{array}$$

$$CO_2 + H_2O$$

Coming from
carotid arteries

Inhalatory
area

Figure 14–14 The chemoreceptive center in the medulla.

ventral, and pneumotaxic respiratory centers in the brainstem are not directly affected by carbon dioxide or hydrogen ion concentrations. Instead, a *chemosensitive* area located bilaterally beneath the surface of the medulla, ventral to the entry of the glossopharyngeal and vagus nerves into the medulla, is the primary receptor for these chemical changes (Fig. 14–14). This area is sensitive to blood carbon dioxide and hydrogen ion concentration, and it sends impulses to other regions of the respiratory center for purposes of excitation, increasing the rate of firing of the inspiratory ramp afferent nerve fibers. Nerve impulses are also transmitted to the glossopharyngeal nerve and dorsal respiratory areas of the medulla.

Pulmonary Stretch Receptors

Frequency of respiration is also regulated peripherally by extent of lung inflation. *Stretch receptors* in smooth muscle located in the walls of the bronchi and bronchioles transmit signals through the vagus nerve to the dorsal respiratory neurons when the lungs are overstretched. These signals affect respiration in the same way as signals from the pneumotaxic center—they limit the duration of inspiration. Specifically, *when the lungs are overinflated, stretch receptors activate an appropriate feedback that switches off the inspiratory ramp signal and thus limits further inspiration.* Inspiratory duration is thereby decreased and expiratory duration increased. This reflex is called the *Hering-Breuer inflation reflex.* However, in humans the Hering-Breuer reflex is probably not activated until tidal volume increases to greater than 1.5 liters. Therefore, this reflex appears to be a protective mechanism primarily for preventing excess lung inflation rather than an important component in control of ordinary respiration. Fig. 14–15 schematically summarizes the location of the respiratory centers, their pathways and functions.

SUMMARY

1. Respiration for speech requires interruption of vital respiration during which a large quantity of air is inhaled rapidly and sustained on exhalation. Subglottic air pressure must be maintained

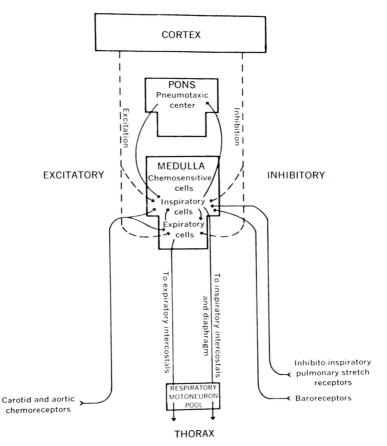

Figure 14–15 Neurophysiologic control of respiration. (*From:* "Neural Control of Respiration." *In* Lambertson, C.J. and Mountcastle, V.B. (Ed.): *Medical Physiology,* ed. 14, St. Louis, 1980, C.V. Mosby Co. Reproduced by permission.

throughout exhalation by a proper balance between the intercostal and abdominal muscles. Reflex chemical control must be temporarily overridden by cortical control.

2. While respiratory disorders cause or contribute to voice disorders, voice disorders also produce respiratory dysfunctions.

3. External respiration, the exchange of air between the lungs and the outside atmosphere, is produced by expansion and contraction of the thoracic cage, which causes air to be drawn into and forced out of lungs.

4. The two main forms of respiration are quiet respiration and forced respiration.

5. The diaphragm is the most important muscle of quiet and forced inhalation, accounting for the major portion of the increase and decrease of the thoracic diameters.

6. Quiet exhalation is brought about primarily by the forces of gravity, untorquing of the rib cage, and return of the abdominal contents to their original position.

7. Forced exhalation, in addition to capitalizing on the return of the thoracic cage to its normal resting position because of passive forces, employs the abdominal muscles.

8. Inhalation occurs when the thorax is expanded and pleural and alveolar pressures become increasingly subatmospheric, causing air to flow into the lungs. Exhalation occurs when the thoracic cage diminishes in size and alveolar pressures exceed atmospheric, causing air to be forced out of the lungs.

9. The lungs expand and contract along with changes in the size of the rib cage during respiration because of their properties of elasticity and compliance.

10. Pulmonary volumes and capacities are determined by the laboratory technique known as spirometry. Pulmonary volumes are defined as tidal volume, inspiratory reserve volume, expiratory reserve volume, and residual volume. Pulmonary capacities are inspiratory capacity, functional residual capacity, vital capacity, and total lung capacity.

11. Average vital capacity for young adult males is approximately 4.6 liters and for females, 3.1 liters.

12. The main neurophysiologic respiratory control centers are located in the medulla and pons of the brainstem. They consist of the dorsal respiratory group, the ventral respiratory group, the apneustic center, and the pneumotaxic center.

13. Oxygen, carbon dioxide, and hydrogen ion concentrations in the body fluid are kept in proper concentrations by the carotid and aortic bodies, feedback mechanisms located at the bifurcation of the common carotid artery and the aortic arch. The ventral medulla is the central nervous system location sensitive to chemical changes in the body fluids.

14. Respiration is also controlled by pulmonary stretch receptors that transmit signals to the central nervous system limiting depth of inspiration, a reflex known as the Hering-Breuer inflation reflex.

SUGGESTIONS FOR ADDITIONAL READING

Guyton, A.C.: Textbook of Medical Physiology. Philadelphia, W.B. Saunders Co., 1986.
  Several chapters in this advanced textbook approach respiration not only from the standpoint of its fundamentals in normal persons, but also discuss respiratory diseases that can affect respiration and phonation.
Lieberman, P.: Intonation, Perception, and Language. Research Monograph No. 38, Cambridge, MA, MIT Press, 1967.
  This small book is one of the most enlightening available on the interrelationships between respiration, intonation, and stress during normal speech. It clearly explains the physiology of speech respiration, including a discussion of subglottic pressures and acoustic data during contextual speech.
Macklem, P.T., and Mead, J. (Eds.): Handbook of Physiology. Bethesda, MD, American Physiological Society, 1986.
  This three-volume work contains more material on respiration than any other single source. They are for the advanced student and contain many graphs and tables showing physiology of respiratory functions.
Minifie, F.D., Hixon, T.J., and Williams, F.: Normal Aspects of Speech, Hearing, and Language. Englewood Cliffs, NJ, Prentice-Hall, 1973.
  The chapter on respiration is well suited as an introduction to respiration, written for the student of communicative disorders before going on to the more advanced textbooks recommended in the section.
Warren, D.W.: Aerodynamics of speech. *In* Lass, N.J., McReynolds, L.V., Northern, J.L., and Yoder, D.E.: Speech-Language-Hearing, Vol. I. Philadelphia, W.B. Saunders Co., 1982.
  Chapter 8 emphasizes the biophysics of respiration, including subglottic and supraglottic pressures. This chapter of intermediate difficulty provides excellent background to the biophysics of airflows and pressures involving the respiratory, glottic, and supraglottic regions of the vocal tract.

Chapter Fifteen

RESPIRATION FOR SPEECH

    Comparison with Vital Respiration
    Respiratory Muscle Action During Speech
    Subglottic Air Pressure
    Laryngeal and Supralaryngeal Valving
    Fundamental Frequency
    Intensity

RESPIRATORY DISORDERS

    Introduction
    Terminology
    Respiratory Diseases Affecting Phonation
    Psychogenic Voice Disorders Implicating Respiration

NORMAL AND ABNORMAL RESPIRATION FOR VOICE

The number of molecules expired per breath by an adult human being is about 10^{22}. The entire atmosphere of the earth contains about 10^{44} molecules. Thus, a single molecule is to a single breath as that breath is to the earth's atmosphere. This calculation would mean that if the molecules expired with the last breath of Julius Caesar were mixed uniformly throughout the atmosphere, then each breath we take should contain on the average one molecule from that historic exhalation.

—Jeans

RESPIRATION FOR SPEECH

Comparison with Vital Respiration

Respiration for speech differs from respiration for life. One difference has to do with *lung volumes*. During quiet respiration, we use 10 to 15 percent of total lung volume, or about 0.5 liters of air during each inhalation and exhalation. For speech, we utilize about 20 percent of total lung volume, or 1.2 to 1.5 liters of air, a moderate portion of the midrange lung volume (Hixon et al., 1973). Lung volumes and airflows are relatively low during speech, as shown in Figure 15–1.

A second difference between vital and speech respiration has to do with *respiratory rate*. The rate of quiet respiration during wakefulness is approximately 16 to 18 cycles/minute, and inhalation and exhalation take from 2 to 3 seconds each. During speech, the frequency of respiration declines dramatically, depending on duration of phrasing. Expiration for speech can extend to 40 seconds with the average number of respiratory cycles decreasing to 8 per minute. The ratio between inhalation and exhalation is approximately equal during quiet respiration, whereas during speech, inhalation consumes only about 10 percent of the total duration of the cycle while expiration occupies 90 percent, as shown in Figure 15–2.

Respiratory Muscle Action During Speech

The muscles of respiration function differently during speech than during quiet breathing. The difference concerns exhalation primarily. During quiet breathing exhalation takes place for the most part due to the passive descent of the rib cage. But, because exhalation needs to be sustained during speech, a greater volume of air needs to be forced from the lungs, which requires activation of the abdominal as well as the thoracic muscles.

Draper et al. (1959) have contributed a landmark study showing the relationship among air volume, pressure changes, and respiratory muscle activity during exhalation for speech. Figure 15–3 shows the sequence of muscular contractions during exhalation for speech as the subject was counting. The figure also shows the relationship between volume of air expended and esophageal pressure, which is analogous to subglottic pressure. In the upper part of the figure we see a normal breath of about 500 ml followed by a deeper inspiration just before speaking and then a steady decrease in volume during counting at a conversational loudness level. A small fluctuation in the air volume curve with a parallel esophageal pressure fluctuation occurs with each stressed syllable.

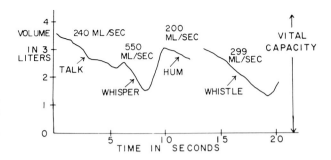

Figure 15–1 Lung volume and airflow changes during speech and related activities. (*From:* Proctor, D.F.: *Breathing, Speech, and Song.* New York, Springer-Verlag, 1980.)

The lower part of the figure illustrates respiratory muscle activity during exhalation and how such muscle activity tries to maintain a steady airflow and pressure as lung volume steadily declines.

1. At the beginning of exhalation, the *external intercostals* remain active, checking the descent of the rib cage and thereby opposing relaxation pressure.

2. As air continues to be expended from the lungs, *external intercostal* muscle activity begins to diminish and stops completely when the lung volume declines to a level slightly less than the volume after normal inspiration. From this point on active muscle contraction is needed to maintain constant subglottic pressure.

3. In order to sustain subglottic pressure, the *internal intercostals* phase into activity with increasing intensity.

4. When lung volumes diminish to a level slightly less than at the end of normal exhalation, action of the *intercostals* is augmented by the *abdominal muscles,* namely, the external oblique and rectus abdominus muscles, and the latissimus dorsi muscle.

The dashed line in the figure indicates that segment of the exhalation during which air is expressed from the lungs without benefit of any muscular contraction. Called the *relaxation pressure,* it is produced by the natural elastic recoil of the lungs and thoracic cage.

Superimposed on the air volume and esophageal pressure curves during exhalation are ongoing, momentary, contractions of the expiratory muscles to increase subglottic pressure for syllabic stress. Studies of subglottic pressure during speech show an increase in subglottic pressure accompanying each stressed syllable (Ladefoged and McKinney, 1963). Knowing the necessity for sudden increases in subglottic pressure to increase pitch and loudness during syllabic stress helps us to understand why patients with respiratory diseases, especially neurologic diseases affecting the respiratory muscles, produce speech characterized by monopitch, monoloudness, and lack of intonation and syllabic stress as, for example, in Parkinson's disease.

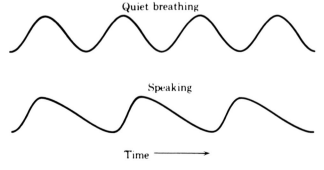

Figure 15–2 Curves showing ratio of inhalation to exhalation during quiet and speech breathing. (*From:* Van Riper, C., and Irwin, J.V.: *Voice and Articulation,* ©1958, p. 348. Reprinted by permission of Prentice-Hall, Inc., Englewood Cliffs, NJ.)

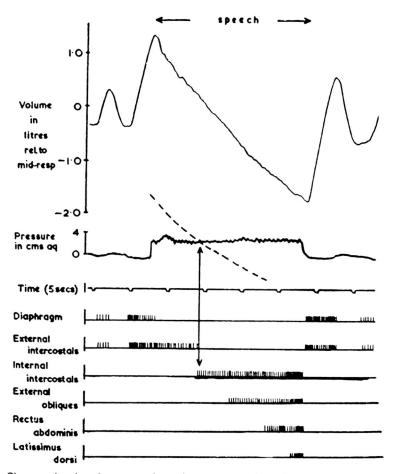

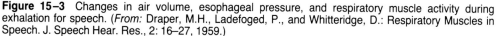

Figure 15–3 Changes in air volume, esophageal pressure, and respiratory muscle activity during exhalation for speech. (*From:* Draper, M.H., Ladefoged, P., and Whitteridge, D.: Respiratory Muscles in Speech. J. Speech Hear. Res., 2: 16–27, 1959.)

Subglottic Air Pressure

Indispensable to exhalation for normal speech is the ability to sustain a constant airflow through the glottis while at the same time maintaining constant subglottic air pressure, as previously illustrated in Figure 15–3. In that figure *air pressure and airflow remain constant despite a steady depletion of lung volume during exhalation*. This curve emphasizes the importance of refined expiratory muscle control in order to maintain constant pressure and flow despite declining lung volume.

Relatively low airflows and subglottic air pressures are required during respiration for phonation in comparison with respiration during physical labor. In fact, subglottic pressure for speech does not even approach the maximum pressures and airflows that can be achieved by the respiratory system under extreme conditions. During quiet breathing, adults use from 30 to 40 percent of their vital capacity, during ordinary conversation, 15 to 35 percent, and during public speaking, 15 to 80 percent of their vital capacity (Wyke, 1974). Subglottic pressures during exhalation for speech range from 6 to 10 cm H_2O, but, subglottic pressures that we are capable of producing under conditions of maximum expiratory effort at various lung volumes can reach as high as 150 cm H_2O when a person uses 80 percent of the vital capacity (Rahn et al., 1946).

Figure 15–4 Effect of supraglottic valving on subglottic pressure and airflow during consonant-vowel repetitions. (a) Lips closed. Intraoral pressure builds up to (b) where the lips separate and pressure drops, at which point voicing begins, (c) followed by lips closed again (d) and pressure rises until they part (e). (*From:* Warren, D.W.: Aerodynamics of Speech. *In* Lass, N.J., McReynolds, L.V., Northern, J.L., and Yoder, D.E. (Eds.): *Handbook of Speech-Language Pathology and Audiology.* Toronto: BC Decker, 1988:196.)

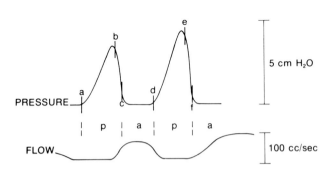

Laryngeal and Supralaryngeal Valving

In addition to the need for maintaining steady exhalatory flow and pressure, the speaker must also be able to alter continuously and momentarily expiratory force and subglottic pressure in order to compensate for changes in the load, or back pressure, imposed on it by laryngeal, velopharyngeal, and articulatory valving. Such supralaryngeal valving needs to be compensated for instantaneously by the respiratory system if subglottic pressure is to be maintained at a constant level. Were this not the case, sound intensity and fundamental frequency would fluctuate erratically, as it, in fact, does in certain neurologic respiratory disorders. The interaction between supraglottic valving on subglottic pressure and airflow is illustrated in Figure 15–4. During utterance of the word /papa/, when the lips are closed at (a), intraoral pressure increases to (b). When the lips separate, pressure falls, and voicing begins at (c). Note an increase in airflow during production of the vowels in this word.

The vocal folds themselves can regulate airflow, depending on the extent to which they are adducted or abducted. During vowel production, subglottic pressures diminish almost to atmospheric, while the vocal folds constrict, maintaining subglottic pressure. Figure 15–5 shows the supraglottal-subglottal pressure differences for vowels, voiced fricatives, and voice plosives. This

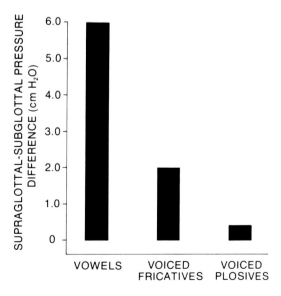

Figure 15–5 Supraglottal-subglottal pressure differences for different phonemes. (*From:* Warren, D.W.: *Aerodynamics of Speech. In* Lass, N.J., McReynolds, L.V., Northern, J.L., and Yoder, D.E. (Eds.): *Handbook of Speech-Language Pathology and Audiology.* Toronto: BC Decker, 1988:196.)

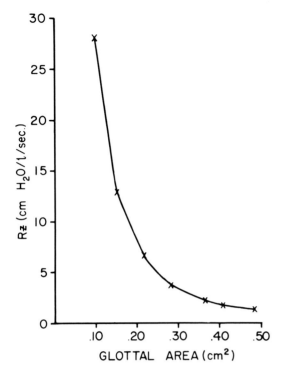

Figure 15–6 Relationship between glottal area and glottal resistance. (*From* Warren, D.W.: Aerodynamics of Speech Production. *In:* Lass, N.J. (Ed.): *Contemporary Issues in Experimental Phonetics*. New York, Academic Press, 1976: 120).

difference is influenced by the oral airway opening. It is highest for vowels, less for voiced fricatives, and least for voiced plosives.

Another laryngeal-respiratory interaction has to do with the ratio of transglottal pressure to airflow through the glottis. The degree of glottal resistance varies with the cross-sectional area of glottal constriction, as illustrated in Figures 15–6 and 15–7. When the area of the glottal opening is larger than 0.5 cm.^{2}, resistance is minimal, as during the production of voiceless consonants,

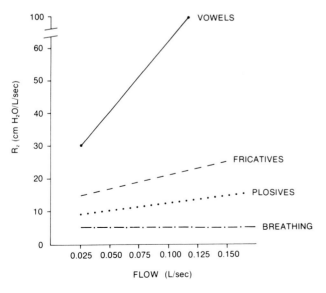

Figure 15–7 Relationship between glottal resistance and airflow rate for vowels, fricatives, plosives, and quiet breathing. (*From:* Warren, D.W.: Aerodynamics of Speech. *In* Lass, N.J., McReynolds, L.V., Northern, J.L., and Yoder, D.E. (Eds.): *Handbook of Speech-Language Pathology and Audiology*. Toronto: BC Decker, 1988:203.)

breathy voice quality, or aphonia. However, the volume rate of airflow also influences glottal resistance; increasing force of exhalation produces higher transglottal resistance.

Clinical experience demonstrates that exhalatory effort is greater not only during voiceless consonants, but also during breathiness and aphonia caused by incomplete vocal fold adduction. During these glottal configurations, air from the lungs is rapidly depleted, requiring more frequent respirations.

Fundamental Frequency

Although it has been established that fundamental frequency is determined to a considerable extent by lengthening and shortening of the vocal folds effected by cricothyroid muscle contraction, fundamental frequency is also regulated by subglottic air pressure. When the pressure is increased, fundamental frequency increases. When subglottic pressure is decreased, fundamental frequency decreases. The interaction between subglottic air pressure and fundamental frequency is illustrated in Figure 15–8. The subject is producing the sentence "*Joe,* ate his soup." The figure illustrates the relationship between subglottic air pressure, fundamental frequency, and air volume. When the patient stresses the word "*Joe,*" a simultaneous increase in subglottic air pressure, fundamental frequency, and expiratory air volume occurs. A relatively linear relationship exists between fundamental frequency and subglottic air pressure, as shown in Figure 15–9.

Intensity

Vocal intensity and its perceptual counterpart, loudness, are also directly proportional to subglottic air pressure. As pressure increases, loudness increases. As pressure decreases, loudness decreases. The higher lung volumes required for increased vocal intensity are shown in Figure 15–10 where a significant increase in lung volumes during loud utterance compared with conversational speech and tidal breathing occurs.

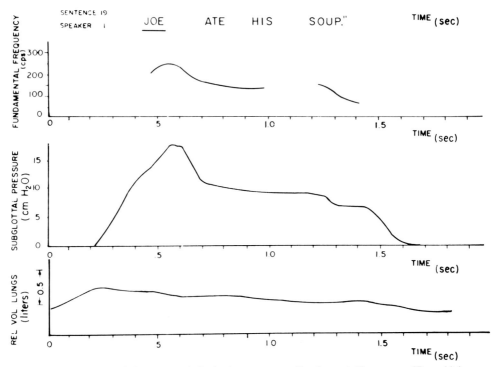

Figure 15–8 Relationship between subglottic air pressure and fundamental frequency. (*From:* Lieberman, P.: *Intonation, Perception, and Language.* Research Monograph No. 38. Cambridge, MA, MIT Press, 1967.)

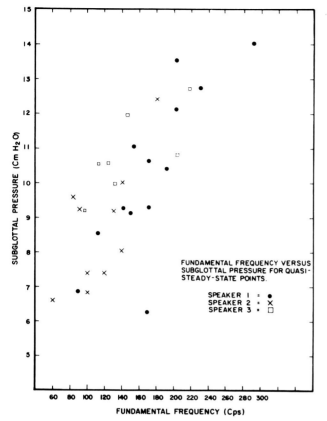

Figure 15–9 Linear relationship between fundamental frequency and subglottic air pressure. (*From:* Lieberman, P.: *Intonation, Perception, and Language.* Research Monograph No. 38. Cambridge, MA, MIT Press, 1967.)

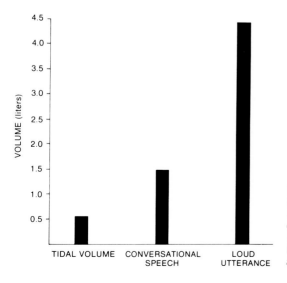

Figure 15–10 Comparison of lung volumes during quiet breathing, conversational speech, and loud utterance. (*From:* Warren D.W.: Aerodynamics of Speech. *In* Lass, N.J., McReynolds, L.V., Northern, J.L., and Yoder, D.E. (Eds.): Handbook of speech-language pathology and audiology. Toronto: BC Decker, 1988:196.)

RESPIRATORY DISORDERS

Introduction

It is an established fact, then, that normal phonation requires that we be able to inhale a sufficient volume of air and to exhale it with sufficient duration and force in order that speech be loud enough and that intonation and stress patterns are capable of being superimposed on the exhaled airstream to accommodate the linguistic and semantic requirements of spoken discourse. Keeping these requirements in mind, we now arrive at certain questions pertaining to respiratory disorders: (1) What respiratory diseases in clinical practice subvert these speech requirements? (2) What laryngeal disorders compromise phonation in such a way that they secondarily cause respiratory dysfunction?

It is a testimony to the adaptability of the respiratory system that respiratory disorders do not cause voice disorders more often than they do. Humans are capable of withstanding a considerable reduction in lung capacity before phonation is affected in any practical way. This observation is based on the fact that normal speech does not require lung volumes in excess of 20 to 25 percent of vital capacity.

Terminology

In discussing the effects of respiratory disorders on phonation, and vice versa, the following terms are commonly used:

- Eupnea = normal breathing
- Tachypnea = rapid breathing
- Bradypnea = slow breathing
- Hyperpnea = a high rate of alveolar ventilation or over-respiration
- Hypopnea = the opposite of hyperpnea and indicates under-respiration
- Anoxia = total lack of oxygen
- Hypoxia = decreased oxygen
- Anoxemia = lack of oxygen in the blood
- Hypoxemia = reduced oxygen in the blood
- Hypercapnia = excess carbon dioxide in the blood
- Hypocapnia = decreased carbon dioxide in the blood
- Orthopnea = sensation of breathing difficulty when lying supine

Respiratory Diseases Affecting Phonation

Categories of respiratory disease that produce phonatory disorders are:

1. Alveolar hypoventilation
2. Increased airway resistance
3. Decreased lung and chest wall compliance
4. General illness producing fatigue and depression
5. Neurologic disease
6. Psychogenic voice disorders implicating respiration

ALVEOLAR HYPOVENTILATION

Diseases that produce alveolar hypoventilation are primarily neurologic, as exemplified by: (1) bulbar poliomyelitis; (2) cervical transection of the spinal cord; (3) myasthenia gravis; (4) Guillain-Barré syndrome; and (5) depression of the respiratory center by anesthetics and drugs.

INCREASED AIRWAY RESISTANCE

Diseases that produce increased airway resistance are asthma, emphysema, pulmonary fibrosis, tuberculosis, infections, and pulmonary edema.

DECREASED LUNG AND CHEST WALL COMPLIANCE

Diseases that reduce the compliance of the lungs and chest wall are silicosis, asbestosis, sarcoidosis, tuberculosis, cancer, pneumonia, scoliosis, and kyphosis.

GENERAL ILLNESS PRODUCING FATIGUE AND DEPRESSION

Patients with weak, breathy, or hoarse voices without laryngeal pathology may have general fatigue owing to chronic and debilitating systemic illnesses. Deep fatigue can also be a sign of reactive depression, but its effects on phonation are essentially the same as fatigue—it *reduces the amplitude and force of respiration for speech.*

Many dysphonic patients have been long suffering from *chronic, borderline illnesses* along with *work stress.* These patients usually have become so accustomed to their fatigue that they are barely aware of it.

In clinical practice, interpersonal conflicts at home or at work are intimately bound up with depression and fatigue. Reduction in respiratory volumes and force during speech in the patient who is chronically depleted of energy proves that speech is work, respiration having to bear the major brunt of accommodating to the physiologic and metabolic requirements of speech. Breathing requires considerable energy to force air out of the lungs against airway resistance and the back pressures induced by supraglottic valving. Following the principle of conservation of physical energy, the fatigued patient breathes for speech only as deeply as necessary for communicative effectiveness. The end result is *shallow breathing.* Shallow breathers do not breathe as much diaphragmatically as they do thoracically, and in extreme cases breathe with the upper thorax only, called *clavicular breathing.* As noted earlier, the thorax moves much less air in and out of the lungs than the diaphragm. Consequently, shallow breathers phonate with *reduced loudness,* and their voices tend to be *flat* and *expressionless,* because of the additional effort required to produce the necessary thoracic and abdominal muscle contractions for normal intonation and stress. A few hours on hospital rounds listening to patients who are chronically ill and whose respirations are shallow because of discomfort, fatigue, and depression will illustrate the deteriorating effects of illness on loudness, intonation, and stress. Even their voices tend to be breathy because of the increased physical effort required for full vocal fold adduction.

For many years, patients with voice disorders due to chronic fatigue from stress and borderline illnesses were labeled "neurasthenics," implying that they were neurotically weak and that their dysphonia and fatigue were trivial. Modern health care requires a more serious approach to this type of patient whose fatigue and dysphonia need to be addressed by the patient's internist and frequently by the psychiatrist or psychologist.

NEUROLOGIC DISEASES

Respiratory disorders from neurologic disease are called *dyspneumias.* Respiratory disorders due to muscular weakness, incoordination, or defects in motor programming are, technically, components of *dysarthria* or *apraxia of speech.*

Flaccid Dyspneumia.   Lesions of the cervical, thoracic, or lumbar spinal nerves anywhere from the cell body in the spinal cord out to and including the muscle can cause weakness or paralysis of the diaphragm, thoracic, or abdominal musculature and thereby cause a reduction in lung volumes and range of respiratory excursions and force. Spinal cord tumors, trauma, vascular, and demyelinating, and myoneural junction diseases are examples of diseases that can cause spinal cord or spinal nerve injuries. Degenerative diseases such as amyotrophic lateral sclerosis can have similar effects. Guillain-Barré disease is an illustration of a viral illness that can completely incapacitate the respiratory system, requiring mechanical assistance. When the cervical spinal cord is transected, all corticospinal tract connections to the spinal nerves are severed, producing complete respiratory paralysis necessitating a respirator to sustain life. Infection or trauma of the phrenic nerve only can produce complete paralysis of the diaphragm, reducing respiratory volumes considerably.

Reduced expiratory force and volume in patients who have flaccid weakness or paralysis of the respiratory musculature causes a drop in subglottic air pressure. *Reduced volume, intonation,* and *stress* result in *monopitch* and *monoloudness.*

Although flaccid dyspneumia can occur in isolation, the remainder of the speech musculature left intact, in most flaccid dysarthrias, dyspneumia and dysphonia coexist. Because of aberrations in laryngeal valving in flaccid dysphonia, these respiratory and phonatory disorders have reciprocally deteriorating effects on the quantity, duration, and smoothness of exhalation. When both the larynx and respiratory musculature are simultaneously affected, it is difficult to separate the phonatory effects of respiratory dysfunction from the phonatory effects of defective laryngeal valving.

In patients with flaccid weakness of the respiratory muscles, it has been established that resting tidal volumes are diminished and frequency of tidal respiration increased. Weakness of the diaphragm and chest wall are responsible for these restrictions, and hypoventilation has been demonstrated in the laboratory in such patients (Newsom et al., 1976a, 1976b; Gibson et al., 1977; Fromm et al., 1977; Parhad et al., 1978). Orthopnea, subjective breathing difficulty when lying supine, is a symptom of which many patients with chest wall weakness complain. In a study of patients with motor neuron disease (amyotrophic lateral sclerosis), it was found that these patients failed to initiate conversation or to read at normal loudness levels using expected lung volumes even though they were able to do so on command. When left to their own devices, they could not sustain normal effort levels because of fatigue or discomfort due to inspiratory muscle weakness. When inspiratory and expiratory muscle weakness coexist, *reduced loudness* and the *flattening of stress patterns* are even more likely as well as the production of *short breath groups* (McNeil et al., 1984).

Spastic Dyspneumia.   Spastic dyspneumia is produced by bilateral corticospinal and corticobulbar tract damage, which usually simultaneously affects the respiratory and phonatory musculature, respectively. Spasticity reduces inhalatory and exhalatory volumes, resulting in shallow breathing. In children with spastic "cerebral palsy," a condition known as *reversed, oppositional,* or *paradoxical breathing* is common. Instead of the abdominal muscles relaxing during inhalation as they ought to, they contract, thereby opposing the downward movement of the diaphragm, restricting the amount of air intake, and producing dysrhythmic breathing.

It is rare to find patients who have lesions of the bilateral corticospinal tracts supplying the respiratory muscles while sparing the bilateral corticobulbar tracts that synapse with Xn nuclei. Consequently, spastic or pseudobulbar dysphonia usually accompanies the spastic dyspneumia and is characterized by hyperadduction of the vocal folds during phonation. The effect is to produce an additional obstacle to exhalation—the *forcing of air through the constricted glottis* requiring abnormally high subglottic pressures.

The combined effects of the reduced expiratory air volume and hyperadduction of the true, and often the false, vocal folds in spastic dysarthria produce a *strained-hoarse, groaning, effortful voice and reduced duration of exhalation.* Typically, the patient will begin to phonate in a highly strained manner at the beginning of exhalation and then, because of the intolerable effort created by the glottic constriction, suddenly release a considerable quantity of air, and the voice becomes breathy prematurely, depleting the remaining air from the lungs. The effect is to require *increased frequency of breathing* for speech and to produce fewer syllables per exhalation. Further interfering with respiration in spastic dysarthria are pseudobulbar *crying and laughter.*

Ataxic Dyspneumia.   Two types of respiratory changes can occur in ataxic dysarthria: (1) Sudden, jerky exhalatory movements that cause abrupt pitch and loudness changes superimposed on exhalation and particularly noticeable during vowel prolongation. This jerkiness owes its existence to sudden movements of the head, shoulder girdle, arms, and thorax. These movements are regarded as postural overcorrections caused by reduced or absent feedback from the respiratory muscles to the cerebellum. These sudden movements cause abrupt changes in intrathoracic pressure that are translated into equally sudden fluctuations in subglottic pressure, which, in turn, are translated into *abrupt changes in pitch and loudness.* (2) Some patients with cerebellar disease have an intention tremor of the laryngeal and respiratory musculature producing a *coarse, slow voice tremor* of approximately 3 Hz.

Hypokinetic Dyspneumia. Parkinsonism produces rigidity and reduced range of motion of musculoskeletal structures and, consequently, can profoundly affect respiration by causing *shallow breathing*. Reduced respiratory volumes result in *reduced loudness*. Diminished control of brief muscle contractions for syllabic stress during exhalation results in *diminishing stress and emphasis patterns* and *monopitch and monoloudness*. Paradoxically, Parkinsonian patients are known for their ability to breathe more deeply and exhale more forcefully on command, a capability that is short-lived once the encouragement is withdrawn. When asked why they are unable to sustain deeper respirations, they will often say that doing so requires too much physical effort.

Hyperkinetic Dyspneumias. The majority of hyperkinetic dysarthrias have respiratory components that implicate phonation.

Organic (Essential) Voice Tremor. Organic voice tremor involves not only tremor of the larynx but, in some cases, the respiratory musculature as well. Both *laryngeal and respiratory tremors are synchronous*. Rhythmic contractions of the *rectus abdominis* muscles have been shown to be synchronous with voice tremor during vowel prolongation and during voluntary, unphonated exhalation, but not during involuntary, rest breathing (Tomada et al., 1987). Jerky movements of the *diaphragm* synchronous with interrupted breathing at the height of inspiration and at the end of expiration during quiet breathing and speech also have been documented in patients with voice tremor (Hachinski et al., 1975).

Sometimes it is clinically difficult to determine whether the tremor is coming from the larynx, thoracic musculature, or both. Whether or not there is a laryngeal component can be determined by laryngoscopy. If the tremor has a laryngeal component, the vocal folds can be seen to oscillate in synchrony with the tremor. Thoracic and abdominal muscle tremor, however, is more difficult to isolate. It can be identified by having the patient exhale silently while the clinician's hands are placed on the lateral walls of the patient's rib cage and abdomen. When thoracic and abdominal tremor is present, the rhythmic movements can be felt along with rhythmic fluctuations of the exhaled whisper.

When organic voice tremor is severe, the vocal folds rhythmically meet in the midline and *momentarily arrest the airflow* through the glottis, producing a tremor form of adductor spastic dysphonia. As in all forms of adductor spastic dysphonia, when the vocal folds meet in the midline and respiration is arrested, the examiner can observe a jerking of the thoracic cage in synchrony with these voice and exhalatory arrests.

Dystonia and Chorea. Dystonic dyspneumia occurs in orofacial dyskinesia, dystonia musculorum deformans, or athetosis. The respiratory disturbance consists of involuntary waxing and waning of muscular contractions of the thorax, producing bending and twisting of the upper torso. These unpredictable, aberrant movements interfere with the maintenance of steady exhalatory pressure during speech. These random muscular contractions produce *sudden changes in loudness, complete voice arrests*, and *shortened exhalation during speech*. A second problem arises in the form of sudden reversals of respiration. While exhaling during speech, the patient may *involuntarily inhale* and thereby disrupt the flow and continuity of exhalation. Some dystonic patients, even while breathing silently, will inhale suddenly with or without inhalatory stridor. These unusual and often startling inhalatory gasps may be mistakenly interpreted as psychogenic but are almost always a variant of respiratory dyskinesia.

Another problem that occurs in the dystonias are intermittent contractions of the laryngeal musculature, which interrupt the flow of exhalation and induce an increase in subglottal air pressure. Acoustically, the effect is to produce an adductor spastic dysphonia of the dystonic variety. The patient, who tries to force air through the constricted glottis, effortfully contracts the thoracic and abdominal musculature.

Similar respiratory arrests occur in patients who have chorea, except that the adventitious respiratory movements are quicker. Changes in loudness and interruptions of phonation produced by thoracic, abdominal, and laryngeal contractions occur more abruptly and are of shorter duration than in dystonia.

Psychogenic Voice Disorders Implicating Respiration

MUTATIONAL FALSETTO (PUBERPHONIA)

Mutational falsetto has a major respiratory component. At the root of the high-pitched, weak, thin, breathy, or hoarse voice lies *shallow respiration*. Clinicians experienced in the diagnosis and treatment of this disorder know that without shallow respiration it is virtually impossible to produce the falsetto. Minimum exhalatory force is characteristic in these patients, and their respiratory volumes are very low during speech. The ultimate purpose of the shallow respiration is to prevent complete vocal fold vibration. Only the medial portions of the vocal folds vibrate, thereby producing the high pitch. As an illustration of how important shallow respiration is to the perpetuation of mutational falsetto, the basic therapy for this disorder is to induce the patient to inhale deeply and exhale with maximum force simultaneous with effort closure of the vocal folds.

IATROGENIC VOICE AND RESPIRATORY DISORDERS

Patients who have been told to rest their voices, or to whisper, that is, to guard their voices, almost always speak with shallow breathing. Consciously or unconsciously, shallow breathing is a reflection of their overcautiousness and anxiety over damaging their vocal folds and their voices. Their overconcern, overattention, and inward rumination about how to produce the voice properly is often the result of overzealous voice therapy and results in excessive musculoskeletal tension, not only in the laryngeal-hyoid region, but in the upper chest as well. A symptom of this elevated tension is the common complaint of pain in the anterior regions of the neck, back of the neck and shoulders, and running down into the clavicular and sternal regions of the upper chest.

PSYCHOGENIC BREATHINESS AND APHONIA

Breathiness and aphonia as a sign of musculoskeletal tension or conversion reaction are produced by incomplete adduction or bowing of the vocal folds. An incompletely closed glottis generates higher than normal transglottal airflow, emptying air from the lungs at a much more rapid rate than normally, and in proportion to the extent of glottal opening. These patients run out of exhaled air rapidly, producing a smaller than normal number of syllables per exhalation. Frequency of respiration for speech can reach such a high rate that patients will complain of fatigue from speaking, breathlessness, and, in extreme cases, may even shown signs of hyperventilation, namely, dizziness and unsteadiness.

Patients with abductor spastic dysphonia have respiratory complaints similar to patients with continuous breathiness and aphonia because of excessive air loss during abductor laryngospasms. The more extensive the abductor spasm, the greater the air loss.

Like patients with neurologic adductor spastic dysphonia, those with the psychogenic form have respiratory repercussions. Each time the vocal folds hyperadduct, the exhaled airstream is partially or completely cut off by glottal constriction. If the laryngospasm is total, not only is phonation arrested, but exhalation momentarily slows or ceases because of the gradual or sudden glottic closure. Following immediately on the heels of the laryngospasm and exhalatory arrest is the patient's effort to maintain phonation. The patient exerts additional, and often extreme, expiratory force to overcome the glottic constriction. The clinician can observe sudden thoracic and abdominal contractions as the patient tries to force air through the constriction. In extreme examples of the disorder in which laryngospasms are constant and powerful, attempts to force air through the constricted glottis can be so intense as to produce distension of the veins of the neck and flushing of the face. Such exhalatory forcing rapidly fatigues the patient, who speaks less and less in order to conserve energy. Some patients find exhalation so difficult and inefficient that they either elect to whisper or to produce breathy voice in an effort to maintain any kind of airflow to support articulation. Some patients discover that if they phonate on inhalation their adductor spasms are less intense and airflow is freer than on exhalation. *The adductor and abductor spastic dysphonias are elegant proofs that aberrant laryngeal valving can profoundly affect respiration during speech.*

SUMMARY

1. In comparing respiration for speech with vital respiration, speech requires greater lung capacity, reduced rate of respiration, and a much longer exhalation phase.

2. Exhalation for speech requires active external intercostal muscles to check the descent of the rib cage and active internal intercostal and abdominal muscle contraction to force maximum amount of air from the lungs.

3. Exhalation for speech requires constant subglottic air pressure in the presence of declining lung volume.

4. Exhalatory force needs to be continuously altered in response to changing back pressures induced by glottic and supraglottic valving.

5. Exhalatory effort is greater for voiceless than for voiced phonemes and in breathy or aphonic voices.

6. Fundamental frequency (pitch) increases with increased subglottic air pressure and falls with decreased pressure.

7. Intensity (volume) increases with increased subglottic air pressure and decreases with decreased pressure.

8. Respiratory diseases that result in phonatory disorders are: alveolar hypoventilation, increased airway resistance, decreased lung and chest wall compliance, general illness producing fatigue and depression, neurologic diseases, and psychogenic voice disorders implicating respiration.

9. Respiratory dysfunction is almost always a direct or indirect cause of dysphonia in neurologic disease and is a component of dysarthria.

10. Neurologic respiratory disorders are called dyspneumias and are of the flaccid, spastic, ataxic, hypokinetic, and hyperkinetic types.

11. Respiratory disorders are deeply implicated in psychogenic voice disorders, particularly mutational falsetto (puberphonia), iatrogenic voice disorders, and psychogenic breathiness and aphonia.

SUGGESTIONS FOR ADDITIONAL READING

Bouhuys, A. (Ed.): Sound production in man. Ann. N.Y. Acad. Sci., 155:1–381, 1968.
    Part II of this volume contains highly worthwhile material on respiratory muscle activity during speech, airflow during phonation, mechanisms underlying subglottic pressure, and linguistic aspects of respiration.
Draper, M.H., Ladefoged, P., and Whitteridge, D.: Respiratory muscles in speech. J. Speech Hear. Res., 2: 16–27, 1959.
    This is one of the most important studies that has been done showing sequence of muscle activity simultaneous with airflow and pressure changes during exhalation for speech.
Lass, N.J., McReynolds, L.V., Northern, J.L., and Yoder, D.E. (Eds.): Speech, Language, and Hearing, Philadelphia, W. B. Saunders Co., 1982.
    Chapter 8, "Aerodynamics of Speech" by Donald W. Warren, is one of the best available on airflow mechanics, airway pressures for speech, upper and lower airway dynamics, effect of glottal activity on air pressure and flow, and methods of measurement.
Lieberman, P.: Intonation, Perception, and Language. Research Monograph No. 38. Cambridge, MA, MIT Press, 1967.
    This special monograph contains information not found elsewhere on the relationship between respiration, intonation, and stress. The book contains many figures that show simultaneous acoustic, respiratory, subglottic pressure, and fundamental frequency values during connected discourse.

REFERENCES

Draper, M.H., Ladefoged, P., and Whitteridge, D.: Respiratory muscles in speech. J. Speech Hear. Dis., 2:16–27, 1959.
Fromm, G., et al.: Amyotrophic lateral sclerosis presenting with respiratory failure. Chest, 71:612–614, 1977.
Gibson, G., et al.: Pulmonary mechanics in patients with respiratory muscle weakness. Am. Rev. Respir. Dis., 115:389–395, 1977.
Hachinski, V.C., Thomsen, I.V., and Buch, N.H.: The nature of primary vocal tremor. Can. J. Neurol. Sci., 2:195–197, 1975.

Hixon, T., Goldman, M., and Mead, J.: Kinematics of the chest wall during speech production: Volume displacements of the rib cage, abdomen, and lung. J. Speech Hear. Res., 16:78–115, 1973.

Ladefoged, P., and McKinney, N.: Loudness, sound pressure, and subglottic pressure in speech. J. Acoust. Soc. Am., 35:454–460, 1963.

McNeil, M., Rosenbek, J.C., Aronson, A.E. (Eds.): The Dysarthrias: Physiology, Acoustics, Perception, Management. San Diego, CA, College-Hill Press, 1984.

Newsom, D.J., et al.: Diaphragm function and alveolar hypoventilation. Q. J. Med., 45:87–100, 1976.

Newsom, D.J., et al.: The effects of respiratory muscle weakness on some features of the breathing pattern. Clin. Sci. Mol. Med., 50:10–11, 1976.

Parhad, I., et al.: Diaphragmatic paralysis in motor neuron disease. Neurology (N.Y.), 28:18–22, 1978.

Rahn, H., Chadwick, L.E., and Fenn, W.O.: The pressure-volume diagram of the thorax and lung. Am. J. Physiol., 146:161–178, 1946.

Tomada, H., Shibasaki, H., Yasuo, K., and Takemoto, S.: Voice tremor: Dysregulation of voluntary expiratory muscles. Neurology (Cleve.), 37:117–122, 1987.

Wyke, B. (Ed.): Ventilatory and Phonatory Control Systems. London: Oxford University Press, 1974.

INDEX

I

J

K

L

COLOR PLATES

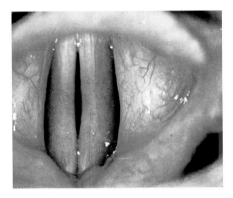

Figure 2–6   Normal larynx during phonation.

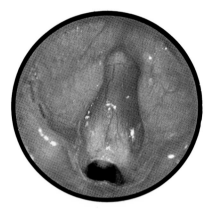

Figure 4–2   Membranous laryngeal web.

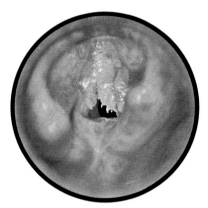

Figure 4–3   Papilloma of the larynx.

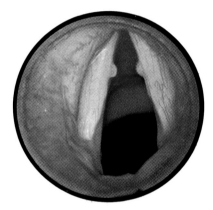

Figure 4–4a   Bilateral polypoid vocal nodules.

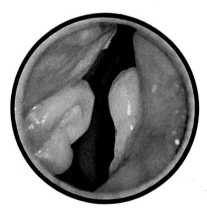

Figure 4–4b   Contact ulcer.

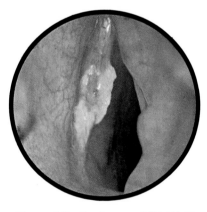

Figure 4–6   Carcinoma of the larynx.